Veterinary Treatment of S

MIX
Paper from
responsible sources
FSC® C018575
FSC
www.fsc.org

I would like to dedicate this book to Gordon Duncanson, a Kentish sheep farmer. He stimulated my interest in farm animals when I was very young, and was all I could have wished for as a father.

Veterinary Treatment of Sheep and Goats

Dr Graham R. Duncanson BVSc, MSc (VetGP), DProf, FRCVS

Equine and Farm Animal Practitioner,
Private Veterinary Practice, UK

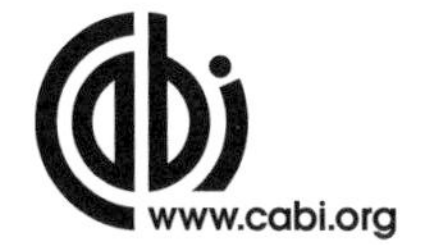

CABI is a trading name of CAB International

CABI
Nosworthy Way
Wallingford
Oxfordshire OX10 8DE
UK

Tel: +44 (0)1491 832111
Fax: +44 (0)1491 833508
E-mail: cabi@cabi.org
Website: www.cabi.org

CABI
875 Massachusetts Avenue
7th Floor
Cambridge, MA 02139
USA

Tel: +1 617 395 4056
Fax: +1 617 354 6875
E-mail: cabi-nao@cabi.org

A catalogue record for this book is available from the British Library, London, UK.

Library of Congress Cataloging-in-Publication Data

Duncanson, Graham R.
Veterinary treatment of sheep and goats / Graham R. Duncanson.
p. ; cm.
Includes bibliographical references and index.
ISBN 978-1-78064-003-7 (hbk : alk. paper) -- ISBN 978-1-78064-004-4 (pbk. : alk. paper)
I. C.A.B. International. II. Title.
[DNLM: 1. Goat Diseases--therapy. 2. Sheep Diseases--therapy. 3. Goat Diseases--diagnosis. 4. Sheep Diseases--diagnosis. SF 968]

636.3'089758--dc23

2011042625

ISBN-13: 978 1 78064 004 4 (pbk)
ISBN-13: 978 1 78064 003 7 (hbk)

Commissioning editor: Sarah Hulbert
Editorial assistant: Alexandra Lainsbury
Production editor: Fiona Chippendale

Typeset by SPi, Pondicherry, India.
Printed and bound in the UK by the MPG Books Group.

Contents

Preface

The author hopes this book will be useful to veterinary practitioners throughout the world who are treating sheep and goats. Obviously there are some differences between wool sheep and hair sheep, and between dairy goats and meat production goats. These differences will be noted in the text. Each species will be described separately with cross-references where helpful. Sheep will be described first in each chapter, followed by goats. Where common names are given for plants, these are generally the names that are used in the UK, but some relate to plants from the USA or Australia.

Veterinary science is evolving at an ever-increasing rate and so some of this information may be out of date before publication. The author apologizes for this and for any inaccuracies. He hopes that these can be corrected in future editions and would be very grateful for any contact from readers via e-mail to vetdunc@btinternet.com.

Foreword

The farming of small ruminants, mainly sheep and goats, has been a major part of global agriculture from the beginning of recorded history. They have become interwoven into our mythologies, our cultures and the development of our civilizations. These cloven-footed animals are classified within the *Bovidae* family in the Subfamily *Caprinae*. Their progenitors, wild mouflon for sheep and wild Bezoar for goats, must have roamed untamed in the ancient grasslands more than 9000 years ago. Both must have been more biddable to domestication than the larger cattle species and would have allowed both women and children to control and nurture them. In many parts of the world, particularly the developing world, this remains the case today. It is estimated that over 1 billion sheep and 450 million goats are presently farmed. Sheep and goats are closely related but are separate species; although they often co-graze, they do not naturally cross mate. Over the years in domestication, a large number of different breeds have evolved and been selected by livestock owners; many of these reflect the major purpose or the geographical location (sub-tundra to tropical) for which they are needed; these major needs have been wool, meat and milk. There are more than 200 breeds of both sheep and goats recorded, respectively. This wonderful variation has been central to the culture and pride of many farming communities, with individual breeds ascribed to the location of their selection, e.g. Devon Longwool sheep and Bagot goats.

However devoted the farmer's selection of individual breeds of these small ruminants has been over the years, all breeds remain vulnerable, sometimes highly vulnerable, to infectious and non-infectious diseases. We have come to recognize that viruses, bacteria and parasites are capable of changing, evolving and emerging themselves and continually presenting new problems for livestock, the livestock keeper and for his veterinary adviser. The scale of such problems may be mild and restricted to a local farm or community, e.g. foot rot, while, on the other hand, they can be of epidemic proportions and of international importance (now referred to as transboundary diseases); a good example of this is peste des petite ruminants (PPR), a viral disease of small ruminants that is presently sweeping across sub-Saharan Africa and Asia.

Ted Hughes reminds us, in his splendid poem 'What is the Truth', that lambs are highly vulnerable to all manner of problems.

> The problem about lambs
> Is that each lamb
> Is a different jigsaw – and each piece
> Is a different problem.

Getting born – one problem
Of many little pieces. The Lamb has to solve it
In the dark, with four fingers.

Once he's born – it's a case
Of which problem comes first. His mother won't have him.
Or he's deficient and won't cooperate.
Or he gets joint-ill
Which sneaks in through the little wick of his umbilical cord before it dries up –
Arthritis for infants.

After that comes Orf – known as Lewer.
Ulcers of the nose, of the lips, of the eyes, of the toes,
All at once,
As you read about in the Bible.

Awful things waiting for lambs.

So, why a new textbook on small ruminants? This concise book places together the skills and expertise needed by veterinarians to care for small ruminants; the conditions and diseases, both infectious and non-infectious, that commonly affect these species and, finally, some Tables and Lists to integrate our present-day knowledge on these matters. Is this book only for veterinarians? Although primarily intended for them, it will be a treasure trove of information for the livestock keeper.

The author, Graham Duncanson, is a farmer's son who qualified from Bristol University as a veterinary surgeon in the mid-1960s. Let me now be honest and declare some familiarity. We first met sitting on a hard bench outside a room waiting to be interviewed for a position on the veterinary undergraduate course at Bristol University. To our surprise, we were both successful and, from the first day of studies, became close friends. His recent switch to authorship, after a lifetime in veterinary clinical work, is marvellous. He has become more eccentric as he matures but remains widely beloved. He writes simply, clearly and with considerable authority. I am delighted to strongly recommend this book; it will appeal greatly to the new graduate, to the veterinarian with farming clients and to the informed stock-keeper. Graham has travelled the world in various guises for nefarious reasons (in fact, for any excuse!) and this experience has been woven into this book; for that reason, this book will be invaluable to global readers. If Ted Hughes is right about sheep, as I suspect he might be, we all need the best information available to maintain the health and welfare of our global populations of small ruminants; with this book in our back pockets, we have a good chance!

Joe Brownlie

Acknowledgements

I would like to thank all my friends and colleagues who have had to stop their mode of travelling while I have taken the photographs for this book:

- my daughter Amelia, who had to ski with me down an extremely steep Alpine ravine;
- her friend George Hall, who had to walk 12 miles in the pouring rain in north Norfolk;
- my great friend Ian Kennedy, who travelled with me overland to Central Asia;
- his wife Judy, who accompanied us up Mount Etna;
- Ann Kent, my boss and travelling companion in Sardinia and Wales;
- Phil and Fearne Spark who drove me all over the Algarve;
- and Professor Joe Brownlie, who took such trouble to take the picture for the back cover of this book.

Glossary

Abortion: the premature birth of young.
Annual: a plant that grows from seed, flowers and dies within 1 year.
Anthelmintics: drugs that expel parasitic worms from the body, generally by paralysing or starving them.
Antigen: a molecule or part of a molecule that is recognized by components of the host immune system.
Awn: a bristle or hair-like appendage to a fruit or to a glume, as in barley and some other grasses.
Bacteraemia: bacteria in the blood.
Biennial: a plant that flowers and dies in the second year after growing from a seed.
Billy goat: a mature male goat.
Billy rag: a piece of cloth rubbed over a mature male goat, particularly its urine-covered front legs, to stimulate a female goat to show signs of oestrus.
Bradycardia: decrease in heart rate.
Bruxism: grinding of teeth.
Buck: a mature male goat.
Calculi: stones formed in the urinary system.
Caprine: the adjective applied to goats.
Cerebral: relating to the cerebrum, the largest part of the brain.
Cestodes: parasitic flatworms, commonly called tapeworms, which usually live in the digestive tract of vertebrates as adults and in the bodies of various intermediate hosts as juvenile stages.
Codon-3: nucleotide sequences that encode a specific single amino acid.
Colitis: inflammation of the colon; often used to describe an inflammation of the large intestine.
Coma: profound unconsciousness from which the patient cannot be roused.
Congestion: the presence of an abnormal amount of blood in an organ or part.
Contusions: bruises.
Convulsion: a violent involuntary contraction of muscles.
Corm: underground bulbous root.
Cryptorchid: *see* rig.
Cull ewe: a ewe no longer suitable for breeding, and sold for meat.
Cystitis: inflammation of the bladder.

Dags: clumps of dung stuck to the wool of the rear and tail of a sheep, which may lead to fly strike.
Dagging: clipping off dags, or clipping the wool to prevent them forming.
Deciduous plants: those that shed all their leaves annually.
Detoxicate: to render a poison harmless.
Distension: the filling of a hollow organ to more than its usual capacity.
Diuresis: excessive urination.
Dysentery: an illness characterized by diarrhoea with blood in the faeces.
Doe: a mature female goat.
Draft ewe: a ewe too old for rough grazing (e.g. moorland or upland), drafted on to better grazing on another farm.
Drenching: giving an anthelmintic dose by mouth.
Dysphagia: difficulty in swallowing.
Dyspnoea: difficulty in breathing.
Dystocia: difficulty at parturition.
Egg reappearance period: the time taken (usually expressed in weeks) for eggs to reappear in faeces after anthelmintic treatment. Usually this is described for drug-sensitive worm populations at the time of product licensing.
Emaciation: excessive body wasting.
Emesis: vomiting.
Emetic: a substance that causes vomiting.
Emphysema: air or gas in the interstices of a tissue.
Enema: rectal injection.
Epidemiology: the study of factors affecting the health of populations and often how diseases are transmitted.
Ewe: a female sheep that has had at least one lamb.
FECRT: a test that measures the effect on faecal egg output of anthelmintic treatment. Generally, efficacy is assessed by comparing faecal egg count (FEC) obtained on the day of treatment with those obtained 14 days after treatment. This is an important tool in detecting anthelmintic resistance in the field.
Flock: the collective word for a group of sheep.
Foetid: malodorous.
Fold: a pen in which flocks are kept overnight to keep them safe from predators.
Genome: an organism's entire hereditary information, encoded either in DNA or, for some types of virus, in RNA. The genome includes the genes that code the proteins and non-coding sequences of the DNA.
Genotype: The inherited instructions that organisms carry in their genetic code.
Gimmer: a female sheep that is mature enough to be served by a ram for the first time; also called a theave.
Glabrous: without hair of any kind.
Goatherd: a person who looks after a herd of goats.
Goatling: a young goat, normally weaned.
Granules: small grains.
Gravid: the pregnant horn of a uterus.
Haematuria: blood in the urine.
Haemoglobinuria: haemoglobin in the urine.
Haemolytic: a substance that causes breakdown of red blood corpuscles.
Hefting: the instinct in some breeds of keeping to a certain heft, or local area, throughout their lives. This allows farmers to graze sheep on different areas without fences. Lambs naturally stay on the area where they were born.
Helminths: a group of eukaryotic parasites that live inside their host. They are worm-like and live and feed off animals.

Hepatitis: inflammation of the liver.
Herbaceous perennials: plants in which the greater part dies after flowering, leaving only the rootstock to produce next year's growth.
Herd: the collective word for a group of goats.
Heterozygous: a genotype consisting of two different alleles at a given locus.
Hogget: a 1-year-old female sheep.
Hogget: a yearling sheep normally destined for meat (also hogg, hog or hoggat).
Homozygous: a genotype consisting of two identical alleles at a given locus.
Iatrogenic: resulting from treatment.
Ileus: failure of peristalsis.
Indigenous: native of the country in which it was produced.
In kid: pregnant goat.
In lamb: pregnant sheep.
***In vitro*:** in the test tube.
***In vivo*:** in the living body.
Jaundice: a disease in which bile pigments stain the mucous membranes.
Kid: a goat in its first year.
Lamb: a sheep in its first year.
Lambing: the process of giving birth in sheep.
Larvae: juvenile forms that many animals undergo before the mature adult stage. Larvae are frequently adapted to environments different from those in which the adult stages live.
Leucocytosis: increase in white blood cells in the blood.
Leucopenia: decrease in white blood cells in the blood.
Linear leaves: those that are long and narrow.
Lumen: the inner space of a tubular structure, such as the intestine.
Mediastinum: space in the chest between the lungs.
Melaena: dark, tarry faeces indicating bleeding high in the intestinal tract.
Metritis: inflammation of the uterus.
Micturition: the passing of urine.
Monoecious: when male and female flowers are separate, but on the same plant.
Mutations: alterations in DNA sequence in a genome that occur spontaneously during meiosis or DNA replication, or are caused by factors such as radiation, viruses or chemicals. Mutations may have no effect, or may alter the product of a gene from functioning properly if at all.
Mutton: the meat of an older sheep.
Myiasis: fly strike.
Nanny goat: a mature female goat.
Narcosis: sleep induced by a drug or poison.
Nematodes: roundworms, one of the most diverse phyla of all animals.
Nodule: a small, round lump.
Non-gravid: the non-pregnant horn of a uterus.
Old-season lamb: a lamb that is 1 year old or more.
Orchitis: inflammation of the testicle.
Ovine: adjective applied to sheep.
Ovoid: egg shaped.
Panacea: a cure-all.
Paracentesis: the technique of puncturing a body cavity.
Pathogenicity: the ability of a pathogen to produce signs of disease in an organism.
Pathognomic: a single specific single sign of a disease.
Pediculosis: lice infestation.
Phenotype: any observable characteristic or trait of an organism such as its morphology, development, biochemical or physiological properties, or behaviour. Phenotypes result from the

expression of an organism's genes as well as the influence of environmental factors and possible interactions between the two.

Polled: inherited hornlessness.

Polydactyly: having an extra limb.

Polymerase chain reaction: a technique to amplify a single or a few copies of a piece of DNA by several orders of magnitude generating thousands to millions of copies of a particular sequence. Polymerase chain reaction (PCR) relies on cycles of repeated heating and cooling of DNA, melting and enzymatic replication of DNA. Primers (short DNA fragments) containing sequences complementary to the target region along with a DNA polymerase (after which the method is named) are key components to enable selective and repeated amplification. As PCR progresses, the DNA generated is used as a template for replication, setting in motion a chain reaction in which the template is exponentially amplified.

Premix: medicine available in a concentrated form to be added to food.

Proctitis: inflammation of the rectum.

Ptyalism: excess saliva production.

Purgative: a strong laxative.

Pyrexia: raised rectal temperature.

Raddle: a colour marker strapped to the chest of a ram, to mark the backs of ewes he has mated.

Ram: an uncastrated adult male sheep.

Recumbency: inability to get up.

Rhinitis: inflammation of the nose.

Rig: a male in which one or both testicles have not descended into the scrotum.

Ringwomb: failure of the cervix to dilate.

Rostral: towards the nose.

Ryegrass: a commonly grown grass, *Lolium perenne*.

Schistosomus reflexus: a deformity of a fetus in which the spine is bent backwards.

Sclerosis: hardening of a tissue.

Septicaemia: pathogenic bacteria in the blood.

Shearling: a yearling sheep of either sex, also called a teg.

Shepherd: a person who looks after a flock of sheep.

Slough: the dropping away of dead tissue from living tissue.

Spasm: involuntary contraction of a muscle.

Staggers: an erratic gait.

Stomatitis: inflammation of the mouth and gums.

Stricture: a narrowing of a tubular organ.

Subclinical: when the symptoms are not evident.

Syncope: fainting.

Syndrome: a group of symptoms.

Tachycardia: increased heart rate.

Tachypnoea: increased respiratory rate.

Teaser: a vasectomized ram.

Tenesmus: straining to pass urine or faeces.

Teratoma: a developmental embryological deformity.

Torpid: sluggish.

Tourniquet: an appliance for temporary stoppage of the circulation in a limb.

Trismus: locking of the jaw.

Tup: a ram.

Tupping: sheep mating.

Twin lamb disease: pregnancy toxaemia.

Tympanic: distended with gas.

Typhilitis: inflammation of the caecum.

Ubiquitous: occurring everywhere.

Udder: mammary gland.
Ureter: the tube connecting the kidney to the bladder.
Urethra: the tube leading from the bladder to the outside.
Urethritis: inflammation of the urethra.
Urine scald: inflammation of the skin caused by persistent wetting with urine.
Urolithiasis: the formation of stones in the urinary system.
Urticaria: an acute inflammatory reaction of the skin.
Vaginitis: inflammation of the vagina.
Vagus: tenth cranial nerve.
Venereal disease: a disease spread by coitus.
Vesicle: a collection of fluid in the surface layers of the skin or of a mucous membrane.
Viraemia: virus particles in the blood.
Volatile: a substance that evaporates rapidly.
Wether: a castrated sheep or goat.
Zoonoses: diseases communicable between animals and man.

Abbreviations

ACP	Acetylpromazine
ad lib.	As much as desired
AGID	Agar gel immunodiffusion
AI	Artificial insemination
AST	Aspartate aminotransferase
BCS	Body condition score
BDV	Border disease virus
BHB	Beta-hydroxybutyrate
BHC	Benzene hexachloride
BHV	Bovine herpes virus
Bid	Twice daily
BSE	Bovine spongiform encephalopathy
BTV	Blue tongue virus
BUN	Blood urea nitrogen
BVD	Bovine virus diarrhoea
Cal	Calorie
CBPP	Contagious bovine pleuropneumonia
CAE	Caprine arthritis and encephalitis
CCN	Cerebrocortical necrosis
CCPP	Contagious caprine pleuropneumonia
CFT	Complement fixation test
CJD	Creutzfeld–Jakob disease
CK	Creatinekinase
CL	Corpus luteum
CLA	Caseous lymphadenitis
CNS	Central nervous system
C-NS	Coagulase-negative staphylococci
CODD	Contagious ovine digital dermatitis
CPD	Contagious pustular dermatitis
CRT	Coproantigen reduction test
CSF	Cerebrospinal fluid
CT	Controlled test

cu	Cubic
Cu	Copper
DEET	Diethyl toluamide
DEFRA	Department for Environment, Food and Rural Affairs (UK)
DIC	Disseminated intravascular coagulation
DM	Dry matter
DMSO	Dimethylsulphoxide
DNA	Deoxyribonucleic acid
EAE	Enzootic abortion of ewes
ECG	Electrocardiogram
EDTA	Ethylene diamine tetra-acetic acid
EHA	Egg hatch assay
EHV	Equine herpes virus
ELISA	Enzyme-linked immunosorbent assay
epg	eggs/g
EU	European Union
FAO	Food and Agriculture Organization (of the UN)
FAT	Fluorescent antibody test
FCE	Feed conversion efficiency
FCR	Feed conversion ratio
FEC	Faecal (worm) egg count
FECRT	Faecal egg count reduction test
FMD	Foot and mouth disease
FPT	Failure of passive transfer
G	Gauge
GA	General anaesthetic
GGT	Gamma glutamyltransferase
GI	Gastrointestinal
GLDH	Glutamate dehydrogenase
GM	Genetically modified
GnRH	Gonadotropin-releasing hormone
GVS	Goat Veterinary Society (UK)
Hb	Haemoglobin
HCN	Hydrogen cyanide
HMD	High mountain disease
IBR	Infectious bovine rhinotracheitis
IgE	Immunoglobulin
IgG	Immunoglobulin
i/m	Intramuscularly
i/p	Intraperitoneally
IU	International units
i/v	Intravenously
LAT	Latex agglutination test
LCV	Large cell variant
LDT	Larval development test
LN	Lymph node
MAP	*Mycobacterium avium* subsp. *paratuberculosis*
MCF	Malignant catarrhal fever
MCH	Mean corpuscular haemoglobin
MCHC	Mean corpuscular haemoglobin concentration
MCV	Mean corpuscular volume
ME	Metabolizable energy

MOET	Multiple ovulation and embryo transfer
MRI	Magnetic resonance imaging
MV	Maedi-Visna
NSAID	Non-steroidal anti-inflammatory drug(s)
NSD	Nairobi sheep disease
OEA	Ovine enzootic abortion
OIE	Office International des Epizooties (World Organisation for Animal Health)
OMAGOD	Ovine mucosal and gum obscure disease
Ov-VH2	Ovine herpes type 2 virus
OxF	Oxalate fluoride
PCR	Polymerase chain reaction
PCV	Packed cell volume
PHV	Porcine herpes virus
PI3	Parainfluenza III
PLR	Papillary light reflex
PMD	Phosphorus magnesium dextrose
pme	Post-mortem examination
PMN	Polymorphic nuclear cell
PMSG	Pregnant mare serum gonadotrophin
PO	*Per os*, orally
ppm	Part(s) per million
PPR	Peste des petits ruminants
PRA	Progressive retinal atrophy
PrP	Prion protein
PUPD	Polyuria-polydipsia
qid	Four times daily
RBC	Red blood cell
RFI	Residual feed intake
RNA	Ribonucleic acid
RPM	Revolutions per minute
RSV	Respiratory syncytial virus
RT-PCR	Reverse transcriptase polymerase chain reaction
RVF	Rift Valley fever
SCOPS	Sustainable control of parasites in sheep
SCV	Small cell variant
SG	Specific gravity
sid	Once a day
SMCO	S-methylcysteine sulfoxide
SNT	Serum neutralization test
SOP	Standard operating procedure
sub/cut	Subcutaneously
TAT	Tetanus anti-toxin
TB	Tuberculosis
TBF	Tick-borne fever
TCBZ	Triclabendazole
TDN	Total digestible nutrients
tid	Three times daily
TMS	Trimethoprim-sulfadoxine
TP	Total protein
TPR	Temperature, pulse and respiration
TSE	Transmissable spongiform encephalopathy
VDS	Veterinary Defence Society

VLA	Veterinary Laboratory Agency
VTEC	Verocytotoxigenic
WBC	White blood cell
WCC	White cell count
ZN	Ziehl–Neelsen

1

Breeds

Introduction

Historically, sheep and goats were at the centre of pastoral life throughout the world. They were important in Roman times (Fig. 1.1), and still are today in Europe; they are even more important with pastoral tribes in Africa and nomads in the Middle East and Asia (Fig. 1.2).

Evolution of the Domestic Sheep

Ovis aries is the domestic sheep. Evidence of its domestication dates back 11,000 years to the 'Fertile Crescent'. The middle of the 'Fertile Crescent' lies over the 'twin rivers', the Tigris and the Euphrates, which run through modern-day Iraq (Fig. 1.3). DNA analysis has shown that domestic sheep are descended from two ancestor species, one of which is *Ovis musimon*, the mouflon (which can still be seen in Corsica and Sardinia), or the ancestral mouflon, *Ovis orientalis* (Fig. 1.4). The second ancestor has yet to be identified. The urial, *Ovis vignei* (a later synonym for *Ovis orientalis* and now called *Ovis orientalis musimon*), which is found in north-eastern Iran, has been ruled out as it has 58 chromosomes whereas the domestic sheep has only 54. The former will actually interbreed with the mouflon. *Ovis ammon*, the argali sheep found in the eastern parts of Central Asia north of the Himalayas, is also ruled out as it has 56 chromosomes. *Ovis nivicola*, the Siberian snow sheep, has 52 chromosomes and so is also excluded.

Structure of the Sheep Industry in the UK

There are many areas in the UK that are really only suitable for sheep farming. These areas are home to a large number of hardy breeds of sheep, which are loosely termed 'hill sheep', although they may not actually have been bred for or live in upland areas. These sheep are kept as purebred flocks. Farmers breed pedigree ewe lambs and ram lambs, the best of which are either kept as replacements or sold. The poor quality ram lambs are castrated and sold for meat. Farmers with better land then buy the pedigree ewe lambs or shearlings. The term 'pedigree' is used loosely, meaning bred to breed rather than actually graded pedigree animals. These are then mated to specific breeds of ram in order to breed crossbreds. These cross breeds, often termed 'halfbreds', are shown in Table 1.1.

The males of these halfbreds are castrated and sold for meat. The females, which are highly prized, are sold to lowland farms. The lowland farms will have these halfbreds as their ewe flock and put them to a terminal

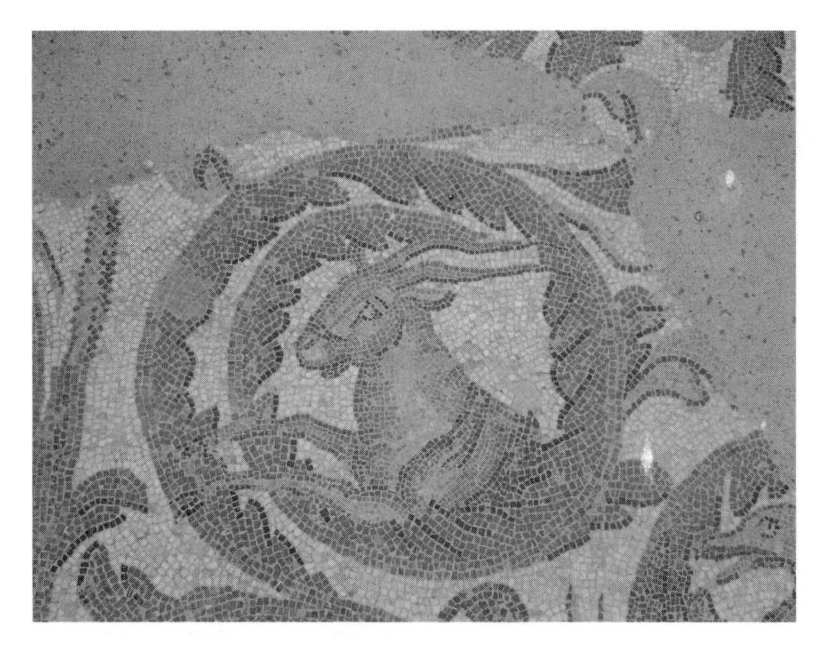

Fig. 1.1. Roman mosaic.

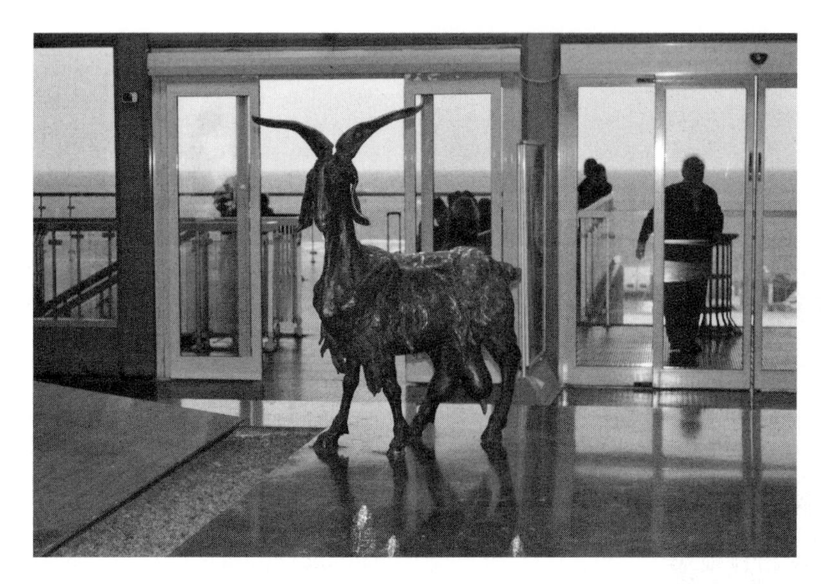

Fig. 1.2. Bronze goat.

sire to produce fat lamb for meat. Traditionally the terminal sire was a Southdown or another downland breed. Nowadays the main terminal sire is still a downland ram but is restricted to the Suffolk (Fig. 1.5), though the Texel and the Charollais are nearly as popular.

Sheep Breeds of the UK

Badger Face Welsh Mountain

These are Welsh Mountain sheep with special colour markings, black with a white belly and a white stripe on their faces.

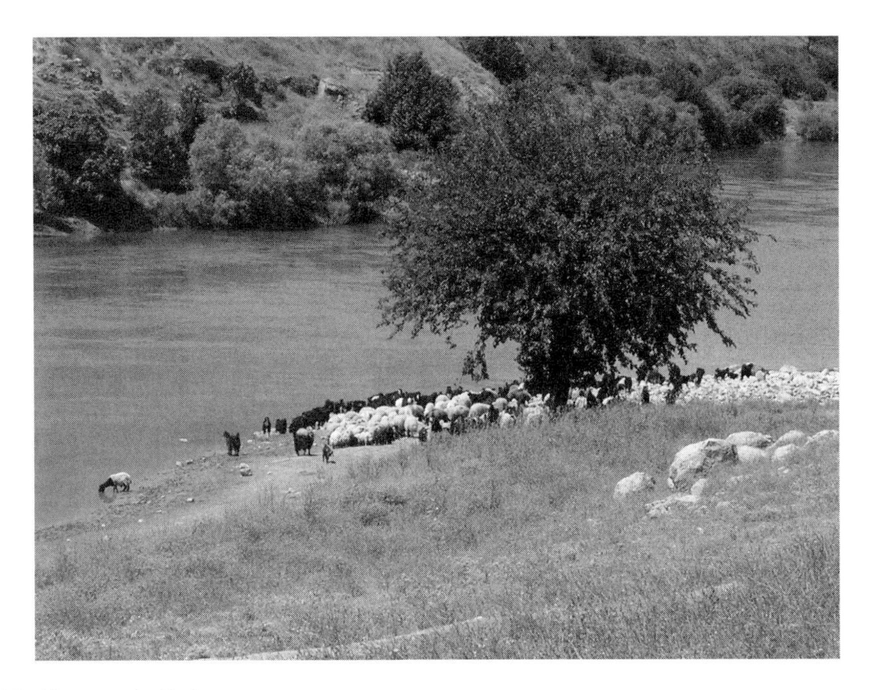

Fig. 1.3. Sheep on the Tigris.

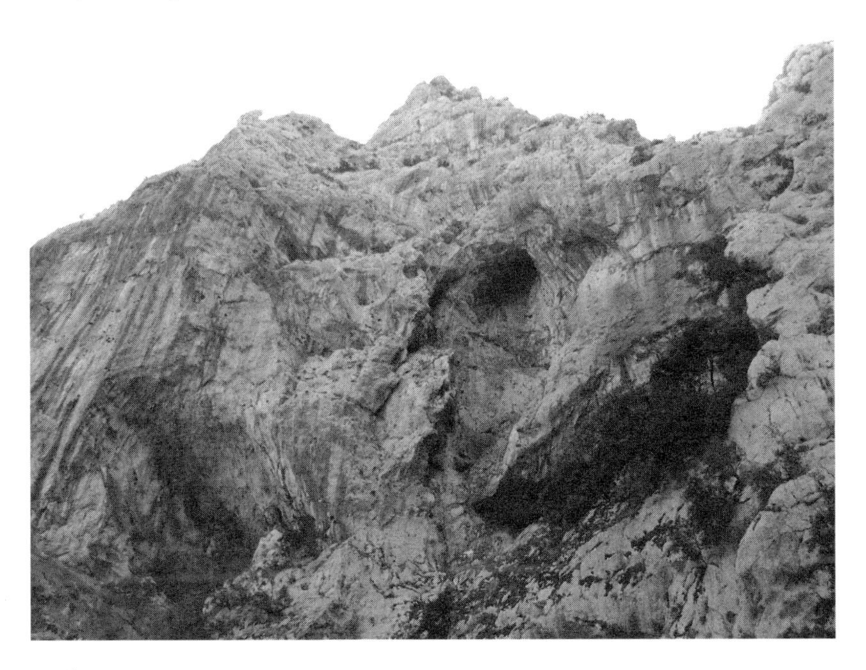

Fig. 1.4. Sardinia.

Balwen Welsh Mountain

These are Welsh Mountain sheep with special colour markings, white with a dark face and belly.

Beulah Speckled Face

These are white sheep with a distinctly patterned black and white face clear of wool. The females are free of horns. This breed originated

Table 1.1. The breeding of well-known halfbreds in the UK.

Breed of ram	Breed of ewe	Name of halfbred produced
Border Leicester	Cheviot	Scottish halfbred
Border Leicester	Welsh Mountain	Welsh halfbred
Border Leicester	Clun Forest	English halfbred
Teeswater	Dalesbred or Swaledale	Masham
Bluefaced Leicester	Swaledale	North of England Mule
Bluefaced Leicester	Scottish Blackface	Greyface
Bluefaced Leicester	Clun Forest	English Mule
Bluefaced Leicester	Welsh Mountain or Beulah Speckled Face	Welsh Mule

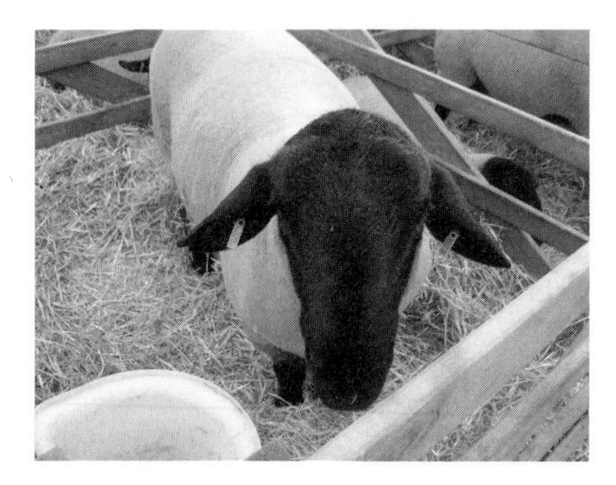

Fig. 1.5. Suffolk.

in Wales over 100 years ago. It is an excellent crossing sheep to breed lowland ewes (see Table 1.1). It is medium sized and hardy, with carpet-quality wool.

Black Welsh Mountain

These are all-black wool sheep that had almost died out by 1975, but since then the breed has made a partial resurgence not only in the Welsh hills but also around the Norfolk Broads. It is a small hardy sheep with a lambing percentage of 150% if carefully managed. A useful but slightly fat lamb is produced if top crossed with a terminal sire, but this is not eagerly sought by butchers. Ideally, Black Welsh Mountain ewes should be crossed with a Border Leicester or a Bluefaced Leicester ram to produce crossbred ewes, which are then served by a terminal sire.

Bluefaced Leicester

These are very similar to the more well-known Border Leicester. However, as the name suggests, they have blue/grey faces. Their wool is not so bright white or quite as good in quality, although breeders may dispute this. The breeders also maintain that they are hardier. The breed is used to sire some excellent halfbreds (see Table 1.1).

Border Leicester

These large white sheep with good wool and conformation make excellent sires to breed lowland ewes (see Table 1.1). The pure-breds have clean white heads and legs and a Roman nose. They have been used throughout the world to breed good crossbred and hybrid sheep.

Boreray

These Scottish meat sheep, also known as the Boreray Blackface or the Hebridean Blackface, have very poor wool, which is brown with flecks of white hair. Both sexes have large horns that curl back.

British Charollais

This breed was developed in the 19th century by crossing the Dishley Leicester with the local breed in central France. It has had a breed society since 1974. It has a very good meat-to-bone ratio and is popular with butchers. It is the third most popular terminal sire. See also under Charollais.

British Friesland

These milk sheep originated in Holland and are common in Germany. Individuals will produce over 500 l of milk a year with a butter fat of over 6.7%. The breed is very prolific with a lambing percentage in excess of 250%. They are large sheep with a distinctive long bald tail and a silky, soft face with pink lips and nostrils.

British Milk

These prolific hybrid milk sheep were first released in 1980. The breed contains East Friesian, Bluefaced Leicester, Polled Dorset and Lleyn. It is extremely fecund, with lambing percentages of over 200% easily obtainable with correct management, and the lambs fatten quickly. However, this was bred as a milking sheep and individuals can produce 900 l in a 300-day lactation. The main numbers of the breed are in Canada.

Cheviot

These bright white hill sheep are very popular for breeding lowland ewes (see Table 1.1), very fecund under the right conditions and also very hardy. They are medium-sized sheep with small clean white heads and legs, and have been used throughout the world to form new breeds and hybrids.

Clun Forest

These medium-sized, polled sheep are exceptionally fecund. Lambing percentages of 180% are easily attainable under the right management. They are ideal sheep to live under rough conditions to cross with a terminal sire, or perhaps better with a Border Leicester, to produce ewes that can then be tupped by a terminal sire. They have a white to grey body with a small black head and black legs.

Cotswold

This long-woolled white sheep breed from the southern Midlands of England dates back to the 1600s. It has been kept and improved in the USA where it is a breed of some importance.

Dalesbred

This breed from the central Pennines has Swaledale and Blackface blood. It is a medium to large hardy sheep, excellent for producing crossbred ewes (see Table 1.1). It is white, with a clean black and white face and carpet-quality wool. Both sexes have horns.

Derbyshire Gritstone

These hardy hill sheep date back to 1770 in the Peak District of England. They are white with black and white faces and good wool. Both sexes are polled. Lambing percentages of 145% are possible with good management. The lambs are quick maturing.

Devon Closewool

This Exmoor meat sheep breed is over 100 years old. It is totally white with a medium-length fleece. Both sexes are polled, of a medium size, very hardy and ideal for open heathland.

Devon Longwool

This breed, recognized for well over 100 years, used to be widespread in the south-west of England. The animals are large and all white with wool on face and legs, and both sexes are polled. The wool has lustrous curls.

Dorset Down

This breed was fixed some 200 years ago by crossing the Southdown with the Dorset Horn. It is polled with a light brown face and legs. It is considerably larger than the Southdown, with a longer body and longer legs. It is more in keeping with modern fat lamb requirements and is therefore an excellent terminal sire. Although it has Dorset Horn blood it does not readily breed out of season. The wool is good quality (Fig. 1.6).

Dorset Horn

The Dorset Horn is a very old breed from southern England, famous for its ability to breed out of season. However in practice the sheep are not bred all the year round and normally farmers are happy to get three lamb crops in two years. As the name suggests, this breed has large curled horns, and it is a white wool sheep with white legs. It has been used to breed many other breeds but is not renowned for its wool quality or fecundity. However, these traits have been added from other breeds to make several excellent breeds such as the Dorset Down and the Dorper.

Easycare

This is a polled white sheep breed which is a true hybrid using mainly Wiltshire Horn and Welsh Mountain blood, and was first bred in North Wales in 1965. It has a good lambing percentage of 180% and produces quick-maturing fat lambs.

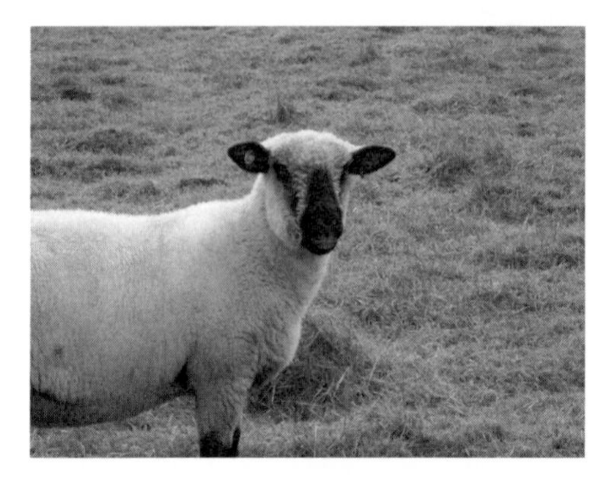

Fig. 1.6. Dorset Down.

Exmoor Horn

This very old breed has been kept on Exmoor for 2000–3000 years. It is a small, hardy, white sheep and both sexes have horns. The face is white with black nostrils and free of wool. It has a medium fleece with the wool coming down the legs, which is sought after by felters.

Faroes

This breed of short-tailed small, hardy sheep, mainly white with a dark face, dates back to the 9th century and is related to Old Norwegian and Icelandic stock. Although the islands are famous for knitwear, the wool is not of high quality and the sheep are now a meat breed. The rams have large curling horns but the ewes are polled.

Greyface Dartmoor

This is a large, long-woolled sheep breed of old lineage. Both sexes are polled and the face is covered in wool. The nose is normally black.

Hampshire Down

This breed was produced by crossing the Southdown and the local Berkshire sheep about 200 years ago. They are polled chunky white sheep with a distinctive black nose in a white wool face and black legs. It has short legs, although not as short as those of the Southdown. The breed is now relatively rare as its progeny are too fat for modern taste. Lambing percentages of 130% are readily attainable and lambs fatten quickly off good grass (Fig. 1.7).

Hebridean

These are very small, exceptionally hardy, black-horned sheep. The wool is very coarse but liked by felters. Twins are rare when kept under rough conditions. They are not wild sheep and are good as crofters' stock (Fig. 1.8).

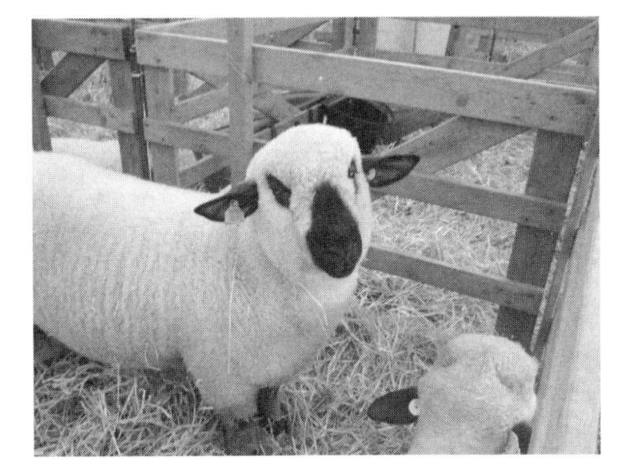

Fig. 1.7. Hampshire Down.

Herdwick

The main base of this extremely hardy breed is in the Lake District. Its lamerotype hairs suggest a Scandinavian origin, as these were only to be found in Scandinavian sheep. Herdwicks will spend their entire lives near the spot where they were born; if they are taken away they will invariably return, a behaviour known as 'hefting'. In consequence Herdwicks are not sold off a farm but are always sold with it. There was considerable concern in the foot and mouth disease (FMD) outbreak in 2001 as the breed was decimated and there was fear that the hefting instinct would be lost. This has not happened, and Herdwicks have been brought back and readily stay on the killed-out farms. Lambing percentages are under 100%. The lambs are born with almost black wool that turns lighter with age (Fig. 1.9), and the breed is noted for its longevity. The rams have white horns. The wool is coarse and full of kemp, a short, hard fibre that sheds regularly and is rarely bought on account of its poor quality (Fig. 1.10).

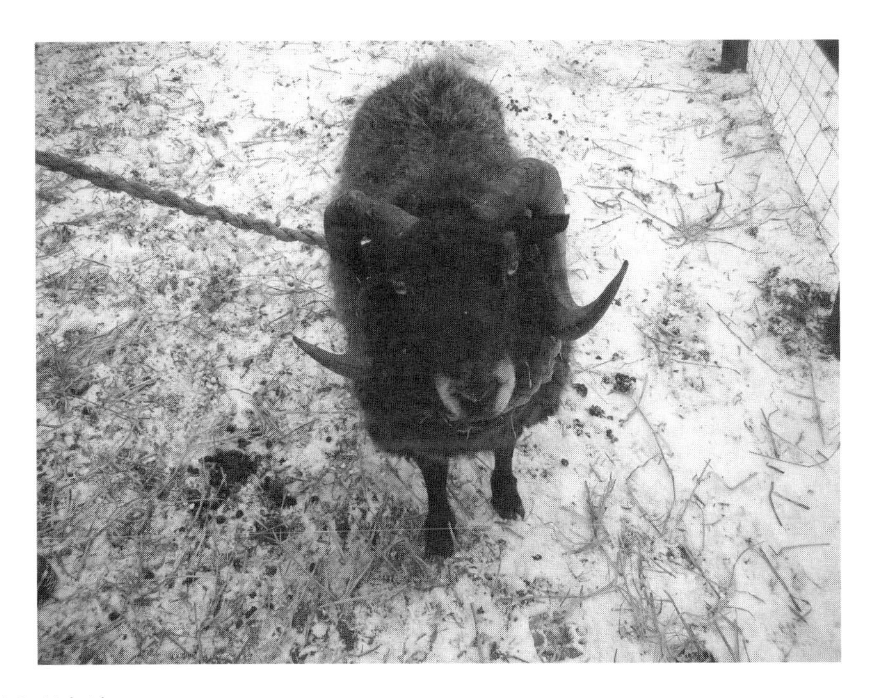

Fig. 1.8. Hebridean.

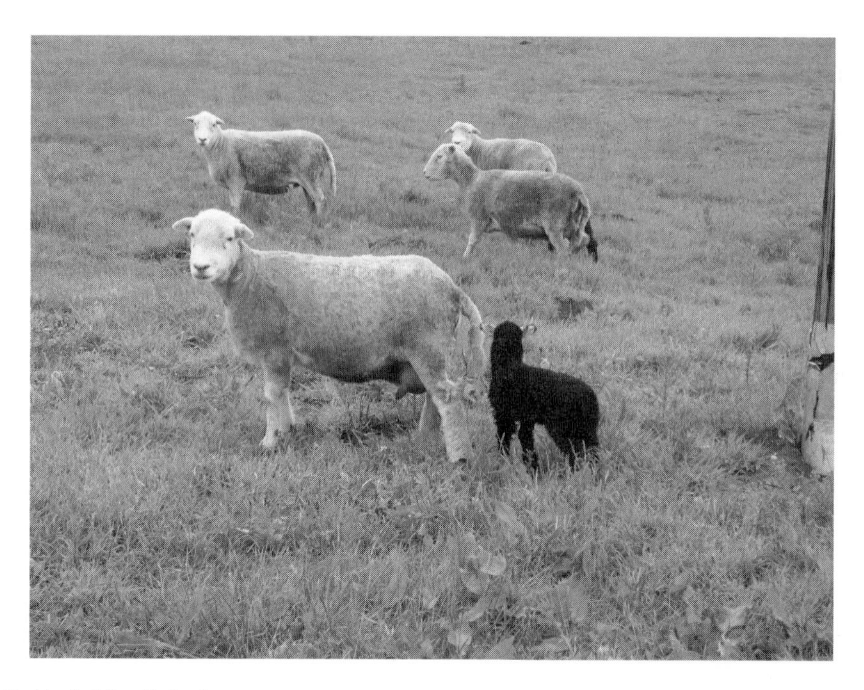

Fig. 1.9. Herdwick with lamb.

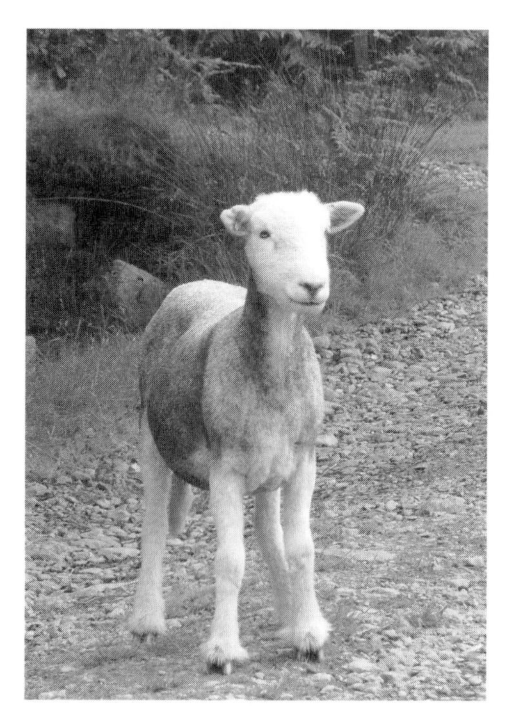

Fig. 1.10. Newly shorn Herdwick.

Hill Radnor

These are hardy hill sheep from Wales, cream in colour with a light brown face and legs. They are medium-sized with coarse wool and relatively low fecundity when kept on the hill. It is a good breed for top crossing to produce ewes for lowland use.

Jacob

These piebald sheep are popular with hobby farmers on account of their colour. They are medium-sized sheep and very fecund in a hobby situation. Both sexes normally have two curled horns, however an inherited gene can give them four spiky horns. This gene has now largely been bred out as it was linked with some detrimental genes such as those producing eyelid defects. The colour is interesting, as when a Jacob is bred to a down ram such as a Suffolk (which is white with a black face and legs), the progeny are all black. If a Jacob is bred to an all-white sheep such as a

Texel, the progeny are either all white or all black. Twins and triplets are common and so single-coloured, mixed litters are seen. The breed will breed out of season. The progeny are too fat for modern tastes.

Kerry Hill

These white sheep with very characteristic black muzzle, ears and eyes originated in Powys in Wales. The breed is hardy and makes a good crossing sheep. Equally, in a lowland situation it can produce a high lambing percentage. Both sexes are polled.

Lincoln Longwool

This is the largest British sheep breed. It has been exported all over the world to increase the size of local sheep. It has long lustrous white wool, and the lambs have good meat but are slow to mature.

Llanwenog

This is a remarkably docile sheep from West Wales. It has medium-length wool that is normally grey or light brown. The faces are usually black. It is very fecund and produces good saleable fat lambs.

Lleyn

As the name suggests, this breed originates from the Lleyn Peninsular in North Wales. It is a very prolific breed producing multiple lambs – often up to five – and milks very well. It will also breed out of season. Traditionally, over 100 years ago, lambs were produced to be fat by Easter. After weaning the ewes were milked for cheesemaking. They are small, white, hardy sheep, once again gaining in popularity.

Lonk

These sheep from Lancashire live up to their name, which means long and lanky. They are white with carpet-quality white wool. Both sexes are polled and have black and white faces. The breed was developed by monks.

Manx Loaghtan

These dark brown sheep are native to the Isle of Man. There is no wool on the face. Normally they have four long horns but some individuals have only two horns and others have six, the horns on the ewes tending to be smaller. The wool is prized by weavers and the meat is a delicacy (Fig. 1.11).

Norfolk Horn

This very old horned breed has been kept for wool in Norfolk for many hundreds of years. They are medium to large white sheep with black head and legs. They can be bred early in the season to produce fat lambs for Easter. They are moderately fecund and with good management can have a lambing percentage in excess of 150%. The breed was the foundation of the Suffolk breed, which was created by crossing a Norfolk Horn with a Southdown (Fig. 1.12).

North Ronaldsay

These remarkable sheep live on the northernmost island of the Orkneys, where they are confined by stone walls to the shoreline. Their main diet is seaweed. They are a small short-tailed sheep with coarse wool.

Oxford Down

This is another down breed created by crossing local Oxfordshire stock with Southdowns. It has good white wool and very light brown face and legs. It is a much bigger sheep than the Southdown, and has considerably longer legs. Lambs can be finished easily in 4 months,

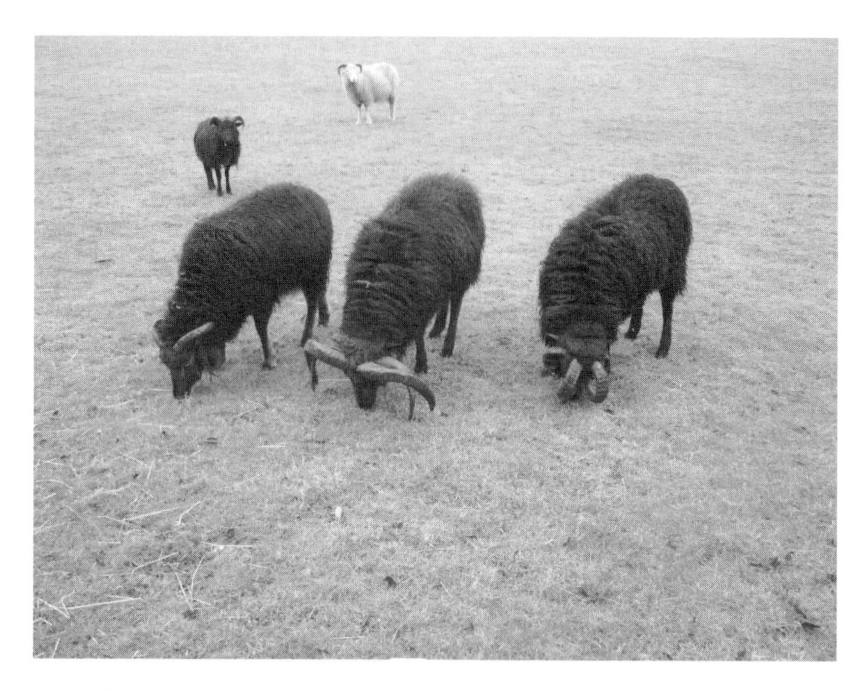

Fig. 1.11. Manx Loaghtan.

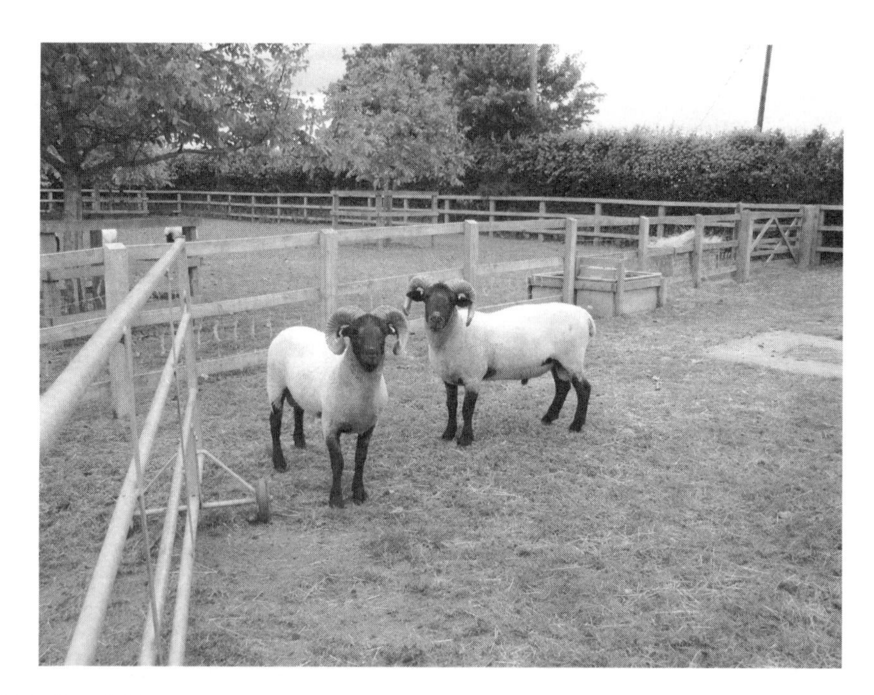

Fig. 1.12. Norfolk Horn.

but it not adapted to breed out of season. It is relatively fecund, with lambing percentages of 130% being the norm. It is polled in both sexes.

Portland

This is a very old white breed of sheep with coarse wool, which was bred on the Isle of Portland off Dorset. The sheep have white faces and both sexes have horns. In the rams these are very large and curled. The wool is long but coarse and is prized by spinners. They are short, stout sheep and do not produce lambs acceptable to modern butchers. They are moderately fecund, and lambing percentages of 120% are attainable.

Radnor Forest

This is a relatively rare breed from a small area on the Welsh borders. It is best described as a cross between a Clun Forest and a Kerry Hill.

Romney Marsh

As the name suggests, these are natives of Romney Marsh in Kent, a low-lying, bleak, exposed area. They are often called 'Kents'. This breed can be traced back to the 13th century and has spread all over the world, being very common in the Antipodes. There are some large flocks in China.

Its importance in large commercial stocks stems from the fact that it can be relied upon to survive and produce lambs under virtually any conditions, whether on bleak marshes or sheltered orchards. It has an unusual habit of spreading out evenly over the available grazing area, thus making the best possible use of the existing pasture (Fig. 1.13).

The lambing percentage is low, rarely over 120%. The wool is of medium quality but yields are over 4 kg and it is all white. Both sexes are polled. On account of the low lambing percentage the ewes can be left to look after their lambs at lambing time with little supervision.

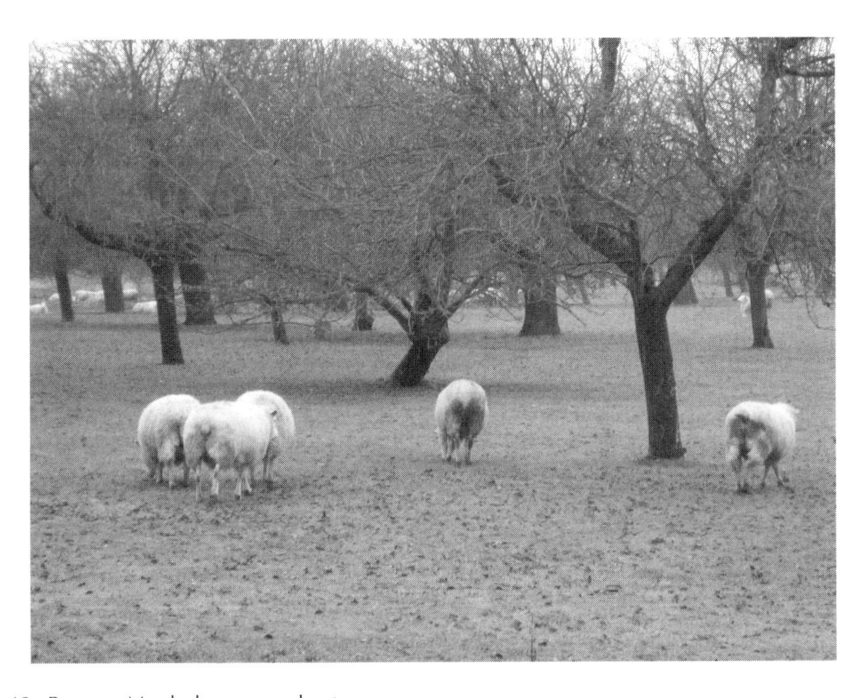

Fig. 1.13. Romney Marsh sheep spread out.

Rough Fell

These very hardy, small- to medium-sized sheep come from south Cumbria. The face is a mixture of black and white and both sexes have horns. The wool is coarse and white.

Ryeland

These are excellent compact smallholder sheep. The wool is normally white but some shades of brown are found. There is tight curly wool on the face, and the muzzle is black. Both sexes are polled.

Scottish Blackface

This Scottish breed was established in 1500. They are very hardy medium-sized sheep with a short tail and long white wool, the face being mainly black with some white areas. As hill sheep they make ideal mothers to breed crossbreds, which can then breed fat lambs on lowland areas. Both sexes are horned.

Scottish Dunface

These medium-sized sheep date back to the Iron Age. They are of variable colours and have short wool. Both sexes have small horns. By the 19th century they had largely been replaced by the Blackface.

Shetland

These small, white sheep, originating from the Shetland Islands to the north of Scotland, have black faces and legs. Many colours are recognized including white, grey, fawn and black, and also colours with Gaelic names such as *Shaela*, *Emsket*, *Mioget* and *Moorit*. The wool is very fine. They are slow-growing sheep that lamb easily and are often used for conservation grazing.

Shropshire Down

These large downland sheep were bred from old Shropshire breeds and the Southdown. They are white with fawn face and legs, and both sexes are polled. The wool is of moderate length and good quality. They breed good fat lambs.

Soay

These small, brown sheep take their name from the Isle of Soay in the Outer Hebrides where they have lived from time immemorial. They are the only living representative of the small primitive sheep that were common in Britain before the Roman occupation. The fleece of about 1 kg is shed naturally in early summer. The lambing percentage is below 100%. They are quite wild, even when kept in domestic situations. They do not flock but disperse in every direction when approached by dogs or strangers. They can leap high, so gathering is a nightmare.

They do not eat clover and so are used in Cornwall to help restore the china clay heaps covered with grass/clover mixture. The clover within the area is never over-grazed. They are also used around the Norfolk Broads as they will eat the young rush shoots and improve the grazing.

Southdown

This breed is thought to have been on the southern downs before Roman times. It was improved by John Ellman of Glynde near Lewes. It was the foundation stock for all the 'down' breeds and 40 years ago was the most chosen terminal sire. It produces one of the finest wools of all the British breeds. The sheep are white with a fawn face, and both the rams and ewes are polled. It is a stocky yet deceptively heavy breed. However it is not in favour with butchers today and is almost a rare breed in the UK, but much more common in New Zealand, the USA and France.

Suffolk

This breed, which is still the most popular terminal sire in the UK, was produced by accident almost 300 years ago by crossing a Southdown ram with a Norfolk Horn ewe. The first cross was so good that the breed was fixed. It is a white sheep with a black head, which is free from wool, and black legs. It produces very quick-maturing fat lambs and is capable of very early out-of-season lambs in January. A lambing percentage of 180% can be achieved.

Swaledale

This hill sheep breed was established in Yorkshire by 1800. It has rough, long wool but a clean neck and head. It is mainly white with a black and white face and legs. Both sexes are horned. It is a hardy, medium-sized animal ideal for breeding crossbred ewes for further top crossing to breed fat lambs (see Table 1.1).

Teeswater

This 200-year-old sheep breed has long, high-lustre, kemp-free white wool that will not felt. The wool is not as long as the Lincoln. The Teeswater is a good meat sheep.

Welsh Mountain

These long-tailed mountain sheep breed excellent crosses (see Table 1.1). They are medium sized, and white with a white, wool-free face.

Wensleydale

These 19th-century hill sheep were bred in North Yorkshire by crossing Leicester and Teeswater sheep. They are good crossing sheep with a blue-grey face and white wool with ringlet-like locks (Fig. 1.14).

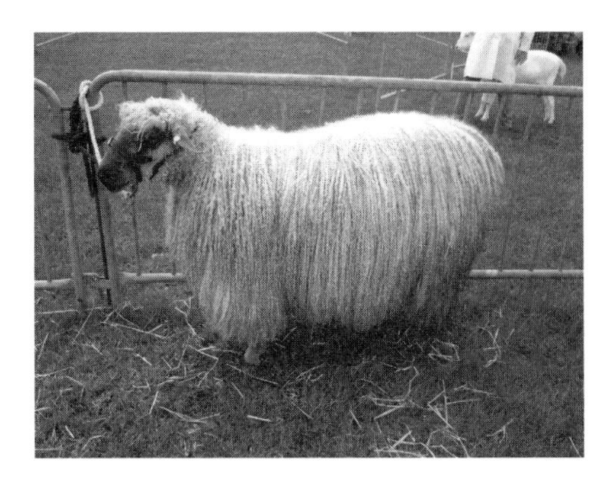

Fig. 1.14. Wensleydale.

Whitefaced Dartmoor

These are all-white hill sheep. Both sexes have horns. The wool is long and the lambs have good meat.

Whitefaced Woodland

This breed is also called the Penistone after the Yorkshire town where it was first bred and sold. It is an all-white large hill sheep with short, fine wool, and produces good meat lambs. Both sexes are horned (Fig. 1.15).

Wiltshire Horn

These white-horned sheep are ideal for smallholders as shearing is not required. They are almost hair sheep. Fly strike is rare. They will breed at any time of the year (Fig. 1.16).

Sheep Breeds of the World

Aclpayam (Acpayam)

This large, white sheep breed has long, coarse wool. It originates from Turkey.

Adal

This breed of small, dark-brown hair sheep with a fat tail originates from Ethiopia.

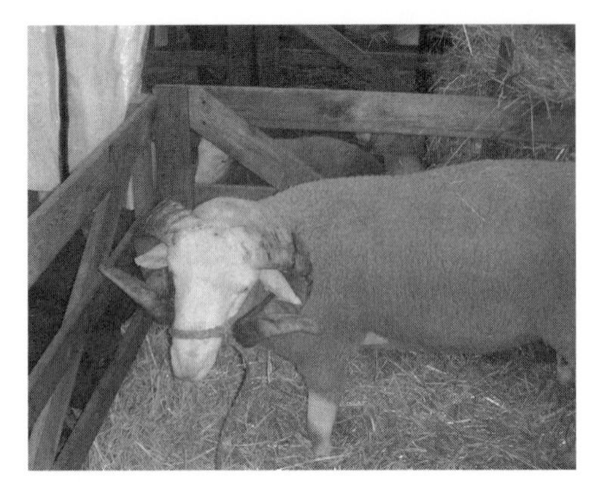

Fig. 1.15. Whiteface Woodland.

Afghan Arabi

This hair sheep breed is kept for meat in Afghanistan, Iran and Iraq. It is black with a white face and long pendulous ears. It is a polled sheep with a fat tail.

Africana

This red-haired sheep breed originally came from West Africa but was developed in Colombia.

Alai

This white wool sheep breed with a fat tail was developed in Kyrgyzstan. Only the rams have horns.

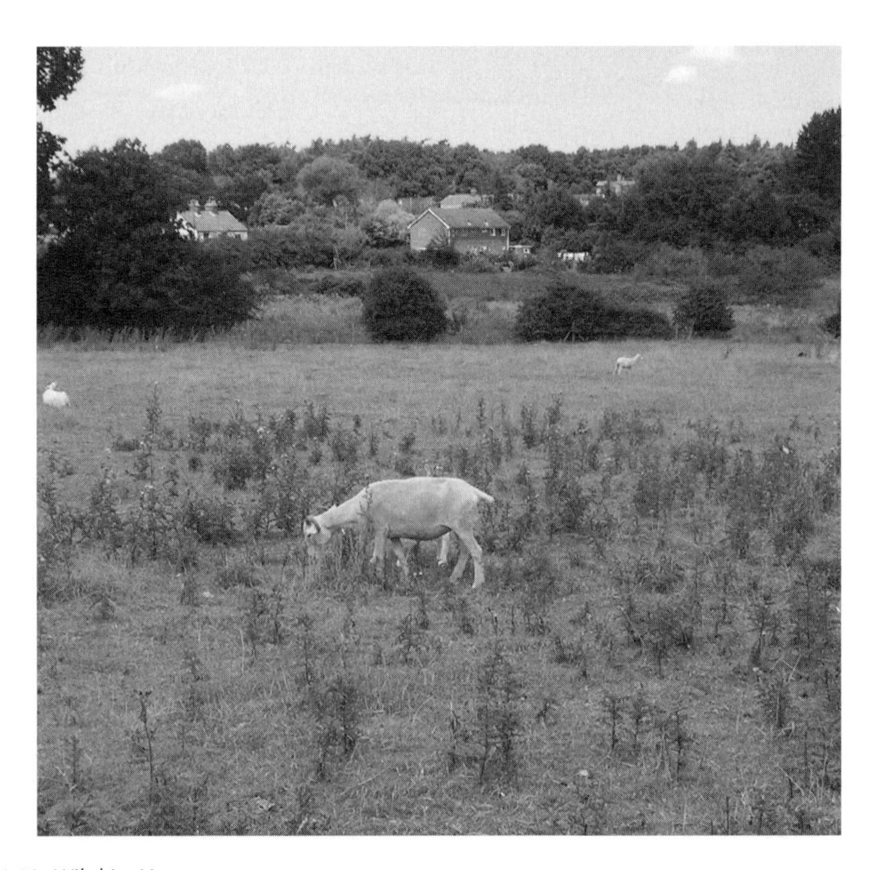

Fig. 1.16. Wiltshire Horn.

Alcarreña

This white-haired, polled sheep breed originates from Spain.

Algarve Churro

This wool sheep breed originates from Southern Portugal. It is white but has black spots on its face and lower legs (Fig. 1.17).

Algerian Arab

This mainly meat sheep breed of various colours has rough wool that is only suitable for carpets. Only the males are horned.

Alpines Steinschaf

This hair sheep breed originated in Germany and is used to improve pastures in the higher alpine regions. They are large, polled sheep with a grey body and black head. The breed has been known since the Middle Ages.

Altay

This rough-woolled sheep breed originates from mountainous regions in China. Animals are polled, with fat tails.

Ancon

This white wool sheep breed, which comes from the USA, is sometimes called the Otter sheep. Only the rams have horns. It is actually an inherited freak with short legs, which has been very closely inbred.

Apennine

This white sheep breed has long rough wool. It is mainly kept for meat in the mountains in Northern Italy.

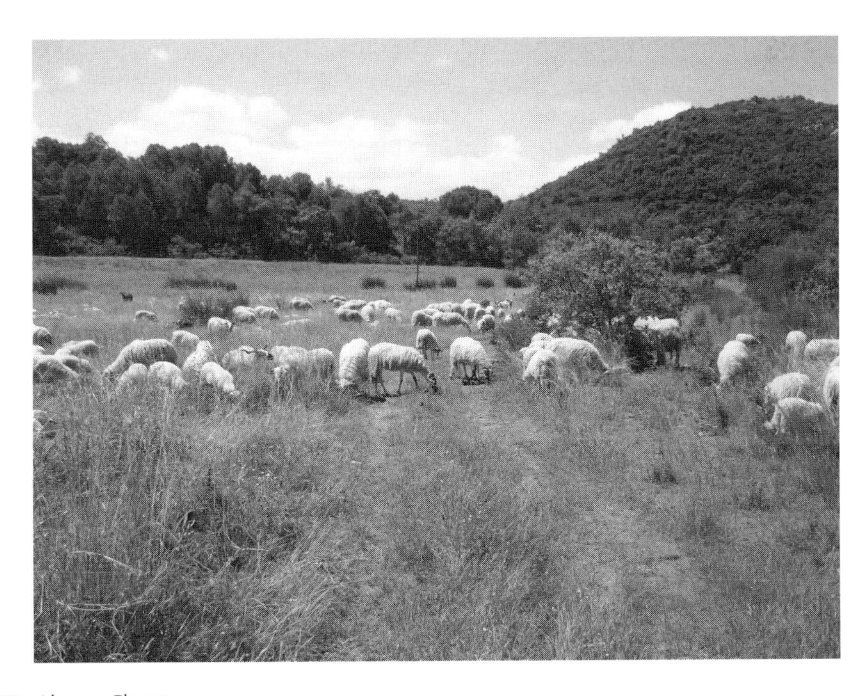

Fig. 1.17. Algarve Churro.

Arapawa Island

This very light brown wool sheep breed has a darker brown face with a wide white blaze and large curling horns. It was bred in New Zealand.

Armenia Semi-coarse wool

This big, white sheep is a dairy breed from Armenia. Its Russian name is Armyanskaya.

Askanian

This white-woolled sheep breed comes from the Ukraine. Its Russian name is Askaniysky.

Assaf

This white-horned, black-faced milking sheep breed is from Israel. It was bred by crossing the Awassi with the Friesian.

Aussiedown

This is a hybrid sheep breed based on the Southdown and the Texel, which was standardized in Australia. It is a very large, meat-producing sheep.

Awassi

These sheep are white with a brown face, and have long wool and strong curved horns. They are milked in Syria and Saudi Arabia.

Badger Face Welsh Mountain

See Sheep Breeds of the UK.

Balbas

This white, milk sheep breed has a black muzzle and spectacles. It produces large amounts of semi-coarse wool. It has a fat tail and is a good meat producer. It is kept in Azerbaijan.

Balkhi

This is a small black-polled sheep breed with coarse wool and a fat tail. It originated in Pakistan and is very commonly seen in the Khyber Pass.

Baluchi

This medium-sized black and white sheep breed has a fat tail and coarse wool. It is very common in the arid areas of Iran.

Balwen Welsh Mountain

See Sheep Breeds of the UK.

Barbados Blackbelly

This very large meat-producing sheep breed is white with a black belly, and is found throughout the Caribbean. Both sexes are polled.

Bardoka

This medium-sized, white sheep breed has a pink skin. Both sexes have horns. It has fine wool and although it is primarily a meat-producing sheep, in certain areas it is milked. It is found throughout the Balkans and was originally bred in Serbia.

Basco-béarnaise

This white dairy sheep breed with a wool-free face is milked in Spain. It is also known as Vasca Carranzana. The nose is slightly Roman and the horns are large in both sexes.

Bellclaire

This is a large, polled, white hybrid sheep developed in Ireland for fat lamb production.

Beltex

This is a very large, polled, white hybrid sheep breed based on the Texel, and was developed in Belgium.

Bentheimer Landschaf

This medium-sized sheep breed has white wool and a wool-free face. It is polled and was specifically bred in Germany to tidy up pastures.

Bergamasca

This large white sheep breed originated in northern Italy but now is found in Brazil. It is a true triple-purpose sheep breed, and is milked, has good wool and produces fine lambs for meat.

Berichon du Cher

This large, white, polled sheep breed is primarily kept for meat and originated in France.

Beulah Speckled Face

See Sheep Breeds of the UK.

Bibrik

This horned sheep breed has coarse wool and is white with a black head and fat tail. It comes from Pakistan and is primarily kept for meat.

Biellese

This coarse-woolled sheep breed is kept for meat in the Piedmont area of Italy. It is white and polled, with lop ears.

Bizet

This is a large white French sheep breed. The rams have horns. The fleece is not too coarse but the wool is not of top quality. It can be bred 'out of season'.

Black Hawaiian

This is a large all-black sheep breed with rough wool. The rams have enormous horns but the ewes are polled. It is only found in the state of Hawaii in the USA.

Black Welsh Mountain

See Sheep Breeds of the UK.

Blackhead Persian

Although this hair sheep breed originated in Central Asia, it was radically improved in South Africa, where its Afrikaans name is Swartkoppersie. As the name suggests, it is a white sheep with a black head. It is polled and has a fat tail and is an excellent breed for producing meat in an arid area.

Bleu du Maine

This excellent meat-producing French sheep breed has good long, thick wool. It is white with blue-coloured head and legs. It is a very good terminal sire, whose progeny are much favoured by today's butchers (Fig. 1.18).

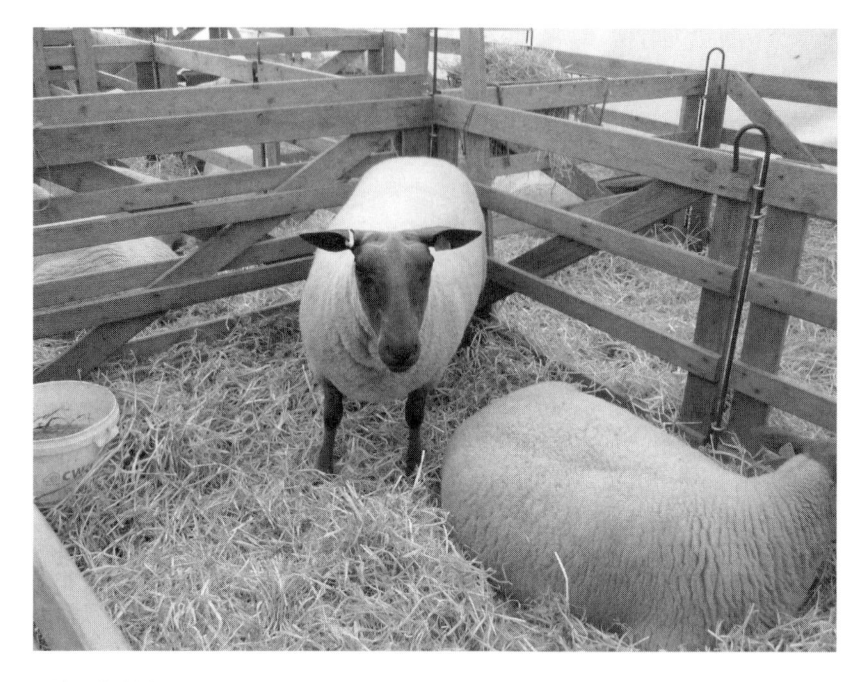

Fig. 1.18. Bleu du Maine.

Bluefaced Leicester

See Sheep Breeds of the UK.

Bond

This is a very large hybrid sheep breed produced in Australia from Merino and Lincoln Longwool stock. It is mainly for wool production, but the lambs make good meat carcasses. It is very popular in Russia and China.

Booroola Merino

These extremely fecund sheep were bred in New Zealand using gene-mapping techniques.

Border Leicester

See Sheep Breeds of the UK.

Boreray

See Sheep Breeds of the UK.

Bovec

These dairy sheep were bred in Slovenia but are now rare. Most are pure white but some have black marks. Both sexes are polled with small ears, thin legs, and a belly free of wool.

Bovska

This extremely rare short-legged sheep breed is used as a milk sheep in Slovenia. It has very small ears and is either white or black and white.

Bozakh

This dairy sheep breed has coarse wool. It can be white, golden or brown but always has a black head and legs. It is found in Azerbaijan.

Braunes Bergschaf

This breed, known in English as the Brown Mountain sheep, is descended from the Tyrolean Stone Sheep. It is used in Germany not only for meat but for managing high, steep, rough pastures. It is brown with long downward-hanging ears.

Brillenschaf

This is a meat-producing sheep breed with saleable wool. It is white with distinctive black ears and black spectacles, and is rare but found in Austria and Slovenia.

British Charollais

See Sheep Breeds of the UK.

British Friesland

See Sheep Breeds of the UK.

British Milk

See Sheep Breeds of the UK.

Bündner Oberländerschaf

This grey sheep breed has a slender wool-free head. The rams are horned but the ewes are normally polled. It is a medium-sized primitive sheep used to manage the vegetation on steep rough pastures in Switzerland.

California Red

This sheep breed was produced on the Pacific seaboard of the USA during the 1970s. The lambs, which make excellent meat, are red. The adults are whiter with red legs and both sexes are polled. The sheep perform well in hot climates and will breed out of season.

Cameroon

A large hair-coated sheep breed from West Africa, producing useful meat. It is fawn with a white rump and thin tail, and has a black underbelly, legs, mandibles, ears and spectacles.

Campanian Barbary

A medium, white, polled wool sheep breed with a clean face and lop ears. It is used for meat and milking. Originally from Tunisia but now found in southern Italy.

Campbell Island

This was a feral breed originating from roughly 5000 sheep left on an island after the farmers had left. Ten of the best specimens were retained in New Zealand in 2005. The blood is mainly Merino.

Canadian Arcott

This all-white wool sheep breed is a hybrid bred from the Île-de-France and the Suffolk. It was standardized in Canada and is primarily a meat-producing sheep, suitable as a terminal sire.

Charmoise

This large, white, polled wool sheep breed was developed in France for meat. It is popular in Ireland.

Charollais

This large, polled, cream sheep breed with a brown face was developed in mid-France several centuries ago. It is an excellent meat-producing sheep.

It is popular in many countries, particularly in the UK, where it is the third most popular terminal sire. Its progeny are sought after by butchers on account of their high killing-out percentage and low fat content.

Cheviot

See Sheep Breeds of the UK.

Chios

This white dairy sheep breed with a semi-fat tail has a black face with a wide white blaze. It was originally from the island of Chios in Greece, hence its name. It is widely found in southern and eastern Europe.

Cholistani

This is a small white-bodied sheep breed with a brown head. It has short ears and a thin tail. It has wool but is primarily bred in Pakistan for meat.

Churra

This dual-purpose sheep breed is often called the Spanish Churro. It is milked in Spain and produces useful fat lambs. It is white with black feet, nose, ears and spectacles, and has soft wool.

Cikta

This small, white mountain sheep was bred in Germany for its wool but the breed is now kept in Hungary as a fat lamb producer. The ewes are polled; the rams have small, white, knob-like horns.

Cine Capari

This small white fat-tailed sheep breed comes from Turkey and is kept for meat; the wool is very coarse.

Clun Forest

See Sheep Breeds of the UK.

Coburger Fuchsschaf

This large, polled sheep breed is often called the Coburg Fox Sheep. It is white with brown legs and a slightly Roman nose. It is used in Germany for pasture management.

Columbia

This is a white sheep breed with good wool properties; both sexes are polled. It was bred in the USA.

Comeback

This is a hybrid sheep breed using Merino and Lincoln Longwool blood, and was developed in Australia for both meat and milk. It is a big, polled sheep very suitable for climates with high rainfall.

Comisana

This is a medium-sized white dairy sheep breed with a red head, and so is often called the Red Head. In its native Italy, it is known as Testa Rossa or Farcia Rossa. Both sexes are polled.

Coolalee

This is a white, hybrid sheep breed bred in Australia for fat lamb production. However, it has quite good wool and a clean face. Both sexes are polled.

Coopworth

This is a white, hybrid sheep breed containing merino blood, from New Zealand. It has excellent wool quality and makes good fat lambs. Both sexes are polled.

Cormo

This white, hybrid wool sheep breed was developed in Australia. It has a large amount of Merino blood. The head is woolly and both sexes are polled.

Corriedale

This famous white wool sheep breed was bred in Australia, not only for its fine wool but also for its excellent fat lamb production. It is now found in hot climates throughout the world. Both sexes are polled.

Cotentin

This hardy longwool sheep breed comes from Normandy in France. It is pure white with a clean head and has excellent meat.

Cotswold

See Sheep Breeds of the UK.

Criollo

This small meat sheep breed with carpet-quality wool is found in highland areas throughout central and south America. It can be black, white or pied.

Dagliç

This white, short fat-tailed sheep breed has black spots on its head and legs. The ewes are polled but the rams have horns. The wool is coarse and only suitable for carpets. It is primarily a dairy sheep but the progeny make good fat lambs. It originated from western Anatolia but is found throughout Turkey, Syria and Lebanon.

Dala Fur

This is a small, white hardy wool sheep breed from Sweden, kept for wool and meat. It has no wool on its tail. The ewes are polled but the rams have horns.

Dalesbred

See Sheep Breeds of the UK.

Damani

This small, white sheep breed has a white body and black head. It is polled and has small ears. It originates from the north-west frontier area of Pakistan and is kept for meat and wool.

Damara

This red- to brown-haired sheep breed was originally from Egypt and is now found throughout Namibia and southern Angola. The rams have large curled horns. It can cope with extremes of climate and still produce and rear twins. It is also content to browse.

Danish Landrace

This medium-sized white wool sheep breed comes from Denmark, as the name suggests. It is also called the Landfar or the Klitfar. It has wool on its face and right down its relatively short legs.

Debouillet

This is a white crossbred sheep breed from New Mexico in the USA. It is a medium-sized sheep containing Merino and Rambouillet blood. The ewes are polled, as are some of the rams.

Delaine Merino

This hardy, white wool sheep breed was bred in the USA. It has a very fine-woolled, oily fleece.

Derbyshire Gritstone

See Sheep Breeds of the UK.

Deutsches Bergschaf

This polled, white, medium-woolled sheep breed has a clean head. Its English name is the White Mountain sheep. It was bred in Germany for wool and meat.

Devon Closewool

See Sheep Breeds of the UK.

Devon Longwool

See Sheep Breeds of the UK.

Dohne Merino

This very large wool sheep breed produces useful fat lambs. It was bred in South Africa but now is common in Australia.

Dorper

This famous white-haired sheep breed is ideally suited to the arid climate of South Africa where it was bred. It produces excellent fat lambs. Both sexes are polled. It was bred from Black-headed Persian sheep crossed with Dorset Horn sheep.

Dorset Down

See Sheep Breeds of the UK.

Dorset Horn

See Sheep Breeds of the UK.

Drysdale

These are small hybrid sheep bred in New Zealand for wool production. Both sexes are horned.

Est à Laine

This French sheep breed is one of the many variations of the Merino, the most predominant breed in the southern hemisphere. Merinos are primarily fine wool producers. However the heritability of wool quality is high, and therefore their crosses will retain this characteristic although obviously the further away from the true Merino, the coarser the wool becomes. It should not be forgotten that although genetics are paramount in producing fine wool, nutrition and housing do play a part.

East Friesian

This excellent milking sheep breed can produce 900 l of milk in a 300-day lactation. It flourishes on the heathland of Northern Germany where it is known as the Ostfriesisches Milchschaf. It is a large, polled, white sheep with a pink nose.

Easycare

See Sheep Breeds of the UK.

Elliottdale

This large white sheep breed is a mutation of a Romney Marsh. It produces large amounts of carpet-quality wool. Both sexes are polled.

Estonian Ruhnu

This is a small, rare white sheep breed with a badger face. Most are polled except a few rams. It is also known as the Eesti maalammas and lives on a single island off Estonia.

Exmoor Horn

See Sheep Breeds of the UK.

Fabrianese

This large, white dairy sheep breed produces good fat lambs. Both sexes are polled. It has coarse wool and a Roman nose and originates from Italy.

Faroes

See Sheep Breeds of the UK.

Finnish Landrace

This is a very prolific breed having litters of between five and seven lambs per lambing. It has been crossed with the Dorset Horn to breed a ewe which is not only prolific but will also breed lambs out of season. It is sometimes called the Finnsheep.

Fuglestad

This polled, white sheep breed has black spots on its face and legs. It has a long tail and is kept in Norway for wool and meat.

Gala

This white wool sheep breed has a black head and legs, and both sexes are polled. It has a fat tail and is a good meat producer. It is kept in Azerbaijan.

Galway

This large, white, polled sheep breed has wool on its face and legs. It is mainly kept in Ireland for meat.

Garadolaq

This is a large, white sheep breed with long legs and a fat tail. It is a good meat producer and can be shorn twice a year. It is bred in Azerbaijan.

Gedebey Merino

This large white sheep breed has a considerable amount of wool and is also is a good meat producer. The rams have large curly horns. It is kept in Azerbaijan.

Godek

This is a small white wool sheep breed with a fat tail. It is a good meat producer and is found in Azerbaijan.

Gotland

This is a very old Northern European short-tailed sheep breed from Sweden. It is grey/brown with a black head, and both sexes are polled. It has good meat. The pelts are often sold and the fleece is sought after by hand-spinners.

Grey Troender

This is a very rare and fecund grey sheep breed from Norway, with distinctive white markings below the eyes. Both sexes are polled. The wool is sought after for handicrafts and the pelts are often sold.

Greyface Dartmoor

See Sheep Breeds of the UK.

Gromark

This dual-purpose, white, clean-headed, lean sheep breed was bred in New South Wales in Australia using half Corriedale and half Border Leicester blood. Both sexes are polled.

Gute

This very primitive Northern European short-tailed sheep breed comes from Sweden. It is grey with large curling horns in both sexes.

Hampshire Down

See Sheep Breeds of the UK.

Hebridean

See Sheep Breeds of the UK.

Heidschnucke

This ancient German horned breed has been changed in recent years by breeding in white polled stock. However, the real breed is a grey animal with a black head and both sexes are horned. It has coarse wool but produces reasonable meat, and is mainly kept nowadays to control and improve pastures.

Herdwick

See Sheep Breeds of the UK.

Hill Radnor

See Sheep Breeds of the UK.

Hog Island

This is a heavy, white-woolled sheep breed with a black head and legs. Both sexes are polled. It is still kept in parts of the USA.

Hu

This is a small, white sheep breed with long wavy wool. It has a clean face and both sexes are polled. It comes from Mongolia where it can breed all year round.

Icelandic

This, as the name implies, was bred and is still found in Iceland. It is a big, white dairy sheep breed with good wool. The lambs are good meat. Both sexes are horned.

Île-de-France

This is really a French Merino breed. It is white with excellent wool and also produces good fat lambs. The breed is very fecund: triplets and quads are common. It has a clean face and both sexes are polled.

Iranian Long-woolled

This wool sheep breed comes from Iran (Fig. 1.19) and is also commonly found in Turkey and Syria (Fig. 1.20). It has a black head with a white forelock. The body is white, as are the legs, except below the fetlocks. It is fecund and produces good mutton.

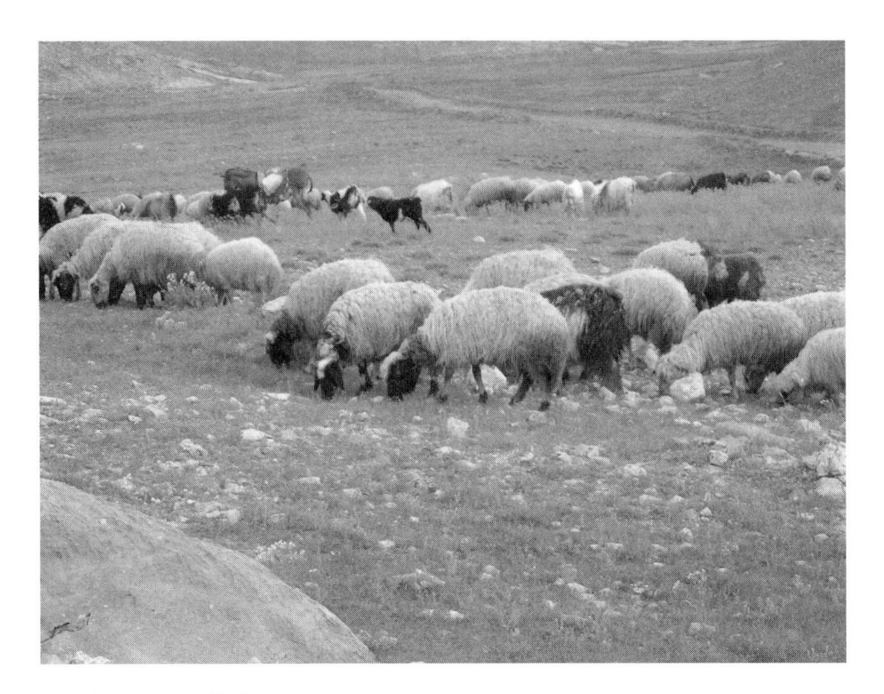

Fig. 1.19. Iranian Long-woolled.

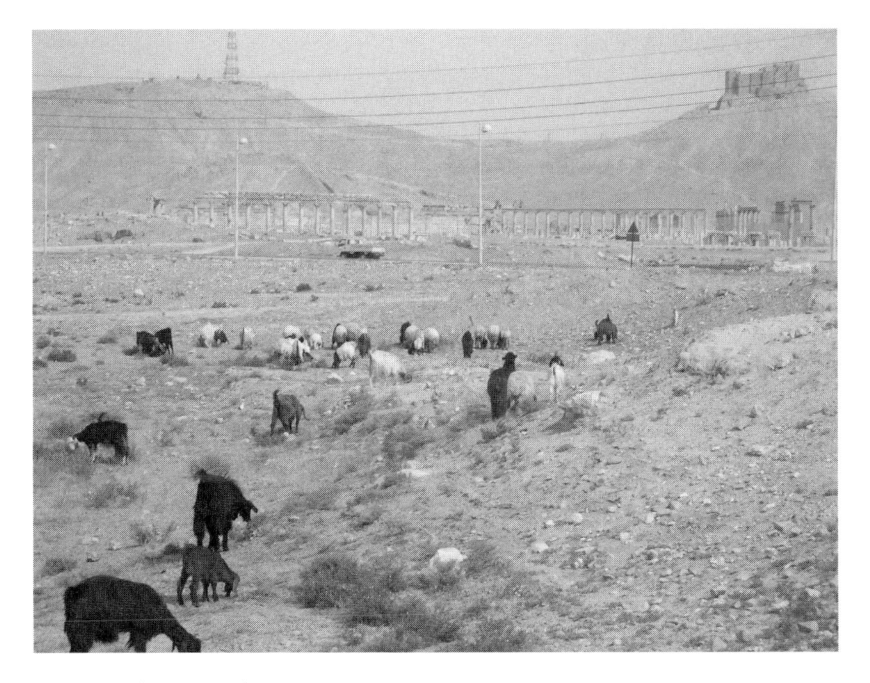

Fig. 1.20. Sheep and goats at Palmyra.

Iranian Red

As the name implies, this sheep breed comes from Iran. The lambs are all red; the adults are cream with red legs and heads. It is really a hair sheep producing good meat. The tail is thin, and both sexes have horns, with the rams having very long spiral horns.

Istrian Milk

This dairy sheep breed of various colours was bred in Italy but is now found in the Balkans. The rams have small curly horns and the ewes are polled. The wool is very coarse.

Jacob

See Sheep Breeds of the UK.

Jaro

This white sheep breed has brown spots on its clean head, brown legs and a fat tail. The wool is coarse. It is kept in Azerbaijan for meat production.

Jezersko-Solcavska

This is a white, mountain sheep breed with long pendulous ears and coarse wool; both sexes are polled. It is found in Slovenia.

Juraschaf

This is a small black or brown mountain sheep breed found in Switzerland. Both sexes are polled. It is a non-seasonal breeder and very fecund. It produces good meat but has coarse wool.

Kachhi

This is a medium-sized sheep breed of variously coloured coarse wool. Both sexes are polled. It has a black head, long floppy ears and a Roman nose. It comes from the Sind area of Pakistan and breeds good fat lambs.

Kajli

This breed from the Punjab area of both Pakistan and India is a big polled sheep of various colours. It has enormous lop ears and a Roman nose. It is a wool sheep, producing good meat.

Kamakuyruk

This is a Turkish white fat-tailed hair sheep breed that produces good fat lambs.

Karabagh

This is an old milk sheep breed that has coarse, light brown wool. It has a fat tail and is a good meat producer. It is found in Azerbaijan.

Karagouniko

This is a dairy sheep breed from central mainland Greece. It is white or black with a thin tail. The wool is coarse but the meat is excellent.

Karakul

This is a medium-sized all-black sheep breed found throughout Central Asia. It is milked and eaten. It produces fine wool and its hide is sought after for leather goods. It is also kept in the arid areas of South Africa. Both sexes are polled.

Karayaka

This is primarily a milk-producing sheep breed found throughout Turkey. It is white with a black head and legs. It has long wool suitable for making carpets and it also produces good meat. Both sexes are polled.

Katahdin

This is a polled, white hair sheep breed bred for rough arid areas in the USA. It is kept for fat lamb production.

Kempen Heath

This is a white, clean-headed, polled sheep breed kept in Holland for meat and wool.

Kerry Hill

See Sheep Breeds of the UK.

Kivircik

This is a white dairy sheep breed with medium-quality wool, kept in Western Turkey. The females are polled but the rams have horns. It produces good fat lambs.

Kooka

This is a white, milk, haired sheep breed from Pakistan. It has a thin tail and long floppy ears. Both sexes are polled.

Krainer Steinschaf

This is a small white, mountain sheep breed from Bavaria in Germany. Both sexes have horns. The wool is coarse so this is primarily a meat sheep.

Lacaune

This is a large, white dairy breed from France. It is renowned for its high milk yield and fecundity.

Landais

This is a medium-sized white sheep breed with black spots, producing coarse wool. The rams have curled horns but the ewes are polled. It was bred in Gascony in France for meat production.

Lange

This small, white dairy sheep breed has coarse wool. It has a clean face with semi-lop ears and both sexes are polled. It produces good fat lambs and is milked in Italy.

Lati

This is a white sheep breed with a clean face but wool down its legs. It has lop ears and a fat tail. It is seen in the Punjab area of India and Pakistan where it is mainly kept for meat production.

Latxa

This breed has cream wool and a fawn face, and is kept for milk production in Spain. Both sexes have small horns.

Leineschaf

This large, white, meat-producing sheep breed is kept in the Hanoverian area of Germany. Both sexes have horns and long ears. The wool is long.

Lezgi

This Russian sheep breed spends the summers high up in the Caucasus Mountains and is moved lower in the winter. It is a white wool sheep with a fat tail and both sexes have curved-back horns.

Lincoln Longwool

See Sheep Breeds of the UK.

Lithuanian Black-headed

This, as the name implies, is a white breed with a black head and comes from Lithuania. The wool is semi-fine and the lambs are good quality. Both sexes are polled.

Llanwenog

See Sheep Breeds of the UK.

Lleyn

See Sheep Breeds of the UK.

Lohi

This is a wool sheep breed from Pakistan.

Lonk

See Sheep Breeds of the UK.

Luzein

This breed is found in the Alpine areas of Germany and Switzerland. It is a white sheep with good wool. Both sexes are polled, and it produces good fat lambs.

Maltese

These red-headed sheep, now found in Malta, were actually from Sicily. They are dairy sheep with silky white wool and produce good fat lambs. Both sexes are polled.

Manchega

This big white dairy sheep breed has a clean face with pink lips and muzzle. It comes from Spain.

Manech

This white sheep breed with long coarse wool and a black head comes from both sides of the Pyrenees. Both sexes have tall curly horns. It is a meat-producing sheep.

Manx Loaghtan

See Sheep Breeds of the UK.

Marco Polo

This famous mountain sheep breed, whose rams have massive curling horns, is not really a domestic sheep. It is found high up in the Pamir Mountains on the Chinese border. It is dark brown with white underparts. It is actually *Ovis ammon polii.*

Masai

This is a medium-sized hair sheep breed found in the Masai areas of Kenya and Tanzania. It has a white body with a red head and neck. The rams have horns but the ewes are polled. It has a fat tail and produces good meat.

Massese

This is a white dairy sheep breed from Italy with good wool that produces good fat lambs.

Meatmaster

This hybrid polled sheep breed has a semi-fat tail. It is of varying colour but produces excellent fat lambs off arid pastures. It was standardized in South Africa.

Mehraban

This light-brown meat sheep breed producing carpet wool comes from Iran.

Merinizzata Italiana

This is a white wool dairy sheep breed from central and southern Italy.

Merino

This breed of world-wide renown is the foundation of a very large number of breeds. It comes from Spain and was developed in the 12th century. It is a good forager with excellent wool with a staple length of 65–100 mm. The wool is always less than 24 μm and from the ultra-fine animals is less than 15 μm. Animals fed solely on 'salt-bush' in Western Australia regularly produce wool of less than 11 μm. Fleeces weigh between 3 and 6 kg. The carcass size is relatively small but in several countries the breed has been perfected to increase this, and excellent fat lambs are produced. It is a white sheep with an almost clean face. Both sexes naturally have long spiral horns close to the head. However, polled animals have been bred and are now much more common. Only in UK is the breed rare.

Moghani

Also known as the Mughan, this is a white sheep breed with good wool. It has a fat tail and produces good fat lambs. Both sexes are polled. It is found in Iran and Azerbaijan.

Montadale

This is a large white hybrid sheep breed from the USA, bred for both meat and milk. Both sexes are polled.

Morada Nova

This is a medium-sized sheep breed from Brazil, bred for meat. It is a red-haired sheep and both sexes are polled.

Najdi

This is a large black sheep breed with a white head and white underside of neck and belly. It has coarse wool and in Saudi Arabia is kept for meat.

Navajo-Churro

This is a white hybrid sheep breed from the USA, bred for wool production. Both sexes are polled.

Newfoundland

This is a medium-sized white sheep breed, mainly polled, bred for meat and wool in Canada.

Nellore

This is a small, hair sheep breed and is mainly white with a black underbelly and legs. The rams have broad horns but the ewes are polled. It comes from the Andhra Pradesh area of India.

Nolana

This is a white hair sheep hybrid breed from the USA for out-of-season fat lamb production.

Norfolk Horn

See Sheep Breeds of the UK.

North Ronaldsay

See Sheep Breeds of the UK.

Northern European Short-tailed

This is really a group of breeds of various colours found in Northern Europe, mainly in Scandinavia, Germany and Russia. They are all meat animals as well as milking animals, with fat tails and coarse wool.

Norwegian Fur

This is a medium-sized, meat-producing, grey sheep breed with a black head and white face, found in Scandinavia. Both sexes are polled.

Ossimi

This is a big white sheep breed with a clean brown head and lop ears. It comes from lower Egypt. The male has horns but the female is polled. It has carpet-quality wool and a fat tail and is mainly kept for meat.

Ouessant

This is a small brown sheep breed with large horns, also called the Breton Island Dwarf. It is largely kept in France as a pet. The wool is used by home spinners.

Oula

This is a native Tibetan meat sheep breed with a fat tail. It comes in a variety of colours.

Oxford Down

See Sheep Breeds of the UK.

Pag Island

This white wool sheep breed comes from Croatia. The rams have horns but the ewes are polled.

Pagliarola

This is a small coarse-woolled sheep breed kept in Italy for meat. It is either red or black, and both sexes are polled.

Panama

This large, white, polled sheep breed is kept in the north-west of the USA for meat.

Pedi

This fat-tailed, polled, meat sheep breed is brown with a white saddle. It is found in South Africa.

Pelibüey

This large red or red and white, long-legged sheep breed is also called Cubano Rojo. It produces good meat but no wool. It is found in the Caribbean, Mexico and South America, and performs well in arid climates.

Perendale

This crossbred sheep breed was standardized in New Zealand to produce fat lambs. It is a white, polled sheep with Romney Marsh and Cheviot blood.

Pinzirita

This white dairy sheep breed has black spots on its head and legs, and coarse wool. It is still milked in Sicily and it also produces fat lambs.

Pitt Island

This very rare black sheep breed with very large horns has thick wool, which is loved by spinners. It is found mainly on the Chatham Islands of New Zealand.

Polish Heath

This is a large, white, short-tailed, meat-producing sheep breed still seen in Poland.

Poll Dorset

This breed was developed in Australia by breeding Dorset Horn ewes with either Ryeland or Corriedale.

Polwarth

This hybrid breed for producing fat lambs and wool was standardized in Australia. It has roughly 75% Merino blood and 25% Lincoln Longwool blood.

Polypay

This hybrid breed was produced in the USA to provide meat and wool. It is a medium-sized white polled animal comprising a large number of breeds.

Pomeranian Coarsewool

This is a large brown wool sheep breed with a clean brown head. In Germany it provides good fat lambs from rough pastures and helps to control the vegetation.

Portland

See Sheep Breeds of the UK.

Priangan

This sheep breed, also called the Garut, comes from Java in Indonesia. It is black or pied and the ewes are polled but the rams have large horns. It is now used for meat but at one time it was used for ram fighting.

Qashqai

This is a brown spotted sheep breed with a fat tail and carpet-quality wool, found in Iran.

Qiaoke

This is a small, black, meat sheep breed found in China.

Qinghai Black Tibetan

This is a large, polled, black sheep breed from Tibet. It has carpet-quality wool and is also used for meat.

Qinghai Semifinewool

This is a hybrid breed standardized in China from crossing Romney Marsh and the local Xinjian breed. The rams have horns but the ewes are polled.

Quadrella

This Italian dairy sheep breed produces some useful meat. Some animals of both sexes have horns.

Quanglin Large-tail

This breed is from the Shanxi region of China. It is a medium-sized brown sheep with a white belly. As the name suggests, it has a fat tail, and is a good meat producer. The rams have large horns but the ewes are polled. The wool is only carpet quality.

Rabo Largo

This pied, fat-tailed, horned, hair sheep breed comes from Northern Brazil. It is a meat sheep.

Racka

This is a very large long-woolled light brown sheep breed. It has amazingly long straight-out horns. It is still milked in Hungary and is a good meat producer.

Radnor Forest

See Sheep Breeds of the UK.

Rambouillet

This breed is the French Merino. It has excellent wool and is pure white with large horns. It also produces good fat lambs.

Rasa Aragonesa

This is a medium-sized white sheep with a clean head. It is a good meat producer. Both sexes are polled. It comes from the Aragon area of Spain.

Red Engadine

This is a dark red Swiss sheep breed with lop ears. It is both a meat and a wool producer.

Red Karaman

This red sheep breed has a fat tail and produces good fat lambs. It originated in Turkey but is also found in the Middle East (Fig. 1.21).

Rhoen

This is a brown, meat-producing sheep breed from Bavaria in Germany. It has coarse wool.

Rideau Arcott

This is a hybrid meat-producing sheep breed standardized in Canada. It is a large, white, polled sheep.

Romanov

This grey sheep breed has a distinctive black head with a white blaze. It is a meat-producing sheep from the Volga valley in Russia.

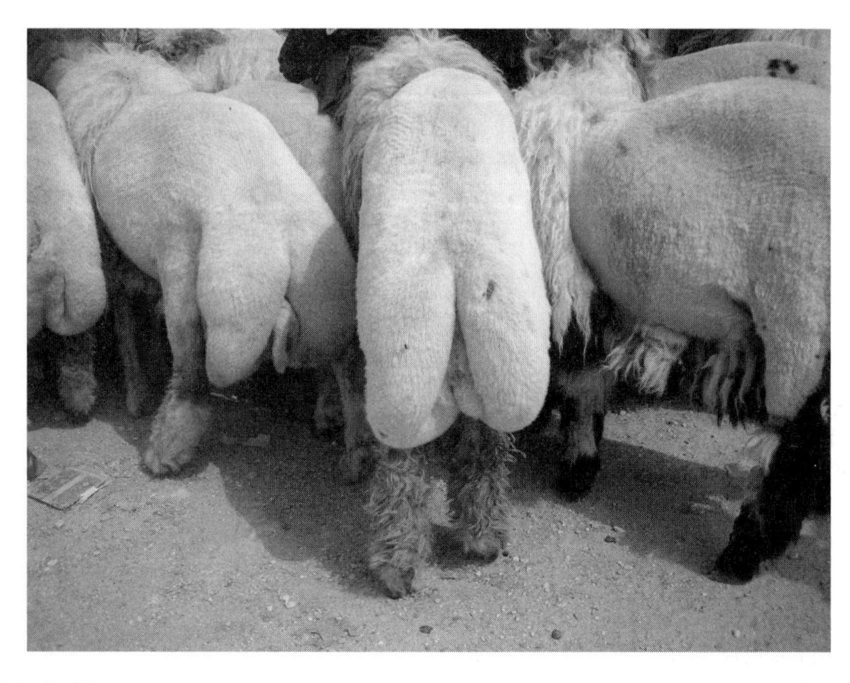

Fig. 1.21. Red Karaman.

Romney Marsh

See Sheep Breeds of the UK.

Roslag

This is a rare sheep breed from Sweden. It produces meat and wool for smallholders. Most are white but about 10% are black. All of the sheep have short tails but only the rams have horns.

Rouge de l'Ouest

This premium sheep breed is cream with a red head, hence its name. It has a very well-muscled rump and is a good terminal sire. The fat lambs are sought after by butchers. It originated in central France but is popular in the UK.

Rouge de Roussillon

This white sheep breed with a red head is kept on the French side of the Pyrenees. It is a good wool and meat producer.

Rough Fell

See Sheep Breeds of the UK.

Royal White

This hybrid, meat-producing sheep breed was standardized in the USA.

Ruda

This rare white sheep breed with pink skin is a good wool producer. It is a small sheep and is found in Albania and Croatia.

Rya

This sheep breed, found in Sweden and Norway, has very short legs. It produces wool for carpets.

Ryeland

See Sheep Breeds of the UK.

Sahel

This hair sheep breed has a red fore-end with a white rump and thin tail. It has small ears, and both sexes have horns that project straight out sideways from the head. It is kept for meat in Chad, Mali, Mauritania and Niger.

Sakiz

This wool sheep breed is kept for milk around Izmir in Turkey. The rams have horns.

Santa Cruz

This white wool sheep breed has long clean legs. It is kept in the USA for wool production.

Sardinian

This white milk sheep breed is found on the Italian mainland as well as in Sardinia. It has coarse wool. Both sexes are polled.

Scottish Blackface

See Sheep Breeds of the UK.

Scottish Dunface

See Sheep Breeds of the UK.

Shetland

See Sheep Breeds of the UK.

Shirvan

This all-white sheep with a clean head has coarse wool but is a good meat producer in arid climates. Both sexes are polled. It is bred in Azerbaijan and Georgia.

Shropshire Down

See Sheep Breeds of the UK.

Sicilian Barbary

This white milk sheep breed has a speckled face and legs. Both sexes are polled. The wool is of medium quality.

Skudde

This small, white, meat sheep breed has a short tail and the rams have curly horns. The wool is of poor quality and is used for felting. It is found in East Prussia and is used for landscape management.

Soay

See Sheep Breeds of the UK.

Somali

This white hair sheep breed has a black head and neck. It is kept for meat in Somalia.

Sopravissana

This milk sheep breed has fine wool and is kept in central Italy. Only the rams have horns.

Southdown

See Sheep Breeds of the UK.

Spælsau

This all-white sheep breed with long coarse wool is kept for meat in Norway.

Spiegel

This medium-sized, white sheep breed has brown areas around the eyes and ears, hence the name. It is kept for meat in Austria.

St. Croix

This tall white sheep breed with very long legs has coarse wool and is kept for meat in the Virgin Islands.

Steigar

This Norwegian wool sheep breed has a clean face. Both sexes are polled.

Steinschaf

This rare, medium-sized sheep breed is grey with a black head. It is kept for meat in the Alpine areas of Austria and Germany.

Suffolk Down

See Sheep Breeds of the UK.

Swaledale

See Sheep Breeds of the UK.

Swedish Fur

This dark grey wool sheep breed has a black head. Both sexes are polled. It is also kept in Sweden for meat.

Swifter

This new hybrid sheep breed, based on the Texel, was developed in Holland for meat and wool.

Taleshi

This hair sheep breed of varying colours is kept in Iran for meat.

Tan

This white wool sheep breed has a speckled nose. It is mainly kept for meat in China.

Targhee

This hybrid sheep breed was developed in Idaho in the USA for wool production. It is a white, polled sheep with a clean face.

Teeswater

See Sheep Breeds of the UK.

Texel

This large, all-white sheep breed with good wool was developed for meat production in the Netherlands, and originally came from Texel Island in the north-west of that country. The breed was started in 1911. It was used in France in 1933, came to the UK in 1970 and is now used in Australia, Africa and South America. It has an excellent conformation with a large rump and with muscle right down to the hocks, and is much sought after by butchers. It is the second most popular terminal sire in the UK (Fig. 1.22). A black animal was bred from two white Texel parents, resulting in the breeding of Blue Texels (Fig. 1.23).

Thalli

This is a very distinctive sheep breed with a large amount of white wool. It is black-headed with a wide white blaze, is polled and has long pendulous ears. It is found in the Punjab in Pakistan.

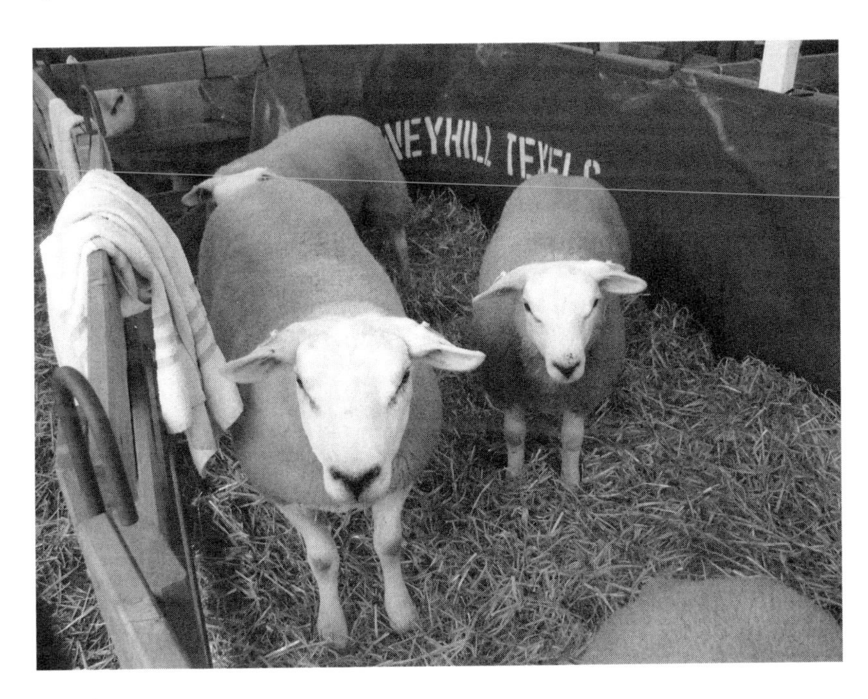

Fig. 1.22. Texels.

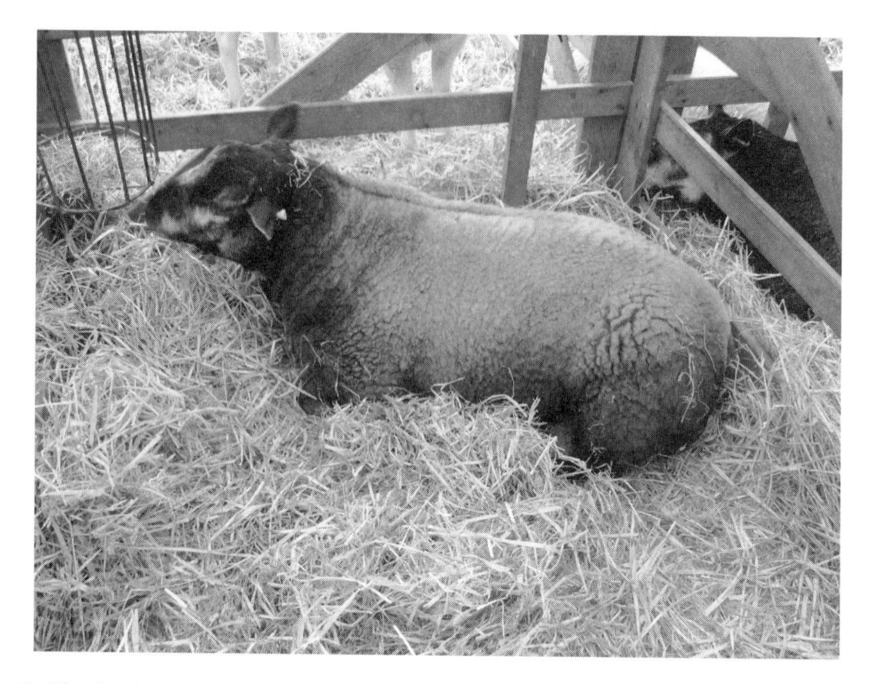

Fig. 1.23. Blue Texel.

Tong

This large, white, polled, hair sheep breed has a very fat tail. It is kept in Mongolia.

Touabire

This is a long-legged sheep breed of various colours with a thin tail. It originated in the Middle East but is now found in Mali.

Tsurcana

This white sheep breed has very long wool. The rams have horns but the ewes are polled. It is found in Romania.

Tuj

The rams of this white hair sheep breed have big horns but the ewes are polled. It has a fat tail and is kept in the Kurdish areas of Turkey, Iran and Iraq for meat.

Tukidale

This hybrid sheep breed was developed for wool production in New Zealand. It is white and grows so much wool that it can be shorn twice a year. The main forebear was the Romney.

Tunis

This is a white, meat-producing sheep breed from Tunisia. The ewes are polled.

Turkgeldi

This dairy sheep breed is white with a clean head. It comes from Thrace in Turkey. Both sexes are polled.

Turki

This large, brown, hair sheep breed has a fat tail. It is kept for meat in Afghanistan.

Tush

This all-white sheep breed has long coarse wool. The rams have curly horns but the ewes are polled. It is a good meat producer and kept in Georgia.

Ujuingin

This white sheep breed has a speckled face, coarse wool and a fat tail. It is kept in China for meat.

Valais Blacknose

This white sheep breed with a black face has thick long wool, but in Switzerland is now kept for meat.

Van Rooy

This all-white hair sheep breed has a clean head. It has a fat tail and is kept in South Africa for meat.

Vendéen

This is a large white wool sheep breed with a brown face, kept in France for meat.

Walachenschaf

This rare white wool sheep breed has spots on its head and long corkscrew horns. It is kept in Slovakia for meat.

Waldschaf

These small Bavarian sheep will breed out of season.

Wallis County

This big white sheep breed with large curly horns is kept in the USA for wool.

Waziri

This white sheep breed with a black head has coarse wool and a fat tail. It is kept in Pakistan for meat.

Welsh Mountain

See Sheep Breeds of the UK.

Wensleydale

See Sheep Breeds of the UK.

White Suffolk

This breed was developed in Australia from the Suffolk. All the black colouring was bred out.

Whitefaced Dartmoor

See Sheep Breeds of the UK.

Whitefaced Woodland

See Sheep Breeds of the UK.

Wiltipoll

This hybrid, meat-producing sheep breed was produced in Australia. As the name implies, it is polled. It is a hair sheep with a large amount of Wiltshire Horn blood in it.

Wiltshire Horn

See Sheep Breeds of the UK.

Xalda

This rare black sheep breed has large curled horns and coarse wool. It is kept in Northern Spain for meat.

Xaxi Ardia

This white sheep breed with coarse wool and curled horns is kept in the Basque region for meat.

Xinjiang Finewool

This large white sheep breed has a black underbelly and long legs, and a fat rump. Both sexes have curled horns. It was standardized in China for wool production.

Zackel

This white dairy sheep breed has a thin tail and carpet-quality wool. The rams have long spiral horns and the ewes are polled. It is kept in Eastern Europe and Western Asia.

Zaghawa

This black hair sheep breed is kept in the Sudan and Chad for meat. Only the rams have horns.

Zaian

This hair sheep breed of various colours is kept for meat in Morocco.

Zaire Long-legged

This white hair sheep breed has lop ears. The rams have horns. It is kept in the Congo for meat.

Zakynthos

This milk-sheep breed of various colours comes from the Greek Island of Zakynthos.

Zeeland Milk

As the name implies, this is a dairy sheep breed from the Netherlands. It is white and polled.

Zel

This white sheep breed with a thin tail has carpet-quality wool. The rams have horns. It is found in Northern Iran.

Zelazna

This wool sheep breed has good meat potential. It is kept in Poland.

Zemmour

This white sheep breed has a brown face. The rams are horned. The wool is carpet quality. It is found on the Atlantic coast of Morocco.

Zeta Yellow

This is a dairy sheep breed with coarse wool that produces good fat lambs. It is white with a brownish-yellow head and feet. It is kept in Montenegro.

Zlatusha

This is a white sheep breed with medium-quality wool. It is bred in Bulgaria.

Zoulay

This sheep breed, of various colours, comes from the High Atlas Mountains in Morocco.

Zwartbles

This brown wool sheep breed has a white blaze, a white muzzle and four white feet. Both sexes are polled. It is kept in the Netherlands for meat.

General Evolution of Goats

Goats are among the earliest animals domesticated by humans, probably 10,000 years ago.

The most recent genetic analysis confirms the archaeological evidence that the most likely area was north-western Iran. Unlike sheep, goats easily revert to feral or wild conditions given a chance. There are many recognized breeds of domestic goat, *Capra aegagrus hircus*. Goat breeds, especially dairy goats, are some of the oldest defined animal breeds for which breed standards and production records have been kept. Selective breeding of goats generally focuses on improving production of milk, meat or fibre. In a few cases goats have been bred for their hides. Certain goats have been selected for traits that improve them as pets. One of the main centres for goat breeding in Europe was in the Alps, mainly in Switzerland. Another key area elsewhere in the world was South Africa.

In 2008 there were 13.4 million goats in the European Union (EU), the majority being in Greece, Spain and France. Obviously this number will increase rapidly when other countries further east are included in the EU. The number in the whole of Europe is only 2.2% of the whole world's population of goats. Only estimates can be made, but there are at least 200 million goats in Africa.

Goat Breeds of the UK

Anglo-Nubian

This large goat breed has been developed in the UK from the Nubian goat. It is a dual-purpose animal with Roman nose and long hanging ears, and is mainly used for milk production. It is usually mahogany with black and white markings, but the colour is extremely variable; spots or marbling are often seen (Fig. 1.24).

Angora

This goat breed produces a fibre known as mohair. It should be noted that the fibre described as angora comes from rabbits. Angora goats originated in Turkey about 200 years ago and were exported to South Africa and the USA, where they were further

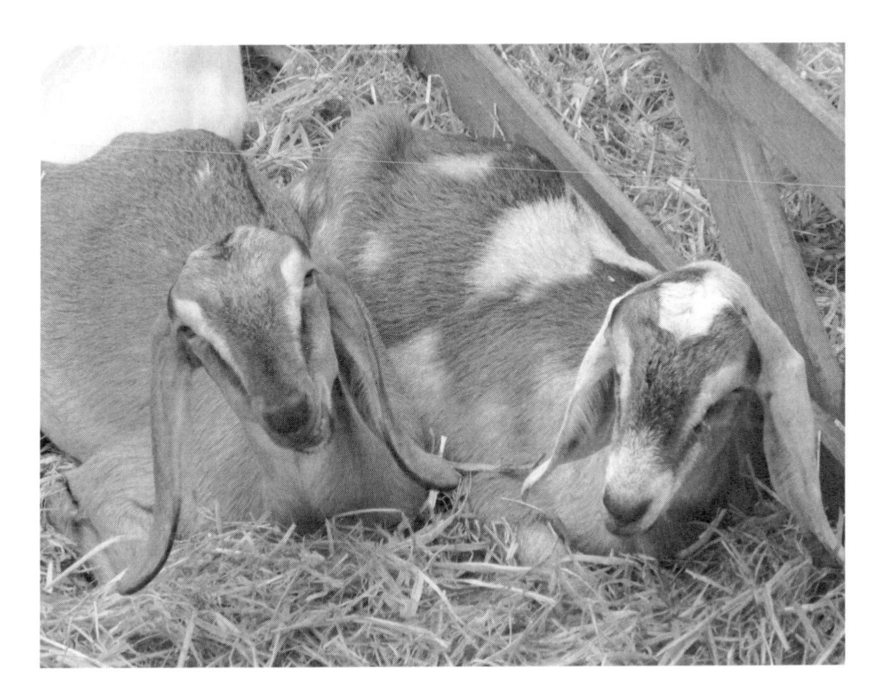

Fig. 1.24. Anglo-Nubian kids.

developed. Only white animals are kept for breeding but coloured 'throw-backs' do occur. In the USA they are mainly found in Texas. They spread to New Zealand and to Australia, particularly to Tasmania, and were imported into the UK from these last two areas in 1981. They have also been imported into Canada and Holland.

Mohair is a long lustrous fibre, which on the animal forms characteristic ringlets or curled staples. In their first year kids produce 1–1.5 kg of fibre, rising to 2.5–3.5 kg in adults. Males, whether entire or castrated, produce more fibre than females. However the fibre quality of the males is not as good, being about 35 μm in diameter whereas in females it is 30 μm. Super-fine kid fibre may be as low as 25 μm. The mohair grows rapidly and so the goats can be shorn twice yearly, with a fleece length of 120–150 mm. The quality of the fibre is also influenced by the quantity of poor fibres. These are either medullated with a hollow core, or kemps, which are more hair-like (Fig. 1.25).

British Alpine

These goats have been bred from the British Toggenburg. They are of similar conformation but are black and white rather than dark fawn and white.

British Saanen

This all-white goat has been bred in the UK from the alpine Saanen but the British breed is larger (Fig. 1.26).

British Toggenburg

This breed has been produced from the Toggenburg, originating in Switzerland. This is a small, pale fawn-coloured goat with a longish coat. Toggenburgs normally have a white stripe on their faces. They have white legs and rumps and are frequently polled. British Toggenburgs are larger and darker than the Swiss Toggenburgs but generally

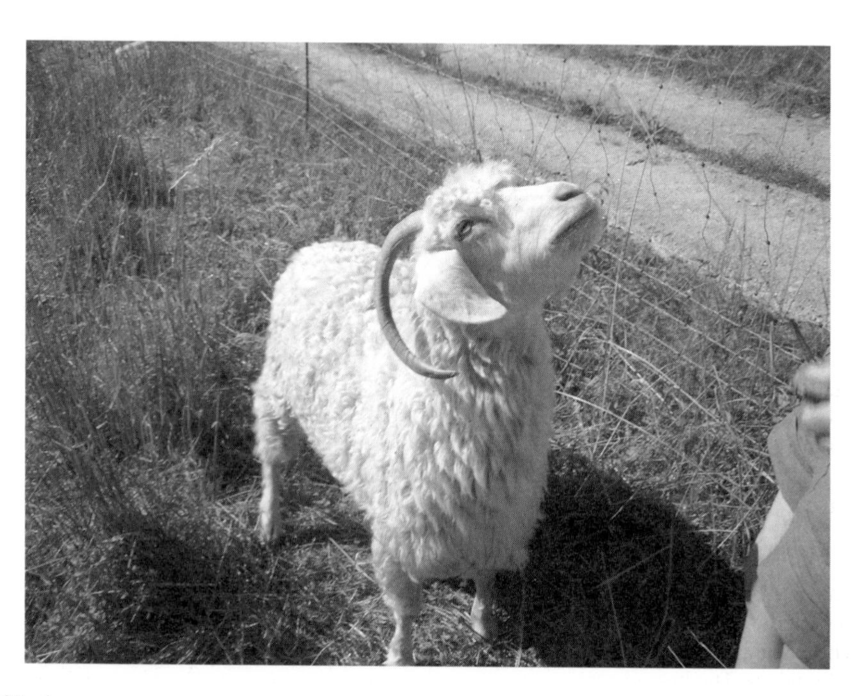

Fig. 1.25. Angora.

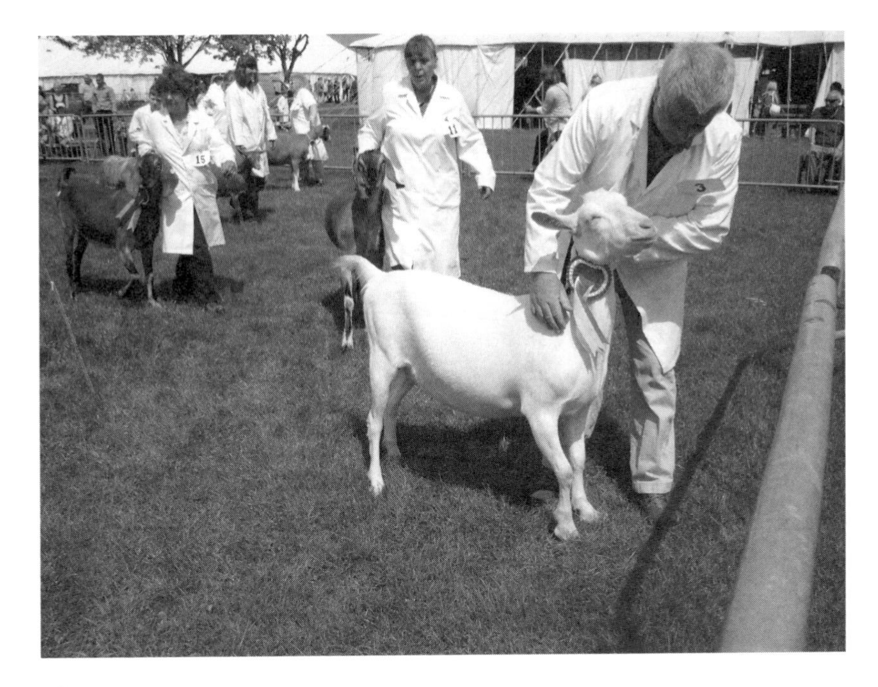

Fig. 1.26. Saanen.

have the same white markings. The British have shorter hair than the Swiss Toggenburgs and nearly always have tassels.

Cashmere

This is a fibre-producing goat that has a double coat. The fleece is made up of a coarse hairy outer coat, which has no commercial value, and a fine undercoat or 'down', which is cashmere, the marketable fibre. This soft undercoat grows seasonally from mid-summer to mid-winter and is shed naturally in late winter or early spring. The original cashmere goats came to the UK from Tibet 300 years ago. However there is actually no specific breed, and cashmere goats have been bred in many countries from feral goats. The main countries where cashmere animals can be found are Iceland, Australia, New Zealand, China, Iran, Afganistan and Russia. The Icelanders have bred a polled cashmere goat.

The cashmere fibre is non-medullated and normally white. The best fibre is under 15 μm. However any fibre below 20 μm is good quality. The goats are only shorn once a year, and the fibre weight of cashmere is 350–400 g.

Golden Guernsey

This breed nearly was lost and is still considered a 'rare breed'. As the name suggests, it originated in the Channel Islands. It is a small, docile breed that can only be golden in colour (Fig. 1.27).

Goat Breeds of the World

African Pygmy

This pet goat breed is black with white patches (Fig. 1.28).

Alpine

This black and white dairy goat breed was developed in Switzerland.

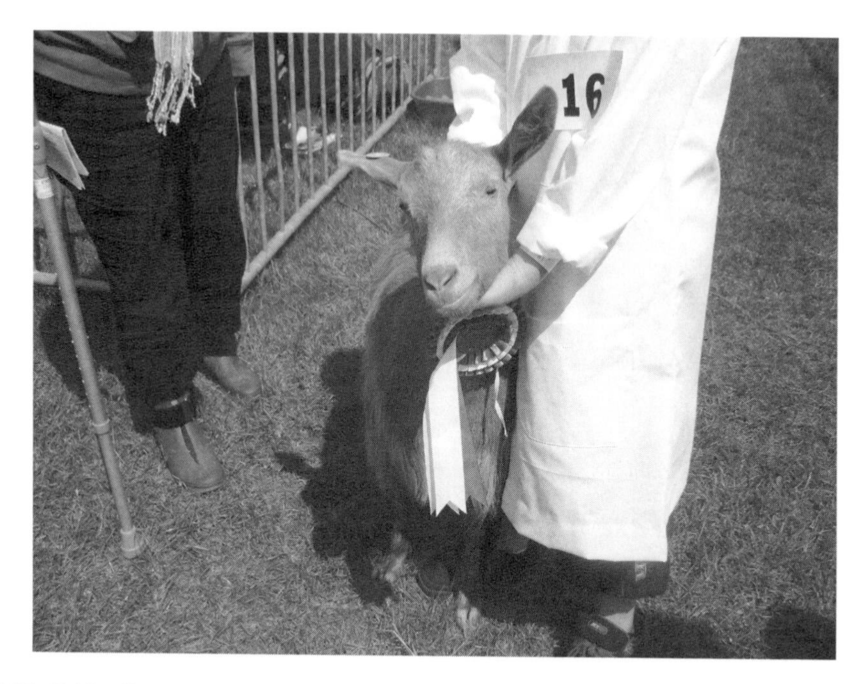

Fig. 1.27. Golden Guernsey.

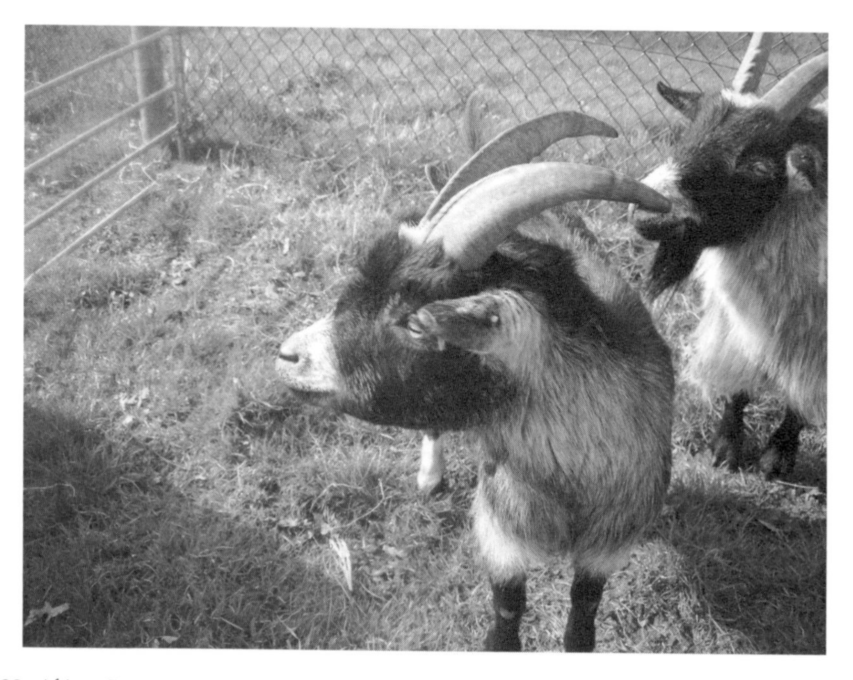

Fig. 1.28. African Pygmy.

Altai Mountain

This dark grey meat goat breed was developed in Russia. It has useable wool.

American Lamancha

This dairy goat breed may be of any colour. It may have originated in Persia and was bred up in Spain for over 2000 years in the La Mancha area. Latterly it has been standardized in Oregon, USA. Its distinctive feature is either the lack of ears or very small ears known as 'elf ears'.

Anatolian Black

This totally black dairy goat breed has long hair, which is shorn. It was developed in Central Turkey, hence the name.

Anglo-Nubian

See Goat Breeds of the UK.

Angora

See Goat Breeds of the UK.

Appenzell

This pure white Swiss dairy goat breed has mid-length hair. It is smaller but stockier than the Saanen, and is hornless.

Arapawa

This rare goat breed is kept in sanctuaries and for showing. It has an elaborate patchwork colour.

Argentata of Etna

This Italian dairy goat breed originated from Sicily. It is silver in colour, hence its name.

Australian Cashmere

This wool-producing goat breed is used worldwide to produce cashmere.

Barbari

This small creamy or golden goat breed originated in India, where it is still kept for meat.

Beetal

This goat breed, which is dual purpose, comes from the Indian sub-continent. It is red, black or pied, with pendulous ears.

Belgian Fawn

This goat breed from France and Belgium, also called the Hertkleurig, is descended from the chamois. It can actually be black or brown. It has lop ears and is mainly a milk goat.

Benadir

This dual-purpose goat breed comes from southern Somalia. It is a red goat with black spots and has lop ears. It is also called the Deguen or Digwain.

Bhuj

This dual-purpose goat breed has been bred in north-eastern Brazil. It is descended from the Kutchi goat of the Sindhi area of India, which has been allowed to die out. It is black with white spots and has lop ears.

Bionda Dell'admello

This light-brown dairy goat breed with white patches was developed in Italy from the

Adany, which used to be milked in Iran, but has now died out.

Black Bengal

This is a small, dual-purpose goat breed from the Bengal area of the Indian subcontinent. It can also be brown or grey.

Boer

This excellent meat-producing goat breed was developed in South Africa and was first imported into the UK in 1987. It is mainly white with a distinctive chestnut/chocolate head and neck. It is naturally horned and has lop ears. Mature does weigh 80–100 kg with bucks being even heavier. It is stocky with shorter legs than dairy goats. It is very fast growing, producing low-cholesterol, lean meat.

Booted

This is a triple-purpose goat breed producing milk, meat and fibre, and was developed in Switzerland. It is mainly brown. It is often called a Suregleiss.

British Alpine

See Goat Breeds of the UK.

British Saanen

See Goat Breeds of the UK.

British Toggenburg

See Goat Breeds of the UK.

Brown Shorthair

This cinnamon or brown-coloured dairy goat breed was developed in the Czech Republic. It is also called the Hnedà Kratkosrsta Koza.

Camosciata Alpina

This dual-purpose goat breed was bred in the Italian-speaking area of the Swiss Alps. It is brown with black stripes.

Canary Island

This dairy goat breed, which can be of any colour, is also called the Güera. The horns can be either sabre shaped or twisted. It was bred in the Canary Islands.

Canindé

This meat-producing goat breed comes from Brazil. It is black with white face stripes and a white belly.

Carpathian

This dual-purpose goat breed is often called a Carpatina or Karpacka. It is white and was developed in south-eastern Europe.

Cashmere

See Goat Breeds of the UK.

Changthangi

This meat goat breed also produces fibre. It was bred in the Kashmir area of the Indian subcontinent and is often called the Kashmiri or Pashmina goat. It is normally black but other colours are seen. It has large twisting horns and is sometimes used as a pack animal.

Chappar

This small black meat goat breed was bred in Pakistan.

Charnequeira

This dual-purpose goat breed is normally pied but can be red. It has twisted, lyre-shaped horns. It was bred in Portugal.

Chengde Polled

As the name suggests, this is a polled goat breed. It was bred primarily to produce fibre but it is suitable for meat. It is white in colour and comes from China.

Chengdu

This is a brown, dual-purpose goat breed, with a dark face and back stripes. It was bred in China and is also known as the Mah.

Chigu

This is a long-haired, white goat breed with long twisted horns. It was bred in India for fibre and meat. It is also called the Kangra Valley Goat.

Chué

This is a long-haired dairy goat breed, often called the Sem Raca Definida. It was developed in Corsica.

Daera Din Panah

This is a black dairy goat breed with long, hanging, twisted ears. It has spiral horns and was developed in Pakistan.

Damani

This is a black and tan dairy goat breed developed in Pakistan.

Damascus

This goat breed is often called the Aleppo or Shami. It is usually brown or grey, although there are also red and pied types. It is a dairy goat found throughout Syria and Lebanon (Fig. 1.29).

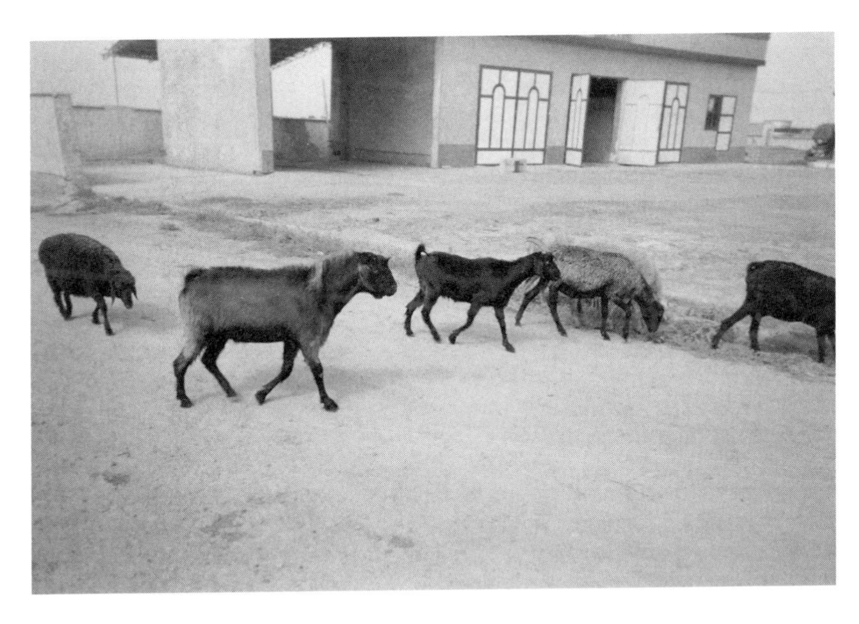

Fig. 1.29. Damascus.

Danish Landrace

This black or blue dual-purpose goat breed is found throughout Scandinavia. The animals make good pets.

Don Goat

This is mainly a fibre goat breed, but can be milked. It is either black or white and has large horns. As the name suggests, it is found beside the Don River in Russia.

Duan

This is a meat goat breed kept in China. It can be various colours: black, pied or white.

Dutch Landrace

As the name suggests, this goat breed comes from the Netherlands. It can be various colours and is normally kept as a pet.

Dutch Toggenburg

This dairy goat breed from the Netherlands is normally fawn in colour (Fig. 1.30).

Erzgebirge

This polled milk goat breed comes from Germany. It is red-brown in colour with black stripes on its face.

Finnish Landrace

As the name implies, this dairy goat breed comes from Finland. It is also called the Suomenvuohi. It is normally grey in colour, but pied or white animals are found.

French Alpine

This dairy goat breed is found in the French Alps. No particular colour has been fixed.

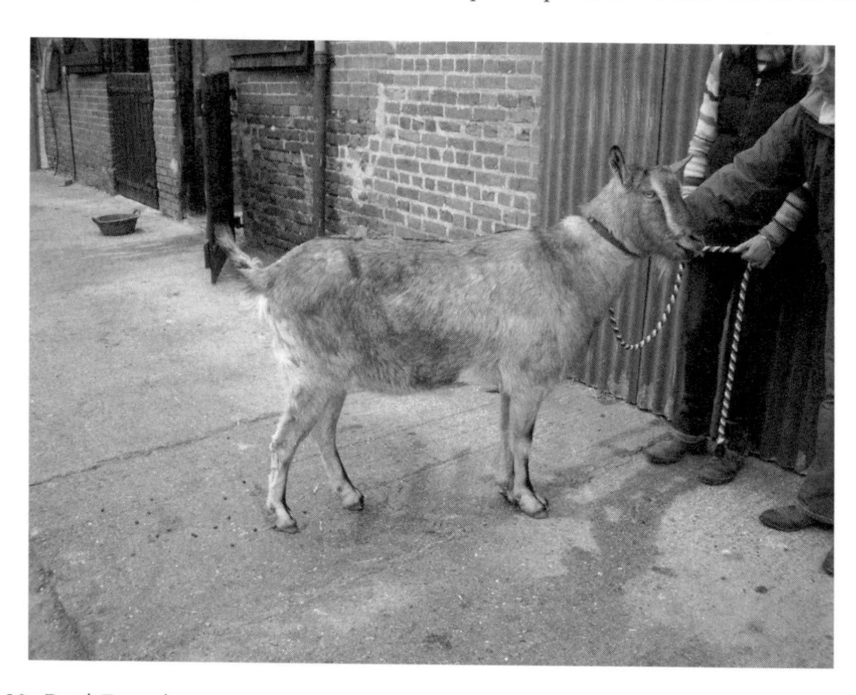

Fig. 1.30. Dutch Toggenburg.

Golden Guernsey

See Goat Breeds of the UK.

Hailun

This dairy goat breed was bred in China. It can be a variety of colours: black is the most common, but grey, brown, pied, white and yellow are also found.

Haimen

This white meat goat breed is found in China.

Hasi

This dual-purpose goat breed is from Albania. It is reddish and has lop ears.

Hejazi

This small black goat breed with long hair is bred for meat in Arabia and other areas in the Middle East (Fig. 1.31).

Hexi Cashmere

As the name implies, this is a fibre goat breed; it comes from China. Black, brown, pied and white colours are found.

Hongtong

This white dairy goat breed is found in China.

Huaipi

This white meat goat breed is found in China.

Huaitoutala

This is a fibre goat breed of no fixed colour, found in China.

Hungarian Improved

The name says it all. This is an improved dairy goat breed from Hungary. Its colour has

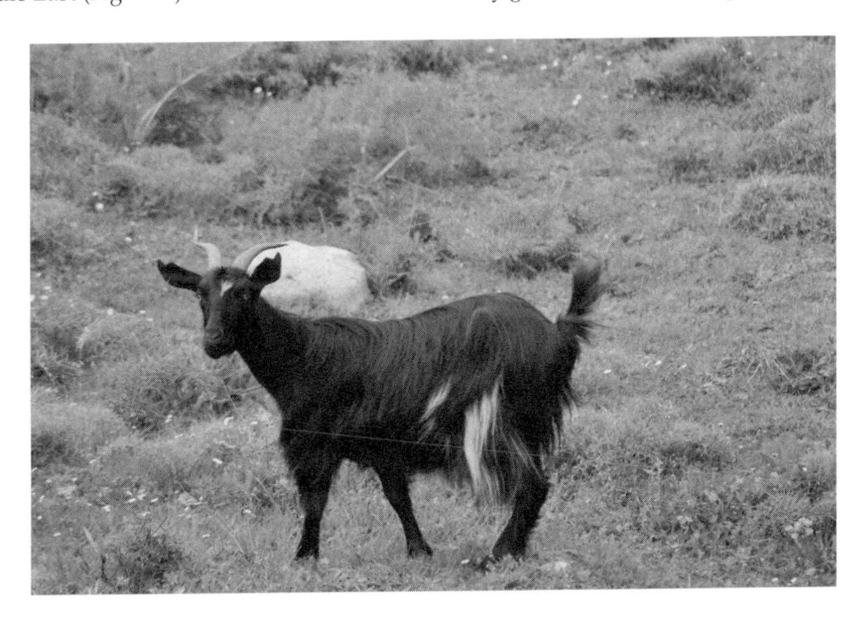

Fig. 1.31. Hejazi.

not been fixed and black, cream, red and white are found.

Irish Goat

This dual-purpose goat breed is found in both Northern Ireland and the Republic of Ireland. The most common colour is white, but grey and black are seen. It is an ideal smallholder goat.

Jining Grey

The name is misleading, as these goats may be black, white or pied, as well as grey. They have been bred in China not only as fibre goats but also for their very fine kid pelts.

Kaghani

This is primarily a fibre goat breed but it produces useful meat. It is bred in Pakistan. The colour is not fixed, and black, brown, grey and white are found.

Kamori

This black spotted dairy goat breed is found in Pakistan. The normal colour is reddish-brown, but white animals are seen.

Kiko

This brown or white goat breed with long horns was bred in New Zealand for meat.

Kinder

This is a hybrid goat breed of no fixed colour, which has been bred in the USA for both dairy and meat.

Loashan

This dairy goat breed of no fixed colour is found in China.

Machi

This black or brown meat goat breed is found in India. It has short rough hair and twisted horns.

Moxotó

This dual-purpose goat breed is from Brazil. It is normally cream with some black markings, but white animals with black markings are found.

Murcia-Granada

This dairy goat breed is also called the Granadina and comes from Spain. It is black or brown.

Nigerian Dwarf

Although this pygmy goat breed originally came from Nigeria, it is now commonly seen in the UK and Europe. It is normally black with white hairs. In Nigeria it is milked, but in the rest of the world it is kept as a pet. It is also called the West African Dwarf (Fig. 1.32).

Norwegian

As the name suggests, this dual-purpose long-haired goat comes from Norway. It is normally blue in colour, but grey, pied and white animals are found.

Nubian

This famous breed was originally bred in north-east Africa and has been improved throughout the world to become an excellent dairy goat. It is polled and has lop ears. The main colour is brown with two black stripes on its face, but other colours are seen. It is

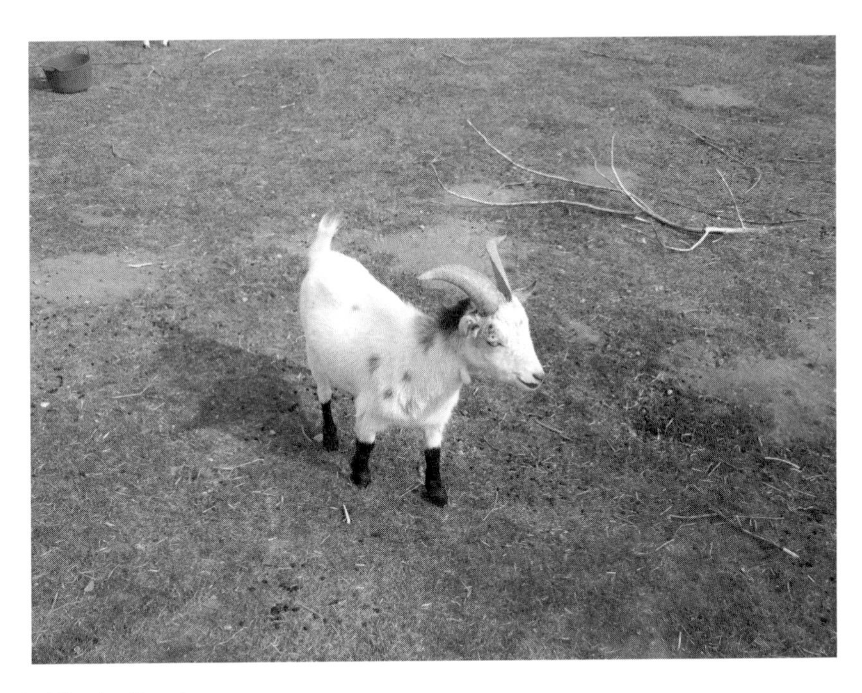

Fig. 1.32. Nigerian Dwarf.

second only to the Alpine breeds as the world's prime dairy breed.

Oberhasli

This Swiss dairy goat breed is also called the Oberhasli Brienzer or the Swiss Alpine. It is a rich red-bay, with black trimmings.

Peacock Goat

This is a Swiss dual-purpose goat breed with distinctive markings. It has a white front, but has black front feet. Its hind end and back feet are black.

Philippine

As the name implies, this meat goat breed comes from the Philippines. There are two types: a horned animal, normally black or brown with a white belt and fine hair; and a polled animal, normally cream, light brown or tan, with coarse hair.

Poitou

Also called the Poitevin, this is a rare breed of long-haired dairy goat from France. It is black-brown with a paler colour below.

Pyrenean

This dual-purpose goat breed from the mountains separating Spain from France is very similar in colouring to the Poitou. It is black or dark brown and paler below, with long hair (Fig. 1.33).

Qinshan

This is a black goat breed from China. It is eaten, but is mainly kept for its high-quality pelt.

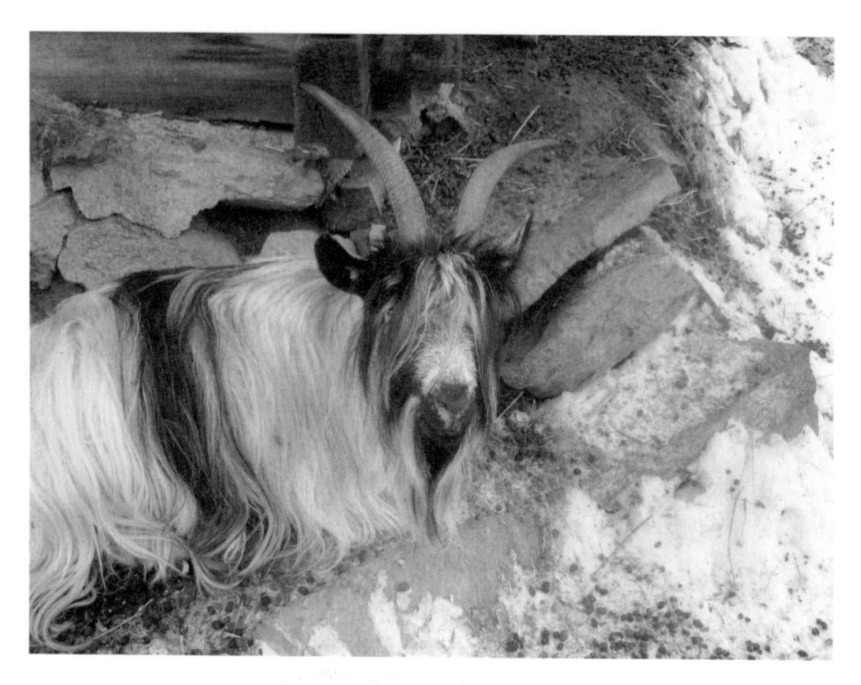

Fig. 1.33. Pyrenean.

Repartida

This mainly meat goat breed from Brazil is milked in smallholder situations. It is brown with black markings on the face. It is also called the Stiefrao.

Russian White

This goat breed from Russia has been improved recently to give considerable quantities of milk. It is also a white fibre animal.

Saanen

This is a prime dairy goat breed from Switzerland. It is normally pure white but may be sable.

Sahelian

This milking goat breed from Mali can be a variety of colours: black, cream, sprinkled with grey, red, white or pied. It is also used for meat and its skin is valued.

San Clemente

This is a rare meat goat breed that was bred in the USA. It is red or tan, with black markings.

Serrana

This dairy breed originating in north-eastern Portugal is also found in Brazil.

Somali

This white meat goat breed is also called the Deghier. It is found in northern Kenya and in Somalia.

Swedish Landrace

As the name suggests, this long-haired dairy goat breed comes from Sweden. It is usually white but can be fawn.

Tauernsheck

This rare dairy goat breed comes from Austria. It is normally black or brown, with white markings.

Tennessee Fainting Goat

This meat goat breed, which is often kept as a pet, is also called the Myotonic goat, because when stressed it will lose all muscle tone and collapse and then fully recover. It is black and white and comes from the USA.

Thuringian

This milk goat breed is also called the German Toggenburg. It is a smallholder goat and is chocolate brown with white markings on the face.

Toggenburg

This very famous dairy goat breed originated in Switzerland. It is brown with white markings.

Uzbek Black

As the name suggests, this black wool goat breed comes from Uzbekistan.

Valais Blackneck

This goat, which is really a dairy breed, produces good meat. It comes from Switzerland and is also called the Wallister Schwarzhals. It has black forequarters and white hindquarters (Fig. 1.34).

Verata

This mainly dairy goat breed is also kept for meat in Spain. It is usually black, but chestnut and grey animals are seen.

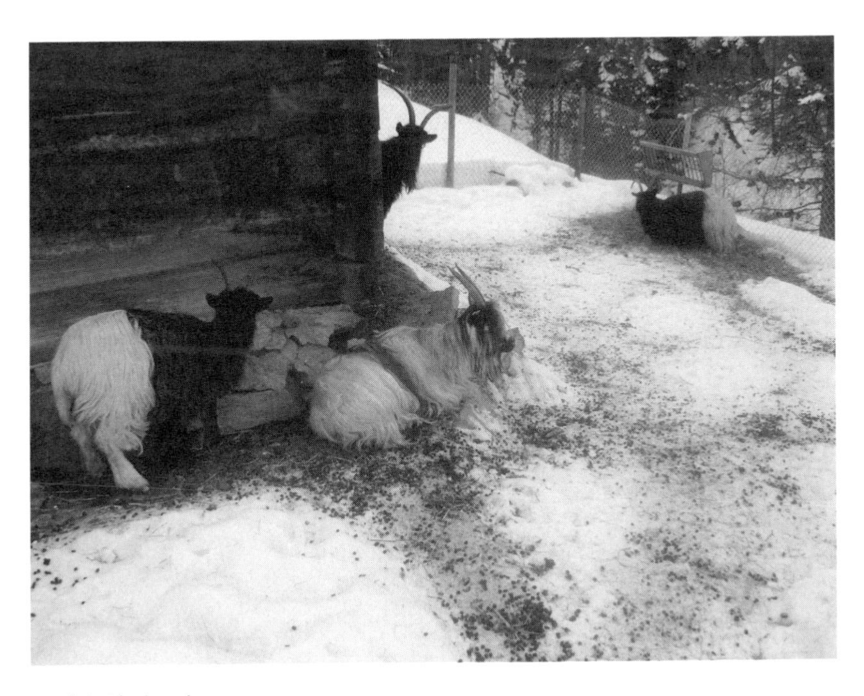

Fig. 1.34. Valais Blackneck.

White Shorthaired

This white dairy goat breed was bred in the Czech Republic.

Xinjiang

This fibre goat breed, which produces beautiful cashmere, comes from China. The goats are also milked and eaten. They can be black, brown or white.

Xuhai

This meat goat breed comes from China.

Zhongwei

This white fibre goat breed, which produces excellent cashmere and pelts, comes from China.

2

Behaviour and Restraint

Biosecurity

In the majority of cases, disease comes from other animals of the same species. If we want to control the risk of unaffected animals becoming infected, we need to stop contact with other animals and not import any new animals. This may occur at the farm level or at the country level. 'The biggest danger to a sheep is another sheep.' If we have to introduce new animals we need to have pre-movement testing, pre-movement certification, and quarantine and vaccination strategies in place. We must also be aware that there is crossover of infections from other animals, mainly from other ruminants, but also from non-ruminants and even from wildlife. Lastly, we must be aware that some infectious diseases are spread by vectors.

Behaviour and Behaviour Problems of Sheep

Introduction

Sheep have been domesticated for many thousands of years, so shepherds have learned their normal behaviour and use that behaviour to good effect. Sheep dogs are admired by all, but in fact the sheep need to be trained as well as the dog. On the whole, sheep will tend to group together when danger threatens and so it is in their nature to form a flock when a dog is put round them. Equally, sheep dogs will naturally round up sheep but not chase them. Sheep will naturally follow other sheep and go through a narrow opening. This trait is used for putting sheep through a race or a foot dip. They will also follow the shepherd, particularly if they have been trained with food (Fig. 2.1).

Behaviour problems

Plenty of trough space is vital when feeding sheep as the more dominant ones will get more. They will become bigger and stronger and so a cycle is established. 'The rich get rich and the poor get poorer.' Over the years farmers rather than shepherds have tried to cut corners to save on labour costs. Large, hard food nuts called 'ewe rolls' were developed so that the sheep feeder could just drive over the field spreading these rolls out of a big hopper on the back of a tractor. This system works well when all the sheep are young and active, but is disastrous if some of the sheep are older and less athletic as they will miss out on the feeding. The disaster is compounded if these older sheep have poor teeth. They will have difficulty chewing these hard

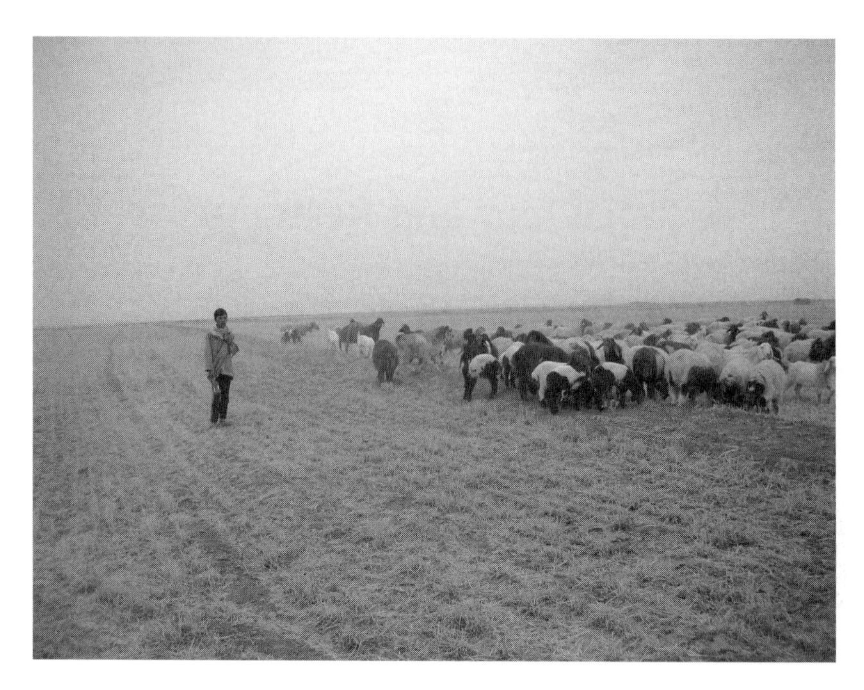

Fig. 2.1. Nomad on stubble.

'ewe rolls'. Minerals need not only to be palatable but readily available. If they are with molasses in a block there should be plenty of blocks, more than one per eight sheep. If the blocks are required to give a daily supply of magnesium it is vital that they are palatable or only 80% of the flock will go to them – magnesium is notorious for being unpalatable. Also it must be remembered they are really licks. They must not be too soft or sheep will break off chunks of them and then get urea or ammonium poisoning if the blocks, which contain urea, are being used to boost the protein in the diet (see Chapter 17).

The rams are kept separate from the ewes and ewe replacements, in a bachelor group, except at tupping time. This system works well except when new rams are added and fighting occurs. Fighting can be dangerous and may be life threatening. The danger can be very much reduced by penning the rams together in a small area for 24 h. They then appear to get the new smells mixed up and are not as likely to fight when turned out into a bigger area, where they can get enough speed up to really damage themselves. Homosexuality will occur in ram groups but does not seem to create problems and is markedly reduced when the rams are put with the ewes.

Extreme bad weather conditions in high-sheep pastures need to be considered from a sheep behavioural stance. Mature sheep will tend to stay in a group, and if they are familiar with the area will tend to go to sheltered places before the really bad weather arrives. Replacements, particularly lambs in their first winter, will not do this and may be lost in snow storms. They will not necessarily follow the mature flock and so should be kept nearer at hand.

Behaviour and Behaviour Problems of Goats

Introduction

In many parts of the world sheep and goats are kept together in large flock/herds with no problems. Their social behaviour in these circumstances is very similar to sheep (Fig. 2.2).

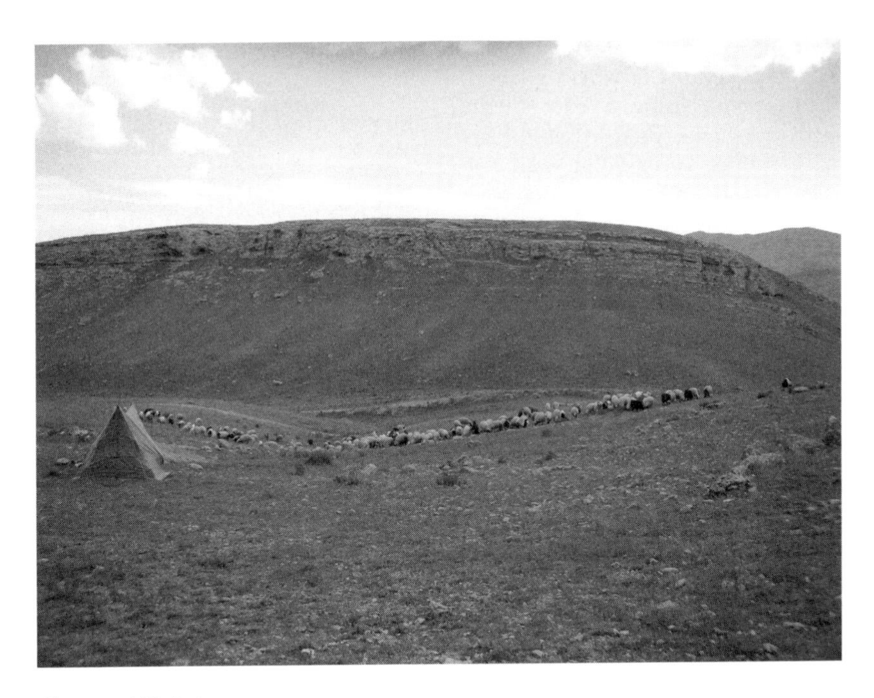

Fig. 2.2. Sheep on hills in Iran.

The major difference is with kids, which will tend to hide when danger threatens, rather than run with their does. When kept with sheep, goats tend to bunch up when danger threatens. When goats are kept just as goat herds they tend to scatter.

Horns tend to play a more major role in male goat behaviour than with horned rams. In fact this is a good trait as bucks tend to stand on their hind legs and wrestle with their horns rather than charging from a distance like rams. Injuries in bucks are less common.

Behaviour problems

Behaviour problems are rare in goats except for self-suckling, defined as an animal suckling on its own teats, and inter-suckling, defined as one animal suckling the udder of another. These are abnormal behaviours observed in dairy goats (Martinez-de la Puente *et al.*, 2011). The occurrence of these behaviours may be affected by feeding management or nutrient deficiencies and may lead to udder and teat damage, causing economic losses due to reduced milk yield. In goats, self-suckling is a habit that is difficult to break and may require culling of affected animals. Self-suckling increases the width of the teat and reduces the milk yield. The frequency of self-suckling can be significantly reduced by feeding wheat straw *ad lib.* in addition to their ordinary feed.

Drug Administration in Sheep

Oral administration of medicines, in the main anthelmintics, is frequently carried out in large numbers of sheep. There is considerable danger in this procedure, not only of causing inhalation pneumonia by drenching the medicine down the trachea but also of causing severe pharyngeal injury. Both can result in death. In a 10-year period the Veterinary Laboratory Agency (VLA) in England recorded 270 cases (Harwood and Hepple, 2011). These cases were confirmed by individual post-mortem examinations, and it is likely, therefore, that many more sheep will have been affected on these and other farms during the same period. In one case investigated by the Scottish Agricultural College, a total of 500 ewes were dosed orally with a vitamin/mineral supplement using a conventional drenching gun. Six ewes died within the first 24 h, and a further 40 or 50 showed submandibular swelling, often extending down the ventral part of the neck. Although some of these ewes did improve, others deteriorated and died or were culled on welfare grounds. At post-mortem examination, there was severe tissue damage to the pharyngeal and retropharyngeal tissue, a direct result of the procedure. A further 500 ewes on the same farm were dosed with the same product by a different stockperson, and these suffered no ill effects. The only difference was the level of skill of the two stockmen who undertook the procedure.

Whenever possible, veterinary surgeons should discuss this procedure with their clients; it is a skilled task and should only be undertaken by a competent stockperson. The dosing equipment used must be well maintained, with no sharp edges, and must not have been bent out of shape. Stock must be suitably restrained to prevent undue movement and held in an appropriate position. If a bolus is being administered it must be the correct size for the sheep in which it is being placed, and sufficient time allowed to prevent operator fatigue or undue hurrying of the technique. Finally, it is worth asking the question 'Is the procedure itself necessary?' Many sheep are dosed as a routine when it may not be required.

Drug Administration in Goats

On the whole, oral administration has the same dangers in goats as in sheep. However, in the UK where many of the goats are kept in very small groups, traumatic oesophageal injuries and inhalation pneumonias are very rare. The one exception to this is at parturition when does may develop hypocalcaemia. It is important when dealing with this condition that all treatment is given by injection. Hypocalcaemia will cause a lessening of the laryngeal reflex and so inhalation at such a time is a very real danger.

Reproductive Anatomy and Physiology of Sheep

General

Sheep are seasonally polyoestrus. In a normal ewe cyclic activity will be stimulated by the shortening of the day length. However some breeds of sheep can breed throughout the year, and the shepherd has considerable control over when parturition is to occur. This is particularly easy in the tropics when the day length is constant throughout the year. The actual mechanism is controlled by the hormone melatonin, which is released by the pineal gland in response to the hours of darkness. Melatonin can be given orally or by implant to circumvent the ewe's natural rhythm.

Mating

Although rams, like ewes, are affected by the day length, most rams will mate at any time of the year. However they produce less ejaculate and their libido decreases out of season. The oestrus cycle normally lasts between 16 and 17 days. This is made up of a luteal phase of 13–14 days when there is a corpus luteum (CL) in the ovary producing progesterone, and an oestrus phase when the CL is reducing and the ovary starts producing oestrogen. Oestrus lasts on average 36 h and ovulation occurs between 18 and 24 h after the onset. Ewes show little overt signs of oestrus. They may seek out the ram and nuzzle his scrotum. They may wag their tails and then stand to be mounted by the ram from behind. Virgin ewe lambs or hoggets may not show any overt signs and therefore it is important to have experienced rams running with them. The oestrus phase is shorter, and indeed the numbers of follicles produced on the ovaries are fewer at the beginning of the breeding season.

Breeding strategies in sheep

The use of a teaser, that is, a vasectomized ram, is very useful at the beginning of the breeding season and may negate the need for hormone treatment (see Chapter 6). Ideally the teaser or teasers should be put in with the ewes 13–14 days before mating is desired. They can then be withdrawn and the entire rams can be introduced a day later. If no hormone treatment has been given to the ewes, the ideal ratio is 3 rams per 100 ewes. This should be increased to 4 rams to 100 maiden ewes. These numbers are only approximate and might have to be increased in flocks which are very spread out on hills. The recommended numbers assume that the rams are not lame and are fully fertile.

Reproductive Anatomy and Physiology of Goats

General

The goat, like the sheep, is seasonally polyoestrus. The onset of cycling is stimulated by the shortening of the day length. Therefore in the northern hemisphere breeding activity will occur between August and March; however many animals are capable of breeding outside of this time. These animals are more commonly found in certain breeds. Obviously female goats will exhibit oestrus throughout the year in the tropics and parturition times can be planned to fit in with food availability. Dairy goats, particularly high-producing animals, may not show oestrus if lactation is occurring when high milk yields are being produced.

Mating

Bucks are also affected by the day length and will show less libido in temperate climates, out of season, but in reality bucks will mate at any time of the year. The oestrus cycle is longer than in sheep and normally lasts 21 days. It is much more variable in length with different breeds. Pygmy goats will cycle between 18 and 24 days. As in sheep the cycle is made up of a luteal phase, which is normally between 17 and 19 days. The period of oestrus is the same as in sheep, 24–48h, but this may be shorter in virgin females and tends to be longer in very mature animals. Does tend to show more overt signs of oestrus compared with ewes, particularly if they smell the presence of a buck. Oestrus can be stimulated in does by the use of a 'billy rag'. This is a cloth which has been wiped over a buck and smells of his urine. The doe will pace her enclosure. There will be swelling of her vulva and constant tail wagging. She will often bleat and show muscle tremors. The vaginal discharge which often occurs will be clear at the beginning of oestrus but become thicker towards the end of oestrus. Both phases of the cycles will tend to be shorter in goats which are suffering from chronic disease, e.g. *Trypanosoma congolense* (Mutayoba *et al.*, 1989).

The buck mounts the standing doe from behind, as in sheep. However, intromission and ejaculation are not as quick as in the ram.

Breeding strategies in goats

Vasectomized bucks can be used to try to synchronize breeding in large herds of goats. However, most mating in goats is controlled and observed, so the number of bucks required is not as large as the number of rams required per 100 animals. Also, it is not vital to have experienced bucks with virgin does.

Shearing in Sheep

There are three reasons to shear sheep. The harvesting of the wool is extremely important with certain breeds such as Merinos. In Australia and New Zealand the wool from these breeds is the main economic reason for keeping sheep. Therefore shearing is not only important but also it has to be done well so that the farmer can get the best return for the wool. The situation in the UK is very different, as sheep are either kept as hill sheep to provide ewe lamb replacements for lowland flocks, or as lowland sheep to produce fat lambs. The wool is only a by-product and in many instances the cost of shearing outweighs the return from the wool (Fig. 2.3). In fact only in lowland, early lambing flocks are the

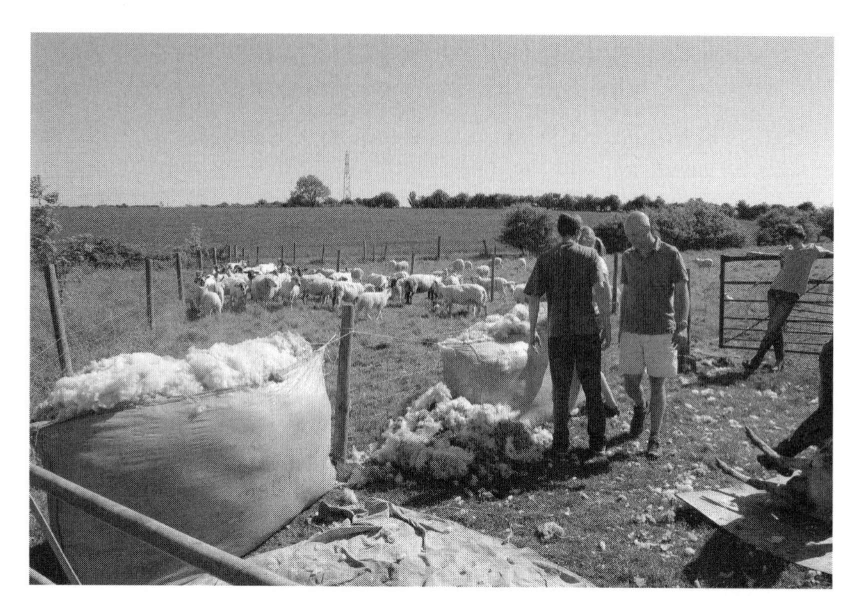

Fig. 2.3. Sheep shearing.

lambs – which have the finest quality wool – shorn at all. The removal of the wool by shearing greatly reduces the dangers of heat stress, but perhaps the most important reason for shearing is to lessen the danger of 'fly strike'. Certainly long wool makes it harder to recognize 'fly strike' until it is very advanced. However it is not the length of wool per se that attracts the flies, but the dirt in the wool. Longer wool does have some advantage in that it retains the chemicals better after dipping if there is a certain length. Certainly the pour-on products require 3 weeks' growth of wool to render them at their most effective as myiasis preventatives.

Shearing in Goats

Angora and Cashmere goats have very fine hair, which is why their fibre is so valuable. However, their fleece is very different from even the finest Merino sheep fleece. The fibre comes from the secondary hair follicle, which produces the under insulating coat or 'down'. The longer fibre from the primary follicle or 'kemp' is in fact a cause of downgrading. Mohair produced from Angora goats grows at about 2.5 cm per month, 30 cm in a year. This is too long for manufacturing, so normally Angora goats are shorn twice a year and some flocks are even shorn three times a year. As with sheep, the kids have the finest wool, and their fleeces are always shorn separately. The comb used to shear goats is different from a sheep comb and has more teeth, usually 20. The speed, however, is normally slower when goats are shorn.

Goats, unlike sheep, do not sit on their rumps very readily when shorn. It is better to lean them further back so in essence they are almost in dorsal recumbency.

Cashmere goats are different from Angora goats. Cashmere goats shed their down in the spring when it was traditionally combed out, although nowadays they are shorn.

Heat Stress in Sheep

In temperate climates, or in the tropics but at altitude, heat stress is not a problem in sheep. However in the tropics at sea level and in the UK in freak conditions sheep may suffer if they have no shade. Certainly hot conditions lessen fertility, and both rams and ewes are

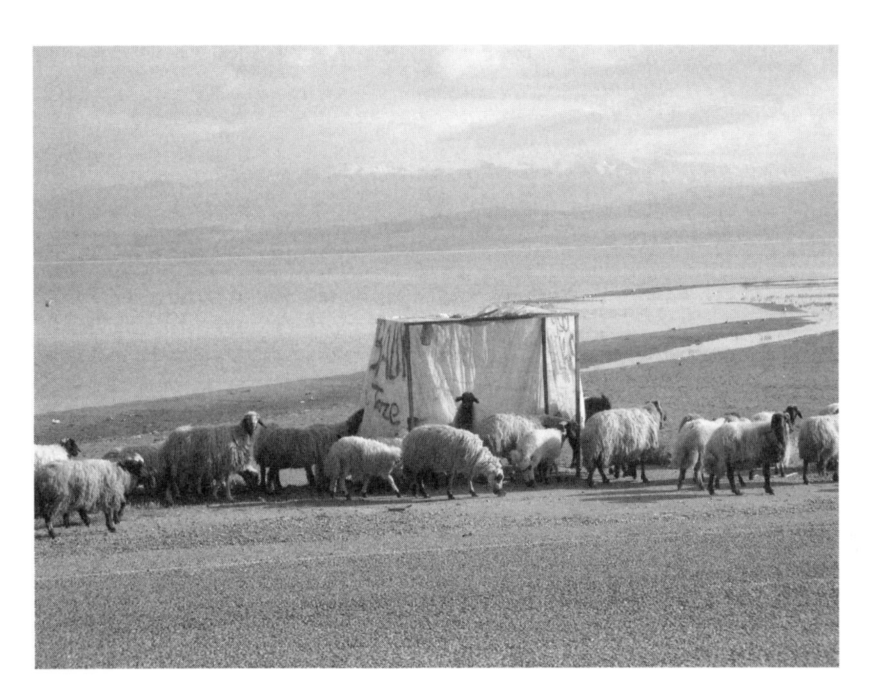

Fig. 2.4. Nomads' sheep by lake.

affected. The treatment is straightforward: shade should be provided (Fig. 2.4); cold water should be freely available to drink; and water can be poured over the animals to saturate the wool. Obviously any air movement is helpful. To lessen the infertility problems, ram numbers should be increased.

Heat Stress in Goats

The timing of shearing to lessen the danger of heat stress in fibre-producing goats is important. It should be remembered that cold stress after shearing can lead to abortion in does and even death in all fibre-producing animals.

3

Vital Signs and Sample Taking

General

Many textbooks assume that vital signs and sample taking are the same the world over. This is not very helpful. This chapter will give a very broad range so that the reader can adapt the guidance in this book by adding narrower ranges for the environment of the individual's practice and from the laboratory available. The term 'reference range' is now widely used, rather than 'normal range'. Classically, a normal animal is said to be within 95% of the normal range. By definition, 5% of normal animals will not appear to be normal. Thus if 20 tests are carried out, every animal is likely to have one value outside of the normal range. Therefore there is a strong argument for only carrying out specific tests for the parameters the clinician is particularly interested in. Laboratories on the whole do not like this arrangement, as they favour a blanket approach, which they find easier and cheaper. Clinicians are urged therefore to work closely with their particular laboratory so that a compromise regarding cost and relevance is reached.

The author is well aware that getting samples to laboratories will not be easy or quick in many parts of the world. High temperatures are likely to be a problem, and the logistics should be considered with the laboratory. Fresh samples may be the most difficult, so swabs for bacteriology should be taken in transport medium. Bacteria can be plated out and grown in the field, and only then be submitted for identification. Equally, smears can be made and microscopic evaluation carried out in the field after appropriate staining, and these slides can easily be referred to a more experienced pathologist. Antibiotic sensitivity testing, too, can well be done in the field, using the relevant antibiotic testing discs. There is little point in knowing the sensitivity of an isolated organism to an antibiotic that is not available. Rather than submitting whole blood, centrifuged serum samples can be sent. Packed cell volumes (PCVs) can be measured easily with a bench hand-driven centrifuge, and thick and thin blood smears can be used to look for protozoal infections. Dung samples can be examined for bowel worms, lungworms and liver fluke eggs. Coccidia oocysts can be included in this screening and their size can be evaluated. Fungi can also be grown.

To help referral pathologists, practitioners can submit photographs of post mortems. If e-mail is available this can be carried out throughout the world. Obviously histological samples will be extremely helpful in tropical climates, as they will withstand higher temperatures than fresh samples. Care should be taken when packing these, as any contamination from the formalin in the latter onto bacteriological samples will be disastrous. Vital signs will vary from climate to climate, as will normal values, and will show a similar bell-shaped distribution curve. Clinicians will obviously carry out a full clinical examination as a matter of routine, building up their own range of normal values. Experience will show how the climatic variations in temperature, air movement and humidity will affect these values. Naturally the physical attributes of the ruminant – such as type, age, gender and pregnancy – will have a marked effect. The state of the individual, whether it is stressed, recently transported, and so on, will cause variation.

Normal Temperature, Pulse and Respiration (TPR) in Sheep and Goats

The rectal temperatures of small ruminants vary enormously. Readings are very helpful if taken over a period of time, but a single temperature reading from an individual animal may not be that helpful. However, if the rectal temperature is linked with a full clinical examination, then it will be more helpful. In any event the rectal temperature should not be neglected. A likely normal range will be 38.3–39.5°C (101–103°F). The normal heart rate for a sheep or goat varies from 70 to 80 beats/min and the normal resting respiratory rate varies from 15 to 35 breaths/min.

Normal Sheep Neonates

In the UK lambs are often faced with very poor weather conditions and may be found very cold and comatose. It is very important that shepherds decide on a protocol or standard operating procedure (SOP) (Table 3.1) to prevent suffering and mortality. The action to be taken will be decided by the age of the lamb and the rectal temperature.

'Hot boxes' can come in a variety of different designs – there is no end to a shepherd's ingenuity. Basically, they need to be draught free with an insulated floor and maintained at a temperature of 40°C (104°F). After treatment the lambs described in Table 3.1 are put into the box until they have recovered and can be returned to their mothers in a small pen.

There are many ways to warm up lambs with hot water bottles or infrared heaters. However, electrical appliances that blow hot air are not recommended as the latent heat of vaporization tends to chill a wet lamb further before the animal has been heated. This chilling can be critical. Microwaves must also be avoided. Shepherds should constantly be aware of the danger of fire. All infrared lamps must be secured with chains, not bailer twine. They must also be high enough not to be knocked by the ewes.

Normal Goat Neonates

Unlike lambs, kids are rarely left to face poor weather conditions in the UK. However if they are found cold and comatose they should be treated in the same manner as lambs. Rejection of neonatal kids is rare. However, multiple births are common, and goat keepers may well have to help neonates to obtain sufficient colostrum in their first 6 h of life. In dairy goats the neonates will be weaned in 2–3 days and will have to be fed milk substitutes. Feeding of cow's milk or colostrum is not to be recommended as it will

Table 3.1. The standard operating procedure for cold lambs.

Under 24 h old and with a rectal temperature of >37°C (99°F)	Under 24 h old and with a rectal temperature of <37°C (99°F)	Over 24 h old and with a rectal temperature of >37°C (99°F)	Over 24 h old and with a rectal temperature of <37°C (99°F)
Give warm colostrum by stomach tube and leave with its mother in a pen for observation	Give warm colostrum by stomach tube and place in a 'hot box'	Give intraperitoneal glucose injection and leave with its mother in a pen for observation	Give intraperitoneal glucose injection and place in a 'hot box'

not contain the nutritional products required by the kid. There is also a danger of spreading disease such as Johne's disease from the cows to the kids.

Examination of the Heads of Neonatal Lambs

The heads of all neonatal lambs should be examined carefully. If there are problems that are going to cause difficulties for the lamb in sucking they need to be addressed as soon as possible. The jaws, incisor teeth and tongue should be checked at the same time as the presence of a sucking reflex is elicited. The eyes should be checked for entropion.

Examination of the Heads of Neonatal Kids

The heads of neonatal kids should be checked in the same manner as lambs, and in addition the presence of horn buds should be recorded. If kids are to be disbudded it is very important that this operation is performed within the first 7 days of life.

Collecting Blood Samples

When collecting blood samples it is important to collect into the right anticoagulant for the type of analysis required. The correct volume of blood for the amount of anticoagulant in the bottle is also important. Blood should be collected from the jugular vein with as little excitement as possible, although this may be difficult with certain individuals. Needles and syringes must be clean and not contaminated with medicines. For haematological samples the anticoagulant required is ethylene diamine tetra-acetic acid (EDTA). (Bottles containing this anticoagulant often come with a lilac-coloured stopper.) Haematological samples will give measures of the haemoglobin and the number of red blood cells. It should be remembered that if a haematocrit tube is not filled from the top of the sample immediately (in other words, before it is allowed to stand) the haematocrit will have a lower reading and there will seem to be fewer red blood cells in the sample than in reality. Anaemia may then be misdiagnosed. Even in profound cases of anaemia, normoblasts are seen in the peripheral blood very rarely. The laboratory will report the number of platelets and the total number of white blood cells, and the latter is then broken down into the total number of neutrophils, eosinophils, basophils, lymphocytes and monocytes. These can be shown as a percentage but this may be misleading. It is better to study total numbers.

Normal Haematological Values

Normal haematological values are shown in Table 3.2.

Table 3.2. The haematological parameters of adult female sheep and goats in the UK.

Parameter	Sheep	Goat
Erythrocytes × 10^9/l	12	14
Size (μm)	5.5 × 5.5	5.5 × 5.5
Lifespan in days	140–150	140–150
Haemoglobin (g/dl)	11.5	11.4
PCV (%)	27–45	25–34
MCV (fl)	34	22
MCH (pg)	10	8.4
MCHC (g/dl)	32.5	39.6
Leucocytes/μl	8000	9000
Granulocyte/agranulocyte ratio	0.5	0.5

Notes: MCH, Mean corpuscular haemoglobin; MCHC, Mean corpuscular haemoglobin concentration; MCV, Mean corpuscular volume.

Erythrocyte parameters

The function of red blood cells (RBCs) is to carry oxygen to the tissues at pressures sufficient to permit rapid diffusion of oxygen. This is particularly important for sheep and goats living at high altitudes in the Himalayas and other high mountain ranges throughout the world. The carrier molecule for oxygen is haemoglobin. This is a complex molecule, formed of four haem units attached to four globins. Iron is added in the last step by the ferrochelatase enzyme. Interference with the normal production of haem or globin leads to anaemia. Causes include copper or iron deficiency and lead poisoning. In the healthy animal red cell mass, and thus oxygen-carrying capacity, remains constant. Mature RBCs have a finite life span; their production and destruction must be carefully balanced, or disease occurs. However, if animals are moved to higher altitudes the red cell mass will increase over a period of 3 weeks. This is a normal physiological process. Pulmonary hypertensive heart disease, often called highmountain disease (HMD), is recorded in cattle but not in sheep or goats.

Erythropoiesis is regulated by erythropoietin, which increases in the presence of hypoxia and regulates RBC production. In sheep and goats the kidney is both the sensor organ and the major site of erythropoetin production, so chronic renal failure is associated with anaemia. Erythropoietin acts on the marrow in concert with other humoral mediators to increase the numbers of stem cells entering RBC production, to shorten maturation time and to cause early release of reticulocytes. Another factor that affects erythropoiesis is the supply of nutrients such as iron, folic acid and vitamin B12. Chronic debilitating diseases and endocrine disorders, for instance hypothyroidism or hyperoestrogenism will suppress erythropoiesis.

A decreased RBC mass (i.e. anaemia) may be caused by direct blood loss, haemolysis or decreased production. In acute blood loss mortality is usually related to loss of circulating volume, rather than actual loss of RBC. Iron is the limiting factor in chronic blood loss. Haemolysis may be caused by toxins, infectious agents or congenital abnormalities. Decreased RBC production is very rarely due to primary bone marrow disease in sheep and goats. It is much more commonly seen from other causes, for example renal failure, toxins or veterinary drugs.

Erythrocyte parameters are very similar in sheep and goats.

Leucocyte parameters

The leucocytes consist of the granulocytes (neutrophils, eosinophils and basophils) and the agranulocytes (lymphocytes and monocytes). Although they are traditionally counted by determining each as a percentage of the total leucocyte white blood cell (WBC) population, meaningful interpretation requires that the absolute number of each type be calculated by multiplying the total white cell count by the fraction attributable to the individual cell type. An increased percentage that is due to an absolute decrease in another cell type is not an increase at all.

Leucocytosis is an increase in the total number of circulating WBCs; leucopenia is a decrease. Changes in WBC counts and morphological appearance of various leucocytes are evaluated by comparison with reference ranges for each of the species. In neonates the total WBC count is more variable and higher than in adults.

Unsegmented neutrophils do not normally appear in peripheral blood. If they are reported it is an indication of a shift to the right; that is, their presence indicates that the neutrophils are young and therefore there is an extra usage of neutrophils. This is likely to be a bacterial infection.

The granulocytes are produced in the bone marrow from the myeloblasts. Neutrophils are the most numerous and in the peripheral blood are normally mature and segmented. Morphological changes in cytoplasm of the neutrophils, including toxic granulation, may occur during systemic bacterial infections or severe inflammation and are referred to as toxic changes. Although all circulating WBCs are exposed to the same systemic diseases, only neutrophils are evaluated for toxic changes. Toxic change is graded subjectively as mild, moderate or marked, based on the number of affected neutrophils and the severity of toxic change. Clinical significance is reflected by the type of toxic change and its severity. Toxic granulation is identified by the presence of pink to purple intracytoplasmic granules within neutrophils; these granules represent primary granules of the neutrophils that have retained their staining affinity. Diffuse cytoplasmic basophilia and cytoplasmic vacuolation frequently occur together. The cytoplasmic basophilia is due to persistent ribosomes, and the cytoplasmic vacuolation is possibly due to autodigestion of the cell.

The magnitude of neutrophilia induced by inflammation is a function of the size of the bone marrow storage pool of granulocytes, hyperplasia of the marrow and rate of WBC migration into the tissues. Neutrophilia, often the cause of leucocytosis, generally characterizes bacterial infections and conditions associated with extensive tissue necrosis, including burns, trauma, extensive surgery and neoplasia. Extreme leucocytosis is seen in blood-borne protozoal infections and closed-cavity infections such as abscesses. The abscess wall inhibits the migration of neutrophils into the site of infection, but does not impair the release of leucocyte chemotactic substances. The net effect is a high peripheral neutrophil count, which often includes a regenerative left shift (i.e. increased numbers of band neutrophils).

Eosinophils contain enzymes that modulate products of mast cells or basophils released in response to IgE stimulation. For example, histamine released by basophils or mast cells is modulated by histaminases in eosinophils. The cytoplasmic granules of eosinophils contain proteins that are involved in killing parasites. Eosinophilia is induced by substances that promote allergic responses and hypersensitivity (e.g. histamine and allied substances) and by IgE. Eosinophils increase in response to parasitic infections, especially those involving tissue migration, due to the contact of parasite chitin with host tissues. Eosinophilia also may occur with inflammation of the gastrointestinal (GI), urogenital or respiratory tracts, or of the skin.

Careful attention to detail should be taken when counting is done manually. If electronic counting is carried out there may well be some strange results, and the number of eosinophils will usually appear as a high percentage of the total number of granulocytes. If in any doubt the sample should be recounted manually. Eosinopenia is commonly reported with corticosteroid-induced (stress) conditions.

Basophils are rare in sheep and goats. Basophils granules contain histamine and heparin as well as mucopolysaccharides. Although basophils and mast cells have similar functions and enzymatic contents, basophils do not become mast cells and there is no proof of a common precursor cell. In sheep and goats normal peripheral blood basophil numbers are low compared with the number of tissue mast cells. In both species numbers of basophils in the peripheral blood are low, so that a basopenia has no diagnostic significance.

Lymphocytes originate from a marrow stem cell and mature in lymph nodes, spleen and associated peripheral lymphoid tissues. Mature lymphocytes consist of two subpopulations, B cells and T cells. B cells are the precursors of plasma cells and produce antibodies for humoral immunity. T cells engage in cellular immunity. A lymphocyte in tissue may return to the vascular bed and recirculate. Some lymphocytes are long lived compared with other WBCs and may survive weeks to years. Care should be taken when evaluating a peripheral lymphocytosis as it may be physiological, but it may also be a result of immune stimulation associated with chronic inflammation. Lymphopenia is a common finding, generally associated with stress or viral disease, but clinicians should be aware that the administration of corticosteroids will cause a lymphopenia.

Monocytes are formed in the bone marrow and enter the peripheral blood for a day and then exit into the tissues. They tend to be fixed or migrate to sites of inflammation. Monocytosis is associated with chronic inflammation and when there are bacteria in the blood stream, such as in an endocarditis. Granulomatous and fungal conditions will also cause a monocytosis. Occasionally there will be a monocytopenia, but this is of no diagnostic significance.

Obtaining Cerebrospinal Fluid Samples from Sheep

Clinicians must be aware that cerebrospinal fluid (CSF) samples are to be drawn from the sub-arachnoid space and therefore full aseptic precautions must be taken. The easiest site is between the most caudal lumbar vertebra (L6) and the first palpable sacral dorsal spine (S2). The area is clipped and shaved with the sheep in sternal recumbency, held by at least two assistants. A skin bleb of 2 ml of local anaesthetic is placed over the small depression in front of S2 in the midline. The area is recleaned and the surgeon is scrubbed and gloved. Using a 2.5 cm (1 inch; 21 G) needle for lambs or a 5 cm (2 inch; 19 G) needle for adults the surgeon directs the needle slowly ventrally in a vertical direction. The surgeon should appreciate the point of the needle passing through the skin, the subcutaneous tissue, and the ligament. A sudden loss of resistance will be felt and CSF will well up through the needle. Great care should then be taken in attaching the totally sterile syringe to the needle to retrieve the sample. In theory blood could be in the sample from a previous haemorrhage into the spinal cord. However, in reality it is likely to be as a result of the technique and should be disregarded.

Obtaining Cerebrospinal Fluid Samples from Goats

CSF in goats is collected at the same site as in sheep. Unless the goat is comatose or paralysed, sedation with xylazine at 0.1 mg/kg is advisable. To help the surgeon, the goat should be held in lateral recumbency on a table.

Analysis of CSF

Bacteriology

The sample should be cultured and a smear prepared. This should be examined under the microscope using oil immersion, after Gram staining.

Protein concentration

In a normal CSF sample this should be very low (<0.4 g/l).

White cell concentration

The normal number of cells in CSF is low ($<0.012 \times 10^9$/l). A differential count is useful. The macrophages should be examined carefully, as phagocytosed RBCs will indicate subarachnoid haemorrhage.

4

Simple Diagnostic Tests

General

It is important with all laboratory tests that practitioners apply two important principles. Each test should have a known 'test sensitivity' and 'test specificity'. Sensitivity is the percentage of diseased animals that test positive and specificity is the percentage of non-diseased animals that test negative. Ideally all tests would be 100% sensitive and 100% specific. However this is very rarely the case, although normally tests have sensitivities and specificities in the high 90s. Practitioners should be aware of the limitations of tests.

No practitioner should be without minimal facilities for initial screening and processing of samples for dispatch. Inevitably none will have sufficient funding to provide all the specialist tests that might occasionally be required. A compromise has to be reached, depending on the availability of trained technical staff, likely throughput of samples, and so on. Here are some hints for internal or external laboratories (MacDougall, 1991):

General (internal or external laboratories):

- DO take samples before any therapy.
- DO examine samples as soon as possible.
- DO dispatch samples as soon as possible.
- DON'T dispatch samples that are unlikely to be diagnostic.

Internal (practice) laboratory:

- DO keep any surplus samples in suitable conditions in case further tests are required.
- DON'T delay in preparing samples.

External (specialist) laboratory:

- DO ensure all samples are adequately labelled, accompanied by full case details and correctly packaged.
- DO be aware of the limitations of the test.
- DON'T send sharps with the material.

Safety in the Laboratory

Unlike large organizations with appointed safety personnel, small businesses such as veterinary practices cannot readily dedicate a large amount of time and manpower to health and safety. However, equally high standards of safety must be maintained. The most efficient means of achieving them is to spend some time identifying all safety hazards. These can be categorized as being due to infection, chemicals or equipment. This should be done by a senior member of the practice who should be designated as 'practice safety officer'. An accident book should be kept for the purpose of recording all injuries, diseases (see Chapter 19) and dangerous occurrences in, or associated with, the work of the laboratory.

High neutrophils and protein concentration are indicators for surgery. The only differential would be a peritonitis which should also give a high rectal temperature.

Anthrax Smears

These are normally blood smears but they may be taken from swellings around the throat. Two microscope slides are required. A drop of blood or fluid is put on the end of one slide. The other slide is just dipped into this drop and drawn down the length of the slide to make a thin smear. This is then dried in the air. The smear is fixed to the slide by passing the slide through a flame with the smear downwards towards the flame. Once cool the slide with the smear is turned upwards. McFayden's stain (old methylene blue) is poured on to the slide and left for 30 s. The slide is then rinsed under a running tap. Once dried, the slide can be examined with an oil immersion objective under a microscope to check for anthrax bacilli. These will take up the stain and have a characteristic purple capsule.

Blood Tests to Monitor Nutrition during Pregnancy in Sheep

To aid farmers on high production farms it is very useful to blood test the ewes 6 weeks before lambing (i.e. at the time of clostridial disease vaccination). Normally farmers will be advised not to flush ewes except on farms under high standards of management. Triplets are not financially advantageous. Farms should aim for ewes with a body condition score (BCS) of 3–3.5. However, scanning the ewes will pinpoint those carrying twins, and particularly those carrying triplets. Both of these groups should be blood tested to monitor their hydroxybutyrate levels. As a rule of thumb, 250 g of barley will provide 3 MJ of energy daily for the last 6 weeks of pregnancy. If there are a large number of uneven twins, this usually indicates poor nutrition earlier in pregnancy. The mechanism is that a triplet has been resorbed, so that there is less placenta available remaining in the horn and the remaining lamb does not develop as well as the lamb in the other horn.

Bronchoalveolar Lavage Technique

This rather specialized technique can be used to diagnose viral and bacterial lower airway disease. The animal should be restrained either in a standing position or in sternal recumbency. The area 5 cm caudal to the larynx should be clipped and surgically prepared. Local infiltration of local anaesthetic solution should be carried out before further surgical preparation. A 12 G 52 × 2.7 mm intravenous catheter should be introduced at 45° to the skin so that the point of the needle is between two trachea rings. A smaller tube of polyethylene with a needle mount is then passed down the catheter for roughly 45 cm, and then 30 ml of sterile isotonic saline is introduced. After 5–10 s some of the saline is withdrawn, and normally 5 ml will be recovered.

Caprine Arthritis and Encephalitis Test

Caprine arthritis and encephalitis (CAE) tests are very sensitive and specific enzyme-linked immunosorbent assay (ELISA) and agar gel immunodiffusion (AGID) tests will identify viraemic goats provided they are over 6 months of age. False negatives will occur below this age and there is the rare goat that will never sero-convert.

Caseous Lymphadenitis Test

The 'gold standard' caseous lymphadenitis (CLA) test is cultured from pus taken from a lesion. The internal wall of the abscess should be scraped if possible, as the organism *Corynebacterium pseudotuberculosis*, which is fairly straightforward to grow, is more likely to be isolated than if only the pus is cultured. There is an ELISA test for sheep but this is not available for goats.

Coccidiosis Oocysts in Faeces Tests

The oocysts are floated in a saturated sodium chloride solution (specific gravity 1.20) using the modified McMaster technique before light microscopic examination; this method is suitable for detecting small coccidia from sheep and goats.

Determination of Passive Immune Status in Neonatal Lambs and Neonatal Kids

Lambs can be tested between 24h of age up to 14 days of age by testing total protein (TP). Blood should be taken into heparin tubes (normally green topped). TP values of less than 65 will indicate failure of passive transfer, in other words insufficient or poor quality colostrum or good colostrum too late. TP can normally be tested simply on a practice refractometer.

Faecal Worm Egg Count

Massively high faecal (worm) egg counts (FEC) are seen worldwide in adult sheep with *Haemonchus contortus* infestation. With thin sheep clinicians should be aware that old ewes with Johne's disease will also show high counts.

Ill Thrift Profiles

These are normally an unnecessary expense in sheep. Obviously the first thing to test in thin sheep is their teeth (see Chapter 10). Other causes are likely to be Johne's disease, chronic parasitism and starvation. Serum protein levels give a useful and inexpensive indicator of health status.

Johne's Disease Test

The 'gold standard' test for Johne's disease in sheep and goats is the identification of the causal organism *Mycobacterium avium* subsp. *paratuberculosis* (MAP) following faecal culture. The main limitation of the test is the timescale, as standard cultures take up to 12 weeks. There are modified liquid cultures that will give strong positive results in 3 days, but these have reduced specificity.

There are polymerase chain reaction (PCR) tests available which give more rapid results and claim similar high sensitivity and specificity but these must be viewed with caution (Kawaji *et al.*, 2011).

Faecal smears can always be examined after staining with Ziehl–Neelsen staining but these will only show acceptable sensitivity values very late on in the course of the disease.

Specific serological tests are available; these are either AGID or ELISA and are prepared for sheep but will give reasonable results in goats. However they are not worthwhile until later on in the course of the disease.

An initial suspicion of Johne's disease can be obtained by numbers of healthy but very small lambs which will fatten. It is important that they are identified as they should be killed fat rather than kept as replacements.

Liver Enzymes

Aspartate aminotransferase

Aspartate aminotransferase (AST) will be raised in liver disease but it is not liver-specific and so will also be raised as a result of muscle cell damage.

Gamma glutamyl transferase

Gamma glutamyl transferase (GGT) is specifically raised in liver disease. Although there high levels in the kidney, it is excreted straight into the urine and does not get into the blood.

Glutamate dehydrogenase

Glutamate dehydrogenase (GLDH) is raised in acute fluke infections and is the most reliable liver enzyme to detect this condition.

Louping Ill Virus Test

A blood sample in heparin (normally in a green-topped tube) is required to isolate this virus.

Lungworm Tests

Normally sheep lungworms eggs will not be seen on the standard FEC. However, in cases of Johne's disease there will be such high levels that eggs will be seen. Lungworms are usually looked for as larvae using the Baermann technique. A sieve and some gauze are positioned in a funnel connected to a tube and a tap. Faeces and some water are placed in the funnel and left for 48 h. The larvae migrate through the gauze and settle in the neck of the funnel. The water in the neck of the funnel is then drained off carefully. This sediment can then be examined under the high power of a microscope to look for first-stage lungworm larvae. A minimum of 50 g of faeces are required for the test.

Paired Samples for Serology

These are useful for retrospective diagnosis for a variety of diseases.

Serum Proteins

These are very simple, cheap tests for sheep practitioners and will give as much information about thin sheep as a full ill thrift profile. However, albumen and globulin levels are required, not just a TP level. The normal albumen level would be 35 and the globulin level 45. In Johne's disease the globulin level will remain normal but the albumen level will drop below 20. A normal level of globulin but with a modest drop in albumen, that is to 35–30, can occur in late gestation, but can also occur with starvation or chronic parasitism. With liver fluke and chronic infections the albumen levels tend to remain normal but there is a large rise in the globulin levels to 55.

Tests for Cerebro-cortico-necrosis

Blood test for transketolase estimation

A blood sample in a heparinized green-topped tube is required to test for cerebro-cortico-necrosis (CCN).

Faeces test for thiaminase

30 g of faeces are required.

Triclabendazole Resistance Test

Researchers have found (Flanagan *et al.*, 2011) that a coproantigen reduction test (CRT) protocol can be used for the diagnosis of triclabendazole (TCBZ) resistance. They suggest that the resampling time is 14 days after treatment (with the inclusion of positive and negative coproantigen samples as controls), and that samples be stored in a fridge or freezer before processing.

Ultrasonography of the Eye

This can be a useful technique to assess the eye in sheep and goats. It is best to use a transpalpedral approach without a stand-off in a horizontal plane. The retrobulbar space can be evaluated to establish the cause of any swellings. Any fine-needle aspirates can be guided by ultrasonography. Tumours and abscesses can be found in this space.

Urine Tests

Normal urine is clear and pale to yellow. Cloudy urine indicates inflammation. The likely causes are:

- urethral rents or trauma;
- pyelonephritis;
- cystitis;
- urolithiasis; or
- urethritis.

Urine may change colour after it is voided due to the presence of oxidizing agents. Pigments in the urine may also stain bedding red. This may be misleading and give the impression that the urine itself is discoloured. Discolouration may be caused by:

- Haematuria – erythrocytes in the urine.
- Haemoglobinuria – haemoglobin in the urine, secondary to haemolysis.
- Myoglobinuria – myoglobin in the urine secondary to nutritional muscular dystrophy and in certain plant poisonings, resulting in muscle necrosis.

A free-catch urine sample is the most appropriate to collect. Catheterization in male animals is not possible and in female animals may cause trauma and give a contaminated sample. After a gross visual examination some urine should be retained in a sterile container for bacterial culture.

The urine should be tested with dipsticks. These reagent strips vary and therefore it is important to read the instructions carefully or a false result may be obtained. Most sticks will give an indication of whole blood or the presence of pigment, either haemoglobin or myoglobin. They will also give an indication of the presence of protein. The likely cause of this will be inflammation. However the inflammation may be occurring anywhere from the kidneys down to the urethral orifice. The presence of sugar indicates a clostridial infection (see Chapter 10). However, sedation with xylazine will also cause glycosuria.

In sheep and goats the specific gravity will range from 1006 to 1015, with an average of 1010. However, rises in the specific gravity must be viewed with caution, as they may just indicate the presence of pigments in the urine.

Centrifugation of the urine and examination of the supernatant may help. It will be clear if red cells are in the sediment. However, if there is haemoglobinuria, the supernatant will remain pink after centrifugation. This should be carried out at 1000 revolutions per minute (RPM) for 5 min, ideally within 30 min of collection. The sediment can be made into smears and examined either immediately or after staining with methylene blue. Cells, crystals and bacteria may be seen. Sperm are a normal finding in the urine of sexually active males.

5

Veterinary Equipment

General

Advances in medical equipment have been very rapid in recent years and progress will continue. The advances in the veterinary field are not very far behind. This chapter will therefore be out of date in some respects before this book has been published. However the whole ethos of this book is for treatment of small ruminants worldwide, and in most parts of the world sophisticated equipment is not available. In fact it is not really required for small ruminants except in specific circumstances, so expenditure on it would certainly not be the best use of resources. Therefore I will concentrate on equipment required for the ambulatory veterinary surgeon, mentioning certain items which are available and which could be included if funds allow.

Equipment for Handling

A small halter and 5 × 1-m lengths of soft 1-cm diameter rope are required to help with restraint of ewes and does during caesarean section.

Equipment for Diagnosis

- Arm-length sleeves are required for internal examinations but are probably not used for actual parturition procedures.
- Blood slides and coverslips are essential.
- Blood tubes are required with different anticoagulants.
- Biopsy punches of the small 8-mm disposable type are useful for skin biopsies. Sophisticated biopsy gadgets are available, and these are vital for certain biopsies (e.g. liver).
- A digital camera is important so that the clinician can download the photographs, label and store them, and send them as attachments to e-mails.
- Faeces sample bottles of sufficient size are required. Clinicians should be aware that quite large amounts of faeces are required for certain examinations. At least 70 g should be collected.
- Haematocrit centrifuge tubes can be used without a centrifuge to get a quick idea of a PCV. However a mini centrifuge is useful and relatively inexpensive. A hand-driven centrifuge for larger tubes is very cheap and can give adequate results.
- Labels, a notebook and a pen are all required for recording cases and sample taking.
- A magnifying glass is useful in skin examination.
- A McMaster slide is required for carrying out faecal worm egg counts. Great care should be taken when handling the cover

slips marked with squares, as they are delicate and expensive.

- A microscope is a delicate piece of equipment. I do not recommend that one be carried in the vehicle as routine. However, the use of a microscope at one's base is vital. It needs to be equipped for oil immersion. Slides already prepared with Giemsa stain are useful. Gram stain, Giemsa and methylene blue are important.
- Sample bottles containing formalin are required for preserving biopsy material. They should be stored separately from swabs required for bacteriological sampling.
- Small strong polythene bags are useful for skin samples and for double sealing various other samples, e.g. faeces sample bottles.
- The stethoscope is the second vital piece of diagnostic equipment after the clinical thermometer. Ideally it needs to be slim so that auscultation is possible under the muscles caudal to the shoulder. Ideally, both a bell and a diaphragm should also be present. Obviously there are sophisticated stethoscopes available, such as Litmans. However the inexpensive models are quite adequate.
- A thin stomach tube is required, passed through a hole in a rectangular piece of wood to act as a gag. This is useful for relieving bloat in sheep and goats and can also be used for obtaining samples of the rumen contents.
- Various types of swab are required, some plain and others with transport media. Sometimes a very narrow swab will be required.
- A clinical thermometer is vital. The traditional glass thermometers will last for years if kept carefully in a plastic case, but are hard to acquire in the UK because of the mercury content. However digital thermometers are available. The thermometer can be calibrated in Celsius or Fahrenheit, depending upon the clinician's personal choice.
- Urine dipsticks are useful occasionally and are relatively cheap.

Equipment for the Feet

Hoof knife

The type of knife is a very individual choice; obviously there are knives for left- and right-handed individuals. Equally, there are double-sided knives, which can be used in either hand. Looped knives are useful for removing the softer parts of the hoof.

Gutter tape

A roll of this tape is very useful for making bandages waterproof in the hoof area and is also useful for covering poultices.

Small clippers for sheep-sized hoofs

These should be kept well oiled.

Equipment for the Limbs

Oscillating saw

This might be considered inessential as a hand-held plaster saw can be used. However, cutting modern plastering materials is seriously hard work. An oscillating saw is quick and accurate.

Splints

Where funds are tight there is no need for sophisticated splints. Smooth lengths of wood and plastic guttering are quite adequate. Any sharp ends can be rasped smooth and covered with gutter tape.

Equipment for the Eyes

Fluorescein strips

These are inexpensive and vital, not only for revealing the presence of deep corneal ulcers, but also for testing the patency of the tear ducts. It should be remembered that in small ruminants it takes up to 30 min for the fluorescein to reach the nasal end of the tear ducts after instillation in the eye.

Ophthalmoscope

This is an expensive piece of equipment but is important to the clinician. Much can be learned by examining the eyes carefully with a small bright torch and a magnifying glass. Sadly, however, without a good ophthalmoscope some pathological conditions will be missed. Although a slit lamp is very useful for examining dogs' eyes, it is not required for small ruminants.

Equipment for Dentistry including Equipment for Sinoscopy

Dental elevators

These are useful, for example for removing wolf teeth in horses.

Dental picks

These should be strong enough to allow the practitioner to pick out food matter compacted between the teeth in diastemata.

Dental rasps

A small diamond-covered rasp is required.

Head light

Some very bright torches with heavy battery packs are available. These are not really required and a light that is easily taken on and off is preferable.

Molar extraction forceps

Two pairs are required. They should be 20 cm long; one should be straight and the other should have the extracting jaws at right angles.

Molar spreaders

A small pair 20 cm long is required.

Mouth washing syringe

A catheter-tipped 60-ml syringe is adequate.

Small ruminant gag

These are hard to obtain.

Steinmann pins

These are inexpensive and useful for making small holes into the sinuses.

Equipment for Stitching

These items are self-explanatory, but I will list them for completeness. The clinician can manage with very few.

Artery forceps

These can be straight or curved. Several pairs are required.

Clippers

These are a luxury. However they make stitching and wound management so much cleaner and easier, particularly in rough-haired animals. The ideal type has a rechargeable battery.

Drapes

A single sterile drape is required as a tray cloth by the ambulatory clinician, although additional drapes will be required for other surgery.

Dressings forceps

The ends of these forceps are important, and can be flat or rat-toothed. A pair of each is required.

Dressings scissors

A pair of curved, blunt-ended scissors needs to be readily available for trimming hair, but a straight pair with pointed ends is required for a stitch-up kit. There are various different sizes.

Needle holders

There are various types. The most convenient for stitching up wounds are the combination of cutting and holding type known as 'Gillies'.

Scalpel blades

These come in different sizes and shapes for different procedures.

Scalpel handle

It is important that the scalpel handle is the same size as the blades.

Stitch-cutting scissors

These small scissors need to be available for removing sutures.

Suture material

This may be absorbable or non-absorbable and may also be either monofilament or braided. On the whole, monofilament, non-absorbable suture material will be required for skin wounds.

Suture needles

These come in various shapes and may be either cutting or non-cutting. On the whole, cutting needles will be required for the skin, and non-cutting for soft tissue.

Tissue forceps

These forceps are for lifting tissue. A minimum of two pairs is required.

Towel clips

These are not normally required by the ambulatory clinician unless surgery is going to be performed under a general anaesthetic (GA).

Swabs

Sets of sterile swabs are required for a variety of tasks.

Equipment for the Reproductive System

Vaginal speculum

These can be disposable and used with a small hand torch. The small duck-billed type affords the very best visibility.

Equipment for Post-mortem

These articles are not normally carried by an ambulatory clinician (see Chapter 18).

Specialist Equipment

I have included these items for completeness, and it would be very useful to have the use of some of this equipment. However within the scope of this book a full description would not be worthwhile. Throughout the text a possible alternative will be suggested wherever possible, to save on financial investment.

- blood analyser;
- centrifuge;
- gaseous anaesthetic machine;
- operating table;
- refractometer;
- ultrasound scanner;
- X-ray machine.

6

Veterinary Medicines

General

The various veterinary medicines will be described in the relevant chapters. In this chapter they are discussed in their therapeutic groups. The chapter ends with a list of medicines that the author suggests should be carried by an ambulatory veterinarian working in the UK. Sheep and goats are all liable to be killed for human consumption and therefore some meat withdrawal times are given. However, as few of the drugs are licensed for sheep, and even fewer for goats, practitioners have to advise their clients to observe a minimum of 28 days before the animal can be killed for human consumption. Sheep and goats are also kept for milk production. Milk withdrawal times are very difficult to state for certain, but an attempt is made to give some guidelines. Clinicians will need to use their judgement, as drugs licensed for sheep and cattle can be used in goats on the cascade principle.

Correct storage of medicines is very important. Practitioners should always follow the instructions on the data sheets. The practice medicine store, the practice refrigerator, the in-car refrigerator and the car itself should have their temperatures monitored constantly. Medicines should never become too hot or too cold. Freezing may lead to the active ingredient coming out of suspension. If this previously frozen product is used subsequently, the amount of active ingredient given may not be consistent, which could lead to both under- and over-dosing. This problem is particularly acute in the winter in temperate climates when products are stored in unheated buildings.

For all sheep and goats that are going for meat for human consumption the safest course of action in the UK is to follow the data sheets and, where there is no specific licence, then to follow the withdrawal times for cattle. Clinicians in other countries should study local regulations. In the UK there is a 28-day withhold time for meat for all unlicensed products.

Antibiotics

Introduction

There are two types of antibiotics. Those that actually kill bacteria are called bactericidal antibiotics and those that limit the replication of bacteria are known as bacteriostatic antibiotics. The actual classification is shown in Table 6.1.

It is important to use a bactericidal antibiotic in young animals and in animals with depressed immune systems.

Tylosin

This antibiotic is available as an intramuscular injection for a dosage of 4 mg/kg, which can be achieved by injecting 1 ml/50 kg. The solution contains 200 mg of tylosin/ml. Higher doses, up to 10 mg/kg, are licensed for cattle. The product has a milk withholding period of 108 h and a meat withdrawal time of 28 days.

Oral antibiotics

These preparations must only be given to young lambs and kids and therefore there are no milk or meat withhold times recommended. Obviously there are many antibiotic tablets prepared for dogs and cats together with boluses prepared for calves. However, listing them would not be helpful for the practitioner treating sheep and goats, as their indications are very few and the oral preparations prepared specifically for lambs are much easier to administer.

Neomycin

This is available combined with streptomycin as an oral solution with each millilitre containing 70 mg neomycin sulfate and 70 mg streptomycin sulfate. The dose is 1 ml/5 kg daily. This product is licensed for lambs in the UK.

Spectinomycin

This is available as a viscous liquid containing 50 mg/ml. The daily dose for a lamb is one measure of 1 ml from the doser. This product is licensed for lambs in the UK.

Streptomycin

This is available combined with neomycin as an oral solution with each millilitre containing 70 mg neomycin sulfate and 70 mg streptomycin sulfate. The dose is 1 ml/5 kg daily. This product is licensed for lambs in the UK.

Other antibiotic preparations

These include topical antibiotics that are available as creams, gels, powders and aerosol sprays. The most usual ingredient is 2% chlortetracycline hydrochloride. Antibiotics are also available as intramammary formulations licensed for cows. These can be used in sheep and goats. If they are used in sheep or goats producing milk for human consumption, then milk withhold times are the same as those recommended for cattle. It is important that if a parenteral antibiotic is used at the same time that this is the same antibiotic as the intramammary preparation. If that is not possible it should be of the same family or at least synergistic.

Antibiotics are also available in ear and eye preparations. One of the most common preparations is eye ointment containing 1% chlortetracycline hydrochloride, which needs to be repeatedly applied, ideally every 6 h. The product 16.67% w/w cloxacillin benzathine has a longer duration of action of up to 48 h. Only one application of cloxacillin benzathine may be sufficient to control contagious ophthalmia in sheep and goats.

Antifungal Agents

These can be divided into systemic agents given either by intravenous injection or orally, and topical agents.

Amphotericin

This is the only injectable antifungal agent. It is active against yeasts, histoplasmosis and blastomycosis. The drug is supplied in powder form to be reconstituted with water or 5% dextrose saline in a very dilute solution to avoid cardiac toxicity. It must always be kept in the dark as it is extremely light sensitive. It is prudent to try a test dose of 0.2 mg/kg initially. This can then be increased slowly over several days to 1.0 mg/kg. Renal function should be monitored. Adverse reactions should be treated with corticosteroids. If kidney damage is suspected then the drug may be given every other day.

Griseofulvin

This is a very effective treatment for *Trichophyton* spp. These are normally caught from cattle. However, it is banned for use in food-producing animals in the UK. Griseofulvin is not very effective against *Microsporum* spp. Care should be taken by pregnant women if they handle griseofulvin, as it is teratogenic. It should be remembered that ringworm, particularly *Trichophyton* spp., are zoonoses (see Chapter 19). Vigorous scrubbing and strong disinfectants, which damage the skin, should be avoided; normal washing with soap is preferable. Women and children are particularly susceptible.

Miconazole

This is a good topical treatment for *Trichophyton* spp. and *Microsporum* spp. It should be used as a shampoo twice weekly.

Natamycin

This is also a good topical treatment for *Trichophyton* spp. and *Microsporum* spp. It comes as a powder to be re-suspended. The suspension is then sponged or sprayed onto the affected area every 4–5 days.

Virkon S

This is actually a broad-spectrum virucidal disinfectant. It is a very effective disinfectant and also can be used to treat *Microsporum* spp. It should be made up as a 1% solution (a 50-g sachet in 5 l of water). This solution can be used as spray or sponged onto affected areas every 48 h. This use is not licensed in the UK but it is widely used off-license.

Antiprotozoal Drugs

These are divided into three groups:

1. To control coccidiosis.
2. To treat blood-borne parasites, mainly in the tropics.
3. To treat other protozoal conditions.

Coccidiostats

Amprolium

This is available as a 9.6% oral solution. Lambs and kids need to be treated daily for 5 days with 3 ml/5 kg. There is a 24-h meat withdrawal period. It is not licensed in the UK.

Decoquinate

This is available as a 6% premix to add to creep-feed to treat lambs. A total of 1.67 kg of the premix can be added to a tonne of feed to provide the recommended concentration of 100 mg/kg. This can be used as a treatment or a prophylaxis during a coccidial challenge. It can also be used in kids. It has a zero meat withdrawal period.

Diclazuril

This is available as a 0.25% aqueous oral suspension that is licensed for use in lambs. It can also be used in goats. The dose is 1 mg/kg by mouth (1 ml/2.5 kg). A single dose should be given and repeated if indicated in 3 weeks. It can be used as a preventative as well as a treatment; that is, it can be given 10–14 days after susceptible stock have been moved onto pasture known to be infected with oocysts. It is safe in lambs from 1 week of age. It has a zero meat withdrawal period.

Toltrazuril

This is available as an oral suspension containing 50 mg/ml of toltrazuril. It is licensed in the UK for the prevention of clinical signs of coccidiosis and reduction of coccidia shedding in lambs on farms with a confirmed history of coccidiosis caused by *Eimeria crandallis* and *Eimeria ovinoidalis*. Each lamb should be treated with a single oral dose of 20 mg toltrazuril/kg. This is equivalent to 0.4 ml of the oral suspension/kg. To obtain the maximum benefit, the lambs should be treated before the expected onset of clinical signs, in other words in the prepatent period. This product has a meat withdrawal period of 42 days.

Trimethoprim-sulfadoxine

The antibiotic TMS is also effective against coccidia. It needs to be given at 30 mg/kg for 3 days.

Drugs to treat blood-borne protozoal parasites

The drugs to treat blood-borne parasites have been developed to treat cattle. They are extremely irritant when injected, and clinicians are advised to use deep intramuscular injections. Some clinicians use the intravenous route, and my personal experience with this route is favourable. However others have reported anaphylactic reactions and death. Local conditions should be investigated so that an informed opinion can be given on the risk to the animal and the likelihood of resistance of the protozoan to be treated.

Diminazene aceturate

This is the most hazardous of this group of drugs. It is extremely effective against *Babesia* spp. However, as less dangerous drugs are available to treat this protozoan, they should be considered. On the other hand it is the most effective drug available to treat trypanosomiasis. This includes *Trypanosoma brucei* (Surra), *Trypanosoma vivax* (acute 'fly'), and *Trypanosoma congolense* (chronic 'fly'). These three trypanosomes are only spread by tsetse fly, so will only be seen in a tsetse area. In areas with a high density of tsetse fly only game animals can survive. Cattle can be kept for short periods with trypanocidal drugs being given prophylactically. Sheep and goats can be kept in the same manner for short periods. If trypanosomiasis is suspected in sheep and goats a diagnosis should be made rapidly from a blood smear. Treatment should only be carried out if the diagnosis is certain. Sheep and goats appear to develop a premunity and do not readily develop the infection. However the organism is very serious in naive animals. Once again, a rapid diagnosis should be made on blood smears and treatment should be carried out. Diminazene aceturate can be used to cure all these infections. It is supplied in 1.05 g sachets for reconstitution in 12.5 ml of water to make a 12.5% solution. This is the normal dose for an adult cow. Often this is made up in a non-sterile manner, which can cause abscesses in cattle. It will cause problems if given in such a manner to sheep and goats. A suitable protocol for treatment of a 50-kg goat is to dissolve the 1.05-g sachet in 50 ml of warm sterile water in the most sterile manner possible. When at blood heat, 5 ml of this solution is then injected as slowly as possible intravenously.

Imidocarb

This is the drug of choice for treating *Babesia* spp. These protozoan parasites are spread by ticks. Imidocarb is supplied in a 12% solution in a 100-ml multidose vial. The risk of abscessation is much less than with Diminazene. The dose for sheep and goats is 1.2 mg/kg by deep intramuscular injection on 2 separate days (this is only 0.5 ml for a 50-kg sheep or goat).

Isometamidium

This used to be a useful drug to treat *T. brucei*, *T. congolense* and *T. vivax* in cattle. Widespread resistance has now been encountered in cattle and so the author would not advise its use in sheep and goats.

Quinapyramine

This drug used to be used in cattle in the form of either the sulfate or the chloride preparation. There is now widespread resistance in infections of *T. brucei*, *T. congolense* and *T. vivax*. Once again the author does not advise its use for these infections in sheep and goats and on no account should it be given intravenously.

Drugs to treat other protozoal parasites

Metronidizole

This can be used to treat protozoal diseases. However its principal use in sheep and goats is to treat anaerobic bacteria topically in wounds or infections in the feet.

Pyrimethamine

This drug can be used to treat toxoplasmosis and to lessen the rate of abortion in sheep and goats. There is a synergism between pyrimethamine and potentiated sulfonamides and so the two drugs are often given together. Pyrimethamine should be given by mouth at 0.1–0.2 mg/kg daily. Sulfonamides should be given at the normal dose rate of 15 mg/kg. This regime may be given from 2 months after service until parturition.

Anthelmintics

General

In the 1960s and 1970s broad-spectrum anthelmintics were developed for ruminants. These products, the benzimidazoles, the imidazothiazoles/tetrahydropyrimidines (levamisole and morantel) and the macrocyclic lactones greatly improved global sheep production. They also improved goat production worldwide. Sadly, rather rapid resistance to these products has developed (Mitchell *et al.*, 2010). In the UK, benzimidazole resistance was first reported in 1982, levamisole resistance in 1994 and macrocyclic lactone resistance in 2001. These reports have been mirrored elsewhere throughout the world. It is vital that effective strategies to combat these resistances are put in place and that farmers should not rely on the recent manufacture of a new class of anthelmintic, monepantel, an amino-acetonitrile derivative.

It is important for clinicians to realize the difference between anthelmintic failure and anthelmintic resistance. Anthelmintic failure occurs due to:

- insufficient anthelmintic dose due to underestimation of animal weight;
- failure to follow manufacturer's instructions;
- poor maintenance of dosing equipment;
- re-introduction of animals onto heavily contaminated pasture; and
- use of incorrect drug for target worms.

In other cases of apparent failure, anthelmintic resistance should be suspected.

There are two anthelmintic resistance detection methods available *in vivo*; the faecal egg count reduction test (FECRT) and the controlled test (CT). The FECRT is the most commonly used field assay for all anthelmintic groups. It has a low sensitivity as there are many false negatives. On the other hand, there are false positives with levamisole. It requires two visits per farm and there is a seasonal variability. The CT is a comparison of parasite burdens in treated and non-treated animals that have been artificially infected with worms suspected of being either susceptible or partially resistant; these two groups are then divided at random into medicated and non-medicated groups. After 14 days the animals are killed and the worms are counted on post-mortem.

There are two anthelmintic resistance detection methods available *in vitro*; the egg hatch assay (EHA) and the larval development test (LDT). These are both cheap and highly sensitive but they are not universally standardized or accepted. Farm visits are not required as submissions can be sent by post. There is a seasonal variability, and the methods are not generally predictive in terms of clinical disease. EHA can only be used for benzimidazole anthelmintics and LDT is not satisfactory for avermectins.

Various factors influence the rate of development of anthelmintics resistance. Farm management and husbandry factors can be affected by owners. Factors include stocking rates, grassland management and anthelmintic usage such as frequency and choice. The climate, with its seasonal range of temperature and rainfall, is a very important factor. The parasitic species – that is, its biotic potential and its proportion in refugia – is an important factor to be considered.

Modes of action of anthelmintic groups

- Benzimidazoles – including fenbendazole, mebendazole, oxyfendazole, albendazole and ricobendazole. They bind to the parasites' tubulin leading to inhibition of

glucose uptake which then leads to glycogen depletion and death.
- Probenzimidazoles – including netobimin. They act in the same manner as the benzimidazoles.
- Imidazothiazoles – including levamisole. They are cholinergic agonists that cause rapid and reversible paralysis.
- Tetrahydropyrimidines – including morantel and pyrantel. They act in the same manner as the imidazothiazoles.
- Avermectins – including abamectin, doramectin, eprinomectin, ivermectin and selamectin. They open invertebrate-specific glutamate chloride channels in the post-synaptic membrane leading to flaccid paralysis.
- Milbemycins – including moxidectin. They act in the same manner as the avermectins.
- Salicylanilides – including closantel and oxyclozanide. They uncouple oxidative phosphorylation, decreasing the availability of high-energy phosphate compounds.
- Substitute phenols – including nitroxynil. They act in the same manner as the salicylanilides.
- Amino-acetonitrile derivatives – including monepantel. They are cholinergic agonists that act on a novel site on the receptor, resulting in spastic paralysis of the worms.

New classes of anthelmintics

At the time of writing monepantel is a new family of anthelmintic, with no resistance problems. It is vital that such new products are used with considerable care. Naturally it may be used as a quarantine dose at the **correct** dose rate and also where triple resistance has been proven. It should **not** be used for routine worming. It is a very safe anthelmintic and the dose is 1 mg/kg. Animals may not be slaughtered for human consumption for 7 days after administration.

Anthelmintics combined with trace elements

Some benzimidazoles are available with the addition of cobalt sulfate and sodium selenate. Clinicians should guide their shepherds carefully on the need for such additives, as they are not commonly required.

Long-acting injectable products

Certain injectable moxidectin products will give a sustained persistency against helminths in sheep. Persistence of 44 days for *Trichostrongylus colubriformis*, 97 days for *Teladorsagia circumcincta* and 111 days for *Haemonchus contortus* is claimed from a single injection of the correct dose. This same preparation claims efficiency against sheep scab for 60 days. The other intestinal nematodes controlled are the adults of *Trichostrongylus axei*, *Nematodirus spathiger*, *Cooperia curticei* and *Chabertia ovina*. The third stage larvae of *Gaigeria pachyscelis* and *Oesophagostomum columbianum* are also controlled. *Dictyocaulus filarial* and *Oestrus ovis* are controlled by the same product. Animals must not be slaughtered for human consumption for 104 days after administration. It should not be used in dairy sheep or in lambs weighing less than 15 kg.

Flukecides

The 34% w/v nitroxynil injection at 10 mg/kg is licensed for use in the UK as a treatment by subcutaneous injection for *Fasciola hepatica* in sheep. It is claimed to be effective against mature and immature flukes, but the age of the immature flukes is not stated. The drug is probably not effective in the UK for the control of acute fascioliasis in sheep in the autumn. However no resistance has been reported, and therefore it is a very useful medicine to use if triclabendazole resistance is suspected. It is also effective against *Haemonchus contortus*. However it is not a broad spectrum anthelmintic and should not be used as such. However, as *H. contortus* and *F. hepatica* are both parasites that cause severe disease and deaths in adult sheep, it is an extremely useful product. It can be used at the same time as levamisole, but in different sites, to provide broad spectrum capability. It has some dangers. The solution contains no preservative so great care must be taken not to introduce a bacterium into the solution, and the discard time of 28 days after broaching should be strictly adhered to. It will stain the fleece so a very careful injection technique is required. It can be used in pregnant sheep but naturally they should be handled with care. It must not be used in sheep producing milk for human consumption. In the event of accidental overdose the symptoms are pyrexia, rapid respiration and increased excitability. Patients should be kept cool, and dextrose saline should be given as a drip. In the normal course of events nitroxynil should be repeated within 49 days. Nitroxynil can be used in goats but is not recommended, as they find the injection painful. The dose rate of triclabendazole is 10 mg/kg in sheep and goats. It must not be used in sheep or goats producing milk for human consumption. The withholding period for meat is 56 days.

Combination fluke and worm products

The liver fluke *F. hepatica* requires the presence of a water snail as the secondary host. Diagnosis is not easy and relies on raised liver enzymes in a serum sample and then very careful floatation of faeces to find the eggs. The presence of one egg is significant. For sheep the following licensed drugs are available: triclabendazole at 10 mg/kg; albendazole at 7.5 mg/kg; closantel at 10 mg/kg; and nitroxynil at 10 mg/kg. There is now a plethora of fluke and worm combination products on the market for use in sheep, and naturally there will be a demand for products suitable for goats. Although convenient, they should only be used if there is a need to target both fluke and worms. As this is a very rare occurrence, they should not be used without considerable thought. This will not only save owners' money but will also lower the risk of drug resistance developing. Combination products undergo extensive testing to ensure that the two components mix evenly and work together properly. It is not acceptable to take two products and mix them together on the farm. The greatest danger to sheep and goats from fluke infection is from acute cases. Not all fluke products will kill immature flukes, and it is vital that sheep and goats are treated early in the course of the disease with a flukecide that will kill immature flukes at the critical time. This is in early autumn in the UK. A second treatment should be given 2 months later to kill any immature or mature flukes that were not killed by the first dose. It takes 10–12 weeks for 2 mm immature flukes to develop into 2–3 cm adult flukes in the liver. These are the only flukes which will be killed by most flukecides. Therefore these products should only be used in the late winter or early spring in the UK.

Anthelmintics for goats

Anthelmintic resistance is commonly reported in goats in many countries where they are kept intensively, and is increasingly reported in the UK, but it should be remembered that there is a limited availability of licensed anthelmintics for goats. However, the nematode species are often identical to those in sheep. Suboptimal dosing is very common in goats. It has been suggested that goats are more susceptible to gastrointestinal nematode infections than sheep because, as principally browsing animals, their resistance mechanisms to these endoparasites are less highly evolved. Modern husbandry methods change domestic goats from browsing animals to grazing ones, increasing their exposure to infective parasitic larvae to a higher level than that experienced by their wild counterparts. As a consequence, when goats are forced to graze at high stocking rates, they carry much heavier nematode burdens than those found in grazing sheep. Evidence can be seen for this from FEC, which can persist at high levels for prolonged periods of time in goats. In goats the post-parturient rise can continue after parturition for up to 18 months. As there is a lack of effective immune response, helminth infection may occur at high levels throughout the life of a goat, unlike a sheep where strong acquired resistance develops at about 1 year of age. Adult goats may show FEC in excess of 2000 eggs/g (epg), indicative of clinical disease, or of 500–2000 epg, suggestive of subclinical parasitism and subsequent reduced production, decreased milk yield or poor weight gains. In the UK the only licensed anthelmintics for goats are ivermectin drenches.

An additional problem in goats requiring anthelmintic treatment is that of milk residues and milk withdrawal periods. Ivermectin drenches have a milk withdrawal period of 60 days.

The Goat Veterinary Society (GVS) in the UK advises that all bought-in goats should be wormed on arrival. Ideally they should be given wormers from two different classes 15–20 min apart. Currently, because of the high risk of wormer resistance in goats, it is acceptable to use the new product, monepantel. If more new wormers are introduced, these can be used as alternatives. After treatment, the bought-in goats should be isolated (ideally indoors) for 2 weeks and FEC should be carried out.

At other times, goats should not be wormed automatically on a regular basis, but as needed. Best practice is to confirm the need for worming by undertaking individual FEC. Whenever a group of goats is wormed, it should be standard practice to carry out a FEC 1–2 weeks later to ensure that the worming has had a satisfactory effect. Ideally, particularly in bigger units, this should be done with multiple classes of wormers at several stages of the year to establish what the levels of wormer resistance are. Because goats metabolize wormers faster than sheep, these tests can be done sooner than recommended for sheep. For benzimidazoles, levamisoles and all macrocyclic lactones (except for moxidectin) these tests should be done 7–10 days after worming. Goats treated with moxidectin should be tested 10–14 days after worming.

At the time of writing, the GVS recommends restricting the use of monepantel to quarantine drenching of bought-in goats only, avoiding its use as a routine wormer. Used in this way, development of monepantel resistance will be slowed and it will remain available for longer in those situations where no other wormer will work. The organization also advises owners to continue to use the wormer they have been using if it is effective, particularly if they are only worming on an as-needed basis. They do not advise rotating between worming classes either annually or for every treatment, because rotation does not slow down the development of resistance. If there is evidence of resistance then a wormer from a different class should be used. This may mean that in some herds it is necessary to swap between wormers during the year as worms in the autumn may have different resistances from those in the spring. Dosages of anthelmintics are different for goats compared with sheep, and are shown in Table 6.3.

Table 6.3. Dosages for anthelmintics for sheep and goats.

Anthelmintic	Dose for sheep	Dose for goats
Benzimidazole	5 mg/kg	10 mg/kg
Levamisole	7.5 mg/kg	12 mg/kg*
Ivermectin	0.2 mg/kg	0.4 mg/kg
Doramectin	0.2 mg/kg	0.4 mg/kg
Moxidectin	0.2 mg/kg	0.4 mg/kg
Monepantel	2.5 mg/kg	5.0 mg/kg

Note: *At this dose, goats will often become mildly ill for 24–48 h after dosing, and in particular may scour.

The best method of worming goats is to use an oral drench, as this exposes the worms directly to the wormer. Injections are second best. Pour-on preparations should not be used in goats.

In the UK there is an automatic minimum milk withhold time of 7 days, and a minimum meat withhold time of 28 days. Clinicians may advise longer withhold periods if appropriate, in keeping with advice given on the data sheet for sheep; for example, monepantel has a 35-day milk withhold for sheep in New Zealand.

Ectoparasiticides

Publications by DEFRA (2005) and Bates (2004) provide some useful views on this subject.

Amitraz

This is available as a clear emulsifiable concentrate for dilution and topical application, containing 5% w/v amitraz for treatment of demodectic and sarcoptic mange; 100ml should be diluted in 10l of water. After the animal has been washed in warm water to remove any dirt it should be bathed in this solution, then removed without rinsing and allowed to dry naturally in warm air. It should not be allowed to drink or lick any of the solution. This should be repeated in 1 week.

Ivomectins and moxidectin

These drugs, which are covered under anthelmintics, do have an ectoparasitic action when given by injection. They do not appear to have any ectoparasitic action when given by mouth.

Benzyl benzoate

This acaricide, which is a lotion, is very effective against mange mites if applied daily to all the affected areas.

Benzoyl peroxide

This acaricide can be used to treat mange.

Coumaphos

This so-called louse powder is not very effective and needs to be applied every 5 days to increase its effectiveness. It has no effect on mange mites.

Alphacypermethrin

This is marketed to control nuisance flies when applied every 14 days. It will control head fly for 4 weeks. Blowfly strike can not only be prevented, but also treated by the pour-on preparation. Sheep and lambs will be given 8–10 weeks' cover. It will also help to control mange mites, ticks and lice. The withhold time for meat is 28 days. It is not allowed for use with lactating animals.

Cypermethrin

This is marketed as a concentrate for dilution to a solution that can be sprayed on with a knapsack sprayer, or sponged on. It will control nuisance flies and lice. It is also marketed for dilution as a plunge dip to control sheep scab and prevent blowfly strike for 8 weeks. It is not permitted for use in the UK in meat-producing animals and so there is no meat withhold period stated. It is also marketed as a pour-on preparation for treating and preventing blowfly strike in sheep. It gives 6–8 weeks' protection, but only in the area of the pour-on sweep. It also gives protection against lice, ticks and head flies. The withhold time for meat is 8 days. It is not licensed for milk-producing animals in the UK.

Cyromazine

This is marketed as a blowfly strike preventative, not treatment. It will last for 10 weeks. The withhold time for meat is 28 days. It must not be used for milk-producing animals.

Dicyclanil

This is a pour-on product to prevent blowfly strike in sheep and lambs. It is available as a 5% solution that offers 16 weeks' protection but has a withhold period of 40 days, which may cause difficulties for marketing summer fat lambs. However, it is also available as a 1.25% solution that protects for 8 weeks but has a withhold period of only 7 days.

Diethyltoludine

This midge repellent is extremely effective, but unfortunately it is washed off by rain and even in dry conditions is rarely effective for more than 6h. It is rarely used in sheep and goats.

Piperonyl butoxide

This can be used to control lice if applied every 14 days. However, if it is required to control midge irritation, it needs to be applied to the affected areas daily.

Deltamethrin

Deltamethrin is prepared in a 1% w/v solution as an ectoparasiticide for the topical treatment and control of ticks, lice, keds and established blowfly strike on adult sheep. It can also be used for the control of ticks and lice on lambs. Although it is not licensed in the UK it can be used on goats elsewhere. It should be used on a single spot between the shoulders after parting the wool and may be used by direct application to a maggot-infested area in established blowfly strike. It should not be used in sheep or goats producing milk for human consumption. The meat withdrawal period is 35 days.

Sheep Dips

General instructions

To prepare the bath:

1. Check that the bath is clean and only use clean water. Prepare the bath and mix in the dip concentrate on the day of dipping. Use a container of known volume to calibrate an approximate volume in the bath. The calibrated volume should be an exact multiple of 150 l.
2. Fill the dip bath with water to the accurately calibrated level. To prevent overspill do not fill the bath to capacity and make sure you allow for water displacement by the sheep. Plunge baffles can help prevent spillage.
3. Follow the instructions for dispensing the dip safely.
4. Follow the instructions for the initial fill carefully and safely.
5. Replenish the bath depending on its size, according to the instructions.
6. Normally sheep will be dipped in the summer to control blowfly strike. This should be carried out at least 3 weeks after shearing to obtain a good residual protection.
7. Treatment for sheep scab can be carried out at any time of year. However, dipping in the winter is not recommended, and another form of control should be used.
8. Treatment to control ticks should be carried out in the spring before lambing. If the infestation is severe then dipping should be repeated in 6 weeks, except for young lambs.
9. After dipping, all sheep should stand in draining pens for not less than 10 min or until they have completely stopped dripping.
10. If a large amount of scum forms on the surface of the bath skim it off and place in a secure container. This must be clearly marked and disposed of safely.
11. Fouling of the dip wash reduces its effectiveness. Therefore, do not dip more than one sheep/2 l of dip wash that was in the bath at the start of dipping. For example, if the total volume of wash in your bath was 1000 l you should not dip more than 500 sheep, no matter how many times you have replenished and topped up the bath. You should then empty, clean and recharge the bath with fresh dip wash.
12. Post-dipping lameness may occur when sheep are dipped in dirty wash or in wash that has stood overnight (see Chapter 15).
13. If dipping of heavily pregnant sheep is essential, they should be gently lowered into the bath and assisted out.
14. Sheep should never be dipped on a full stomach, when the wool is wet or when they are heated, tired, thirsty or suffering from wounds or open sores.
15. If possible, dipping should be carried out on a cool day early in the morning.
16. Rams and fat sheep should be assisted through the bath and lambs dipped separately from the ewes.
17. Care should be taken to ensure that the sheep do not swallow or inhale any wash.
18. The manufacturer's instructions should be studied and followed carefully regarding the administration of any other veterinary medicine within 2 weeks of dipping.
19. Different dipping products should not be mixed.
20. Sheep should not be taken through a foot bath on the same day as dipping.
21. The meat and milk withholding times for each dip should be carefully followed according to the manufacturer's instructions.
22. Health and safety regulations and recommendations should be followed exactly according to the manufacturer's instructions.

23. Care must be exercised when disposing of the finished dip and all the dip containers.

Diazinon

This is supplied in a 60% w/w solution for further dilution to a 0.04% w/w solution to control blowfly strike, ticks, keds, lice and scab infestations. The sheep should remain in the solution for at least 0.5 min and have its head plunged twice for treatment of sheep scab. This can be reduced to 0.5 min and one head plunge for all other infestations. Sheep may not be slaughtered for human consumption for 70 days. Diazinon is not suitable for milking sheep.

Dipping of goats

There are no licensed dips for goats in the UK. However, goats may be safely dipped in sheep dips in other parts of the world. All the safety instructions and recommendations as for sheep should be followed. It should be remembered that most dips are not suitable for milking goats and that most have considerable meat withdrawal times.

Non-steroidal Anti-inflammatory Drugs (NSAIDs)

Special consideration has to be given to the treatment of milking sheep and goats. None of the medicines listed in Table 6.4 is licensed for milking sheep or goats. In the UK, however, and using the cascade system, flunixin could be used and the milk withdrawn for 12h; tolfenamic acid could be used and the milk withdrawn for 24h; and meloxicam could be used and the milk withdrawn for 120h. Following the model for dairy cows there is no milk withdrawal on ketoprofen. Clinicians in other countries should study the local regulations.

For all sheep and goats which are going for meat for human consumption the safest course of action in the UK is to follow the data sheets and, where there is no specific license, then to follow the withdrawal times for cattle. Clinicians in other countries should study local regulations. In the UK there is a 28-day withhold time for meat for all unlicensed products.

Other Useful Drugs in Sheep and Goats

Oxytocin is vital to aid the third stage of labour and milk let down. The dose is 10–20 IU given intramuscularly. If given intravenously it must be diluted with at least 20 ml of water or the animal will show quite severe colic. Remember that it should be carried in a car fridge. The other drug that needs to be carried in the car fridge is tetanus anti-toxin (TAT). The dose is empirical; however the author recommends 3000 IU for an adult (given subcutaneously), and 1500 IU for lambs and kids.

Goats are very sensitive to the toxic effects of local anaesthetic. Local blocks, such as those

Table 6.4. Dosages of both NSAID and opiates for injection into sheep and goats.

Agent	Dose	Route	Duration (h)
Pethidine	1 mg/kg	i/m	2
Butorphanol	0.5 mg/kg	Sub/cut or i/v	4
Buprenorphine	10 μg/kg	Sub/cut or i/v	8
Flunixin meglumine	2.2 mg/kg	i/v or i/m	24
Carprofen	1.4 mg/kg	Sub/cut or i/v	24
Meloxicam	0.5 mg/kg	Sub/cut or i/v	24
Ketoprofen	3 mg/kg	i/v or i/m	24
Tolfenamic acid	4 mg/kg	i/v	24

Note: i/m, intramuscularly; i/v, intravenously; sub/cut, subcutaneously.

for caesarean section, should be given with care. You should not exceed the maximum recommended dose of 4 mg/kg. A dose of 1 ml is quite sufficient for epidural anaesthesia.

Sheep and goats may suffer from CCN. Thiamine can be given daily either subcutaneously or intravenously at 15 mg/kg.

Miscellaneous Medicines

Intra-vaginal devices

Sponges impregnated with 30 mg cronolone (flugestone acetate) can be used in sheep to synchronize oestrus and hence lambing. They can also be used to facilitate artificial insemination (AI) and to induce oestrus during the non-breeding period in sheep. The sponge is inserted approximately 10–15 cm into the cleaned vulva using a lubricated tube applicator. The sponge has a small string attached to it, which is left hanging out of the vulva. Licensed disinfectant is supplied with the sponges, as alcohols, cresols, phenols or sheep dips should not be used to clean the vulva. The operator should wear rubber gloves. The progestogen is absorbed through the wall of the vagina while the sponge is in the ewe. The optimal time before removal is 14 days, and the ewe will come into oestrus 48–72 h after removal. Occasionally the string of the sponge cannot be found. In these cases the sponge has usually been lost early. However the vagina should be investigated with a small speculum and a torch to make sure it has been withdrawn (Fig. 6.1).

Synchronization can be carried out at any time during the breeding season. It should be remembered that the ratio of rams to ewes has to be increased to 1 per 10 ewes. The ewes and rams should be kept on a relatively small paddock to aid fertility. Ewe lambs should not be synchronized. If the devices are being used outside of the breeding season they should be withdrawn after 12 days and each ewe should receive an injection of 500 IU of pregnant mare serum gonadotrophin (PMSG) at the time of removal. Ewes may not be slaughtered for human consumption until 14 days after the sponges have been removed, nor may their milk be used for human consumption. Great care should be taken with the disposal of the removed sponges as they are very attractive to dogs.

Melatonin

Melatonin is a natural secretion of the pineal gland and is the day-length messenger by which all animals recognize different seasons. The pineal gland only produces melatonin during the hours of darkness. As days shorten in temperate areas, the amount of melatonin secreted increases and this signals the reproductive system to increase activity in sheep and goats, producing a natural peak in breeding performance in the autumn. Melatonin is supplied as a cylindrical implant containing 18 mg melatonin, which is licensed for use in the UK for sheep. The implant slowly releases melatonin over an extended period, mimicking the natural effect when the day length shortens. It improves the reproductive performance of purebred and crossbred lowland sheep, which are to be mated early in the season before the usual peak of reproductive activity. It is recommended for particular use in Suffolk and Suffolk cross flocks that are intended to start lambing between early December and mid-January, and in Mule and half-bred flocks starting lambing between late December and mid-February.

The implant should be inserted subcutaneously near the base of the ear. In Suffolk and Suffolk cross types it should be used from

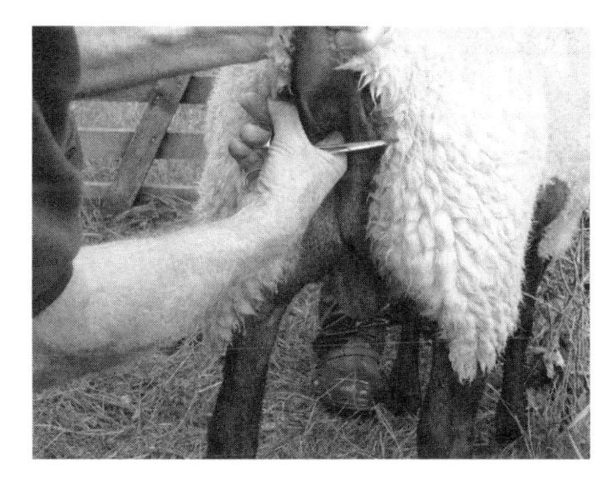

Fig. 6.1. Retrieving an intra-vaginal sponge.

mid-May to late June for ram introduction in late June and July. In Mule and half-bred flocks the implant should be administered from early June to late July for ram introduction from mid-July to late August. It should not be used at other times in the UK, but of course it can be used at different times in the southern hemisphere. Before receiving the implant, ewes should be isolated for more than 1 week from the sight, sound and scent of rams and buck goats, as their presence will interfere with the ovulatory process. The rams should be reintroduced no less than 30 days and no more than 40 days after implantation. There is normally a delay of 14 days before cycling starts, so an introduction of vasectomized rams for these 14 days is beneficial to tighten up the lambing pattern. The peak mating will occur between 25 and 35 days after reintroduction of the rams. Melatonin should only be used in adult ewes or shearlings. It will be ineffectual in immature sheep or in ewes suckling lambs. It has a zero milk and meat withdrawal period. It can be used in goats, but careful adjustment needs to be carried out with the timing.

Pregnant mare serum gonadotrophin (PMSG)

This serum gonadotrophin is supplied as a freeze-dried crystalline plug containing 5000 IU of hormone with a solvent, which when reconstituted gives a solution containing 200 IU PMSG/ml. PMSG is a protein hormone that acts on the ovary to stimulate the production of follicles. The number of follicles produced can be influenced by the dose of PMSG administered. This must be taken into account when calculating the dose for a particular flock when used in conjunction with progestogen-releasing sponges out of the normal breeding season. In general, the further out of season that breeding is attempted and the lower the normal prolificacy of the flock, the more PMSG that will be required. An average dose of 500 IU per ewe is recommended as a useful starting point but doses ranging from 200 to 750 IU have been used on occasion. It is therefore recommended that accurate flock records are kept of breed, dose given, time of injection and lambs produced, so that in future seasons the amount can, if necessary, be adjusted for optimum results. There is a nil milk and meat withdrawal period.

PMSG can be used in goats during the transition period, that is, between the anoestrous and breeding seasons, to bring does into oestrus. However, in common with prostaglandin injections, it does not seem effective in the real anoestrus period. The 'buck effect' may be helpful when used in conjunction with PMSG, or photoperiod manipulation can be tried. Herds can be subjected to 2 months of artificially lengthened days, providing 20 h of light per day.

Trace Element and Vitamin Injectable Products

Cobalt/vitamin B12

Cobalt can be given orally either separately or with an anthelmintic. Vitamin B12, cyanocobalamin, can be given subcutaneously or intramuscularly. It is supplied in a solution containing 1000 μg in 1 ml. The dose is 1 ml/adult sheep, and it can be repeated in 7 days. There is a nil milk and meat withhold period. It is also available at a quarter of this strength in a 0.025% w/v solution. The dose for a sheep is 1–3 ml. This injection is also suitable for goats.

Copper

Copper toxicity is a very real danger in sheep (see Chapter 17) so copper supplementation should be carried out with care and only in sheep known to be copper deficient, or in areas known to be either low in copper or – more commonly – high in molybdenum, sulfur or iron. In the UK the only supplementation available is hard gelatine capsules containing copper oxide. These are marketed as 4 g capsules for ewes and 2 g capsules for lambs. These give a sustained release of copper for 3 months and so administration should be delayed until 2 months after tupping in very low copper areas. Lambs should not be given the smaller capsules until they are over 5 weeks of age, and must weigh more than 10 kg. The mode of action is that some of the copper oxide

Table 6.5. Veterinary drugs to be carried for ambulatory practice carrying out work with sheep and goats.

Drug	Dosage	Comments
Acepromazine	0.02–0.05 mg/kg i/v, i/m	For milk letdown and urethral relaxation
Barbiturate solution	Triple strength	Only for euthansia
Butorphanol	0.1 mg/kg i/v, i/m	Analgesia
Calcium borogluconate	20% solution sub/cut or slow i/v	50–80 ml daily
Calcium borogluconate + 5% magnesium hypophosphite	20% solution sub/cut or slow i/v	50–80 ml daily
Cloprostenol	0.5 ml i/m	Repeat in 24 h
Dexamethazone	0.1 mg/kg i/m, i/v	Not in pregnant animals
Enrofloxacin	5 mg/kg sub/cut	Double dosage for 48 h
Florfenicol	10 mg/kg sub/cut	Double dosage for 48 h
Flunixin meglumine	1 mg/kg sub/cut, i/v	Oral not effective
Ketamine	Various i/m	Anaesthesia
Ketoprofen	2 mg/kg sub/cut, i/v	NSAID for pain relief
Lidocaine 2%	4 mg/kg max. dose	1 ml epidural
Magnesium sulfate 25%	50–80 ml daily	Only sub/cut
Oxytetracycline	Vary i/m i/v	Higher dosage for longer action
Oxytocin	10 IU i/m	Dilute for i/v
Penicillin	22,000–44,000 IU/kg	Often with streptomycin
Thiamine	15 mg/kg sub/cut, i/v	Every day for 5 days
Xylazine	0.3 mg/kg i/v; 0.6 mg/kg i/m	Sedation

Note: i/m, intramuscularly; i/v, intravenously; sub/cut, subcutaneously.

lodges in the folds of the abomasum. Owners should take care when administering the capsules using a specially designed gun. To avoid injury, the dosing gun should be used without force, and each animal should be checked to see that the capsule has been swallowed. The capsules have no meat or milk withdrawal period and are suitable for goats.

Magnesium

In the UK magnesium bullets are available that are licensed for sheep. These contain 15g of magnesium and are intended to lie in the reticulum, slowly releasing magnesium over a 3-week period. They are suitable for goats. Great care should be taken when administering these bullets to avoid damage to the oesophagus.

Selenium

There is a long-acting preparation licensed for use in sheep in the UK, which lasts for 12 months. It is supplied in an aqueous suspension containing 50 mg/ml of selenium (175 mg/ml barium selenate). It should be given by subcutaneous injection only in the neck area to aid removal at slaughter. The dose is 1 ml/50 kg, so normally an adult sheep will require 1–2 ml. Lambs at weaning will require 0.5 ml. There is a nil milk and meat withholding period. The preparation is suitable for goats.

Vitamins B and C

There is a licensed preparation of four B vitamins and vitamin C available for sheep in the UK. It can be used in any deficiency related to these five vitamins including cerebrocortical necrosis (see Chapter 14). Each millilitre contains 35 mg thiamine hydrochloride (vitamin B1), 0.5 mg riboflavin sodium phosphate (vitamin B2), 7 mg pyridoxine hydrochloride (vitamin B6), 23 mg nicotinamide and 70 mg ascorbic acid (vitamin C). The dose is 5–10 ml, which can be given subcutaneously, deep intramuscularly or slow intravenously. There is a nil meat and milk withhold period. It is suitable for goats.

Suggested medicines to be carried by the practitioner are shown in Table 6.5.

7

Vaccines

General

The availability and the need for vaccination against an individual disease will vary between countries and species. It would be hard to cover such eventualities in this book. However, as a rule of thumb, vaccines prepared for virus diseases tend to be more effective than vaccines prepared for bacterial diseases. Equally, live vaccines, which have been stored and used correctly, tend to be more effective than dead vaccines. It should be remembered that if a live vaccine has been used it would be difficult for a serum sample to differentiate between a vaccine titre and that of active disease, unless the vaccine is a 'marker' vaccine.

Storage of vaccines is extremely important. It is not only live vaccines that have to be stored at controlled temperatures. Practitioners should read the data sheets carefully for storage instructions before reconstitution of the vaccine and after reconstitution. Vaccines that require reconstitution with a diluent normally have a very short life after this has been done, and this period should be strictly observed. Refrigeration storage should be monitored, with maximum and minimum temperatures recorded on a regular basis. It should be stressed that it is vital that expensive vaccines are stored and used in the correct manner, as otherwise they will not only be ineffective but also may cause reactions in the animal. It is also important that the correct technique is used for administration. Most vaccines must be given subcutaneously, so a short needle of 1.5 cm (⅝ inch) can be used. The gauge of the needle is important. In essence the smallest gauge is best especially for small young animals (e.g. 23 G). However a larger gauge (e.g. 21 G or 19 G) will be more appropriate for adults. Practitioners should be aware that small-gauge needles are more likely to break at the hub; immediate retrieval of the broken needle is vital. Contamination of the vaccine container must be avoided, and only a sterile needle should be used to draw out the dose of vaccine. A different needle should then be used to inject the animal. It is quite reasonable for an assistant to be drawing up doses of vaccine using the same needle in the bottle of vaccine. The same second needle can be used to vaccinate a number of animals, but this needle should be changed at regular intervals. The use of multidose syringes is widespread and should be encouraged, as on the whole there is less contamination. However it is important that they are calibrated for the correct dose of vaccine. Once again the needle should be changed at regular intervals.

It is also important to consider the animals to be vaccinated. They should not be unduly stressed, and this is particularly important for pregnant animals. Often there is a need for careful timing of vaccination in pregnant animals so that the risk to the pregnancy is kept to a minimum but the level of immunity in the colostrum is at a maximum. The practitioner should give careful advice to the owner on the timing of vaccination in young animals. If the dam has not been vaccinated, then quite young animals can receive their first dose of vaccine. On the other hand, if the dam has received a booster during her pregnancy, the first vaccination should be delayed. There is no harm in vaccinating animals too early, it is just that the first dose may be ineffective and so an extra dose will need to be given. Having vaccinated the female animals, it is important to remember to vaccinate the male animals at the correct time so their immunity is maintained.

In general, wet animals should not be vaccinated as there is a much greater risk of needle contamination. This is particularly important in fibre-producing species. It is worthwhile stressing that dates of vaccination and groups of animals should always be recorded carefully.

There are various types of vaccine. Live modified vaccines usually stimulate high levels of solid immunity from a single inoculation. Inactivated vaccines usually contain weaker antigens and require an initial course of two doses. Vaccines often use multiple antigens. There is no evidence to suggest that there is diminution in the individual antigen protection or less protection in the face of field challenge. These vaccines are more economical to produce and also mean that sheep and goats have to be handled less frequently.

Most vaccines are licensed to be given subcutaneously. An ideal place is 10–15 cm below the ear or over the ribs behind the shoulder. Data sheets should always be consulted, as some vaccines need to be given intramuscularly. An ideal place in sheep and goats is in front of the shoulder, well above the jugular grove.

With most vaccines circulating antibodies fall to apparently non-protective levels fairly quickly, but are raised rapidly by a challenge in the field. Most inactivated bacterins and toxoided vaccines require annual boosters in the sheep for which they were specifically prepared. Normally this annual vaccination is timed to coincide with a need to booster colostral levels of antibody and so is given in the last 6 weeks of pregnancy. It is prudent to boost the rams and the replacements at the same time. In goats, there is some confusion as the sheep vaccines are not licensed for this species and there is no data sheet available. To make sure these animals are adequately covered most clinicians give boosters twice a year. The practice of giving twice the dose only once a year is unlikely to be sensible.

To allow the mother time to produce adequate colostral antibodies, booster doses need to be given a minimum of 2 weeks prior to parturition. There is little information available to advise clinicians on the extent of the period of maternal or so-called passive immunity. In both sheep and goats it is likely to be 3–4 months, although there are many question marks with each condition.

Therefore, if clinicians are in any doubt when dealing with sheep or goats, it is prudent to give vaccines earlier and an extra dose later. Most vaccines prepared for sheep are relatively inexpensive so cost is not an issue, only the handling problems and the fact that many pet sheep and goats are kept in small groups and therefore some vaccine has to be discarded. Certain vaccines (e.g. those for orf) do not create maternal antibodies and therefore there is no benefit in using the vaccine late in pregnancy. In fact in the case of orf vaccine this should definitely be avoided as the vaccine strain may cause lesions on the mouths of young lambs, which in turn will spread to the teats of the ewes, with disastrous effects.

Clinicians may be consulted when there appears to be a failure of vaccination. Careful detective work together with great tact will be required. There are a large number of factors that need to be considered:

1. Incorrect storage. Obviously this can occur at any place along the chain from manufacturer to wholesaler, merchant, and farmer, to animal. As a veterinary surgeon one hopes that the route to the farmer is not at fault. The manufacturers are normally extremely helpful when there are problems. Clinicians should make 100% certain that their controls (e.g. fridge temperature monitoring) are in place before blaming the farmer or shepherd.
2. The method of administration should be checked. Not only must the route be correct but also the actual technique; that is, the vaccine must actually go into the animal.

3. We have discussed earlier the influence of maternal immunity. Vaccines given during the period of high maternal antibody circulation will not be effective and will have to be repeated.
4. Vaccination can be ineffective if disinfectants contaminate any of the equipment and needles. Equally, vaccination will not be accomplished if there is bacterial contamination and abscessation.
5. Naturally the vaccine must be the correct choice for controlling the disease in question. If sheep are dying from braxy (*Clostridium septicum*), for example, they will continue to die if given Lambivac™ (Intervet/Schering-Plough Animal Health, Milton Keynes, UK), which has no activity against *Cl. septicum*.
6. The animals must be healthy when they receive the vaccine. Animals in very poor condition or suffering from a deficiency will not be able to respond to the vaccine.
7. Animal owners should obtain advice when giving several injections at the same time. On the whole the less the animals are stressed by continual handling the better. However, giving anthelmintics, antibiotics and several vaccinations at the same time may place too much stress on the animal.
8. Off-licence vaccines, i.e. vaccines prepared for sheep that are given to goats.
9. Vaccination is a numbers game. The majority of a group of animals may respond but certain individuals may not make an antibody response. They may actually be immune, or of course they may not be immune.

When using more than one vaccine there are no hard and fast rules. However, following these guidelines constitutes a good code of practice:

1. If possible separate the two vaccines by at least 2 weeks.
2. If this is not possible it is better to inject them at the same time rather separate them by only 2 or 3 days.
3. If two vaccines are to be given it will take longer, so stress should be minimized by providing adequate food and water to waiting animals.
4. Always use separate vaccinators and needles.
5. Inject at different sites (e.g. left and right side of neck).
6. *Clostridium/Pasteurella* vaccines should not be given at the same time as *E. coli* vaccines.
7. Erysipelas vaccine can be given with either *Clostridium/Pasteurella* vaccine or with *E. coli* vaccines.

Vaccines for Sheep

Akabane

This vaccine is available in Japan. Two doses of the inactivated vaccine should be given 4 weeks apart, ideally before the ewes are put to the tup. A booster dose should be given annually.

Blackleg

This disease is often covered by multicomponent *Clostridium* vaccines. However there is a single component vaccine available which gives very good immunity to *Clostridium chauvoei*. Ideally sheep should receive two doses given subcutaneously, separated by at least 6 weeks with the second dose given 3–4 weeks before lambing. Sheep only require an annual booster after the primary two doses. The annual booster should be given 3–4 weeks before lambing. There is no milk or meat withdrawal period.

Blue tongue

There are many serotypes of the virus and the single serotype vaccines are very rarely cross-protective to other strains. In the UK only vaccines against serotype 8 have been licensed. They provide immunity after 25 days of a single injection, or with some preparations after two doses separated by 3 weeks. The most sophisticated are purified by liquid chromatography. They are safe in pregnancy and can be used along with other treatments. Immunity lasts in excess of 1 year. Booster doses should be timed 2 weeks before the major risk periods of warm weather in summer and autumn. Lambs born to ewes that have been vaccinated for a second time against serotype 8 of the blue tongue virus receive enough antibodies in colostrum to protect them against the disease until at least 14 weeks of age. Vaccination in ewes may be given at the same time as clostridial disease vaccination without any lessening of the immunity levels generated for both diseases. There have been no adverse reactions reported. However, when vaccination has been carried out against two serotypes of blue tongue virus – namely 1 and 8 – at the same time, adverse reactions have been noted.

Botulism

There are two vaccines that are approved for vets to import into the UK under special licence. One, Ultravac Botulinum®, is from Pfizer Animal Health (Sandwich, UK); and the other is Botulism Vaccine™, from Onderstepoort Biological Products (Pretoria, South Africa).

Brucella melitensis

A live vaccine is available for this condition, although it is not licensed in the UK. A single 1-ml injection needs to be given to 4–6-month old lambs. It is not a marker vaccine and therefore vaccinated animals cannot be differentiated from animals which have seroconverted from the live bacterial infection.

Campylobacter

A vaccine for this is available on its own or in combination with vaccine for enzootic abortion of ewes (EAE). It should be given before tupping, with a second dose halfway through pregnancy in animals that have not received the vaccine before. It is not licensed for use in the UK.

Caseous lymphadenitis

Vaccination is available for this disease but it is not licensed in the UK. When the disease is endemic a combination of vaccination and clinical examination reduces the prevalence of infection more quickly than just treating or culling diseased animals alone.

Clostridial diseases

Most of these vaccines are multicomponent. Their good protective response has been demonstrated in sheep (Kerry and Craig, 1979) and it is just as good as single components. *Clostridium* spp. are ubiquitous; that is, they are found throughout the world in soil, sewage, decaying animal/vegetable material and in the gut/organs of other animals. Locally, they excrete extremely potent toxins into the bloodstream, causing toxaemia. The sheep may be found dead or be *in extremis*. It is often difficult to make a diagnosis and therefore multivalent vaccines are often used. There are now vaccines available against ten diseases containing ten different toxoids: *Clostridium perfringens* type A, B, C and D; *Cl. chauvoei*; *Cl. novyi*; *Cl. septicum*; *Cl. tetani*; *Cl. sordellii*; and *Cl. haemolyticum*. The vaccines need an initial course of two injections separated by 4–6 weeks followed by a booster injection annually. They should be given subcutaneously. Lambs can be injected from 2 weeks of age. However the vaccine is normally given to the ewes from 8 to 2 weeks before parturition and will then provide 3 months of passive immunity provided the ewes have had a full primary course of 2 vaccinations. If lambs have received this passive immunity, the start of their primary course can be delayed until they are 8–10 weeks of age. The vaccine can cause some reaction at the site and a clean vaccine technique should be used. There is a nil milk and meat withdrawal.

There are a large number of vaccines with varying components made for *Cl.* spp. in sheep. It is important that practitioners guide shepherds on the suitable vaccine for their disease situation.

If lambs are born to unvaccinated ewes, or if lambs have failed to receive adequate colostrum, they can be treated with a suitable vaccine soon after birth and given a second dose at 4 weeks of age. As there is little immunity conferred by a single dose of vaccine, lambs at risk can be given a dose of clostridial antiserum at the same time as the first dose of vaccine.

Contagious agalactia

The live vaccine for this condition requires only a single 1-ml subcutaneous injection, but it needs to be given under very strict circumstances. It must not be given to any sheep with active infection or which are incubating the disease. It must not be given in the last 2 months of pregnancy or in the first 2 months of lactation. It is not licensed for use in the UK.

Erysipelothrix

This organism causes joint-ill in lambs. Some degree of protection can be conferred to lambs by passive protection via the colostrum. Pregnant ewes should be given two doses 2–6 weeks apart, with the second dose at least 3 weeks before lambing. Pregnant ewes that have received these two doses in a previous pregnancy only need to be given a single dose. If post-dipping lameness is a problem, the lambs can be vaccinated with two doses 2–6 weeks apart with the second dose at least 2 weeks before dipping. However, this condition can be prevented by not allowing the dip solution to become contaminated. Made-up dip solution should not be allowed to stand for several days between batches of sheep.

Escherichia coli

This organism causes problems in young lambs. Some protection can be afforded to lambs by transfer of passive immunity via the colostrum. Ewes should receive two doses of the vaccine 4–6 weeks apart, with the second dose being given at least 4 weeks before lambing. In ewes that have received these two doses in a previous pregnancy, only a single dose of vaccine needs to be given, at least 4 weeks before lambing.

Foot rot

Vaccines for this condition are multicomponent, covering the ten serogroups of *Dichelobacter nodosus*. Some authorities consider there are only nine strains classified as A–H and M, and that there are two sub-strains of B. B is certainly the most common. A characteristic of *D. nodosus* is the pili, which are carried on the surface and determine the serotype. The vaccines are oil adjuvanted and often cause quite severe post-vaccination reactions. Clinicians should be careful when advising vaccination in show animals and should warn pet sheep owners. Sheep do not mount an immune response to foot rot, which is why the condition persists in a flock. However, a single dose of vaccine elicits a high level of circulating antibody, which lasts for approximately 4 months. Doses need to be given strategically as the vaccine is both protective and curative. Sheep are most at risk in the UK in spring and autumn. Sheep worldwide are at risk on housing.

Johne's disease

There is an oil-based, inactivated vaccine for this condition, which after a single dose produces a long-lasting cellular immunity. It should be administered early in life, or in the face of an outbreak to the whole flock. Vaccinated animals subsequently exposed to *Mycobacterium paratuberculosis* will create an immune response preventing the bacteria from establishing in the small intestine. In animals that may already be infected, vaccination will delay the onset of clinical signs, thereby reducing mortality and morbidity rates. Faecal shedding is greatly reduced. This helps to stop the source of infection, as the bacteria will survive for over a year in the environment, withstanding extreme natural conditions. The disease is commonly transmitted by ingestion of feed, soil and water.

Louping ill

The vaccine for this condition is prepared from louping ill virus grown in tissue culture. It is inactivated with formalin and emulsified in a mineral oil. Because of this shepherds should read the data sheet carefully as it needs to be warmed before use. It is for active immunization of sheep. Immunity occurs 4 weeks after a single dose of vaccine and lasts for over 18 months, so ideally animals should be revaccinated every 2 years at least 4 weeks before the high-risk period related to tick feeding. There are no specific studies on its use in pregnancy or lactation, but no adverse problems are cited. It is prudent to avoid the last month of pregnancy.

Orf

Vaccines for orf need to be used with considerable care as they are live, mild field strains, which produce a local mild reaction at the site of scarification. They are never fully protective, due to the incomplete immune response elicited. They are described as only an aid to control of the disease.

Ovine enzootic abortion

Vaccine strains of *Chlamydophila abortus* have been isolated in large enough numbers to have actually caused abortion. Gene-sequencing techniques have shown that only the vaccine strain was present in aborted fetuses. Two vaccines are available in the UK to control EAE, both based on the 1B strain, which differs slightly from the wild-type strains but which gives a strong protective immunity. The extent of the problem is not known. However with the current state of knowledge, farmers are urged to continue to use the vaccine.

The most common vaccination programme in sheep is with these live, modified, heat-sensitive *Chlamydophila* vaccines. They should be used in ewes before tupping and should not be given to pregnant animals. Ideally there should be a 4-week period between vaccination and tupping. They are likely to give life-long immunity from a single dose, although company data only guarantee immunity for 3 years. Practitioners should check the data sheets. Ideally they should not be given within 4 weeks of any other live vaccine. The vaccine should not be given while the ewes are being treated with antibiotics, particularly oxytetracyclines. Ewe lambs may be vaccinated as early as 5 months of age. Animals may not be slaughtered for human consumption within 7 days of vaccination. There is an inactivated *Chlamydophila* vaccine which is in a water-in-oil adjuvant that can be given to pregnant sheep. Proven immunity only lasts for 18 months.

Para-influenza 3

Vaccination for this condition is available in the USA as a nasal spray for young lambs. It gives rapid immunity. It is not licensed in the UK.

Pasteurellosis

There are vaccines available to offer some degree of immunity to *Pasteurella haemolytica* ('A' types) and *Pasteurella trehalosi* ('T' types). The former will affect all ages of sheep but the latter is normally restricted to lambs between 6 and 9 months of age. Most *Pasteurella* vaccines are combined with clostridial disease vaccines and so the timings are confusing. Practitioners and shepherds should decide where the real risks lie and vaccinate accordingly. The vaccine that is solely for pasteurellosis has to be given as two doses separated by 4–6 weeks. If there is an early threat to younger lambs, the first dose should be given at 2 weeks of age and the second at 6 weeks of age. Otherwise the timing should be adjusted so that the second dose is given a few days before the time of greatest threat. Shepherds should be made aware that the *Pasteurella* component is much more expensive than the clostridial component of the combined vaccine, and so should only be given if there is a real need.

Peste des petits ruminants

There is a live, single injection vaccine available for peste des petits ruminants (PPR), and 1 ml should be given subcutaneously to lambs between 4 and 6 months of age and then repeated in another 3–6 months. After that an annual vaccination is recommended. It is not licensed in the UK.

Rabies

There is a vaccine available for rabies, but it is relatively expensive and therefore unless there is a grave risk its use is probably not justified. It is not licensed in the UK.

Rift Valley fever

There is a live attenuated vaccine for Rift Valley fever (RVF). It should be given as a single injection to non-pregnant sheep and gives a lifelong immunity within 1 week. The entire flock should be vaccinated in areas where the disease occurs. Formalin-inactivated vaccines are available for use in pregnant sheep.

Salmonellosis

Many *Salmonella* species will infect sheep, including *S. abortus ovis*. The only worthwhile *Salmonella* vaccine is one prepared for cattle against *S. dublin*. This is not licensed for sheep in the UK but it appears to be effective, although only against infection from this species of *Salmonella*.

Sheep pox

A live vaccine is available for this disease. Great care needs to be taken with the use of this vaccine as lambs require only 0.2ml between 6 and 12 weeks. Older sheep require 0.5ml. Booster doses are required every second year. Injections should be given subcutaneously. The vaccine is not licensed for use in the UK.

Toxoplasmosis

A live vaccine containing the S48 strain of *Toxoplasma gondii* is available to treat this condition. Vaccination should be carried out with a single dose given at least 3 weeks before tupping. Ewe lambs may be vaccinated from 5 months of age. The vaccine lasts 2 years and so needs to be carried out every other year. This vaccine may be given at the same time as certain enzootic abortion vaccines.

Vaccines for Goats

Akabane

There is a vaccine available in Japan. Two doses of the inactivated vaccine should be given 4 weeks apart, ideally before the does are put to the billy. A booster dose should be given annually.

Blackleg

A single component vaccine licensed for cattle and sheep against *Clostridium chauvoei* (blackleg) can be given safely to goats to provide good immunity. Goats require two doses separated by 6 weeks, boosted by a single dose annually. To obtain passive immunity in kids, does should receive the second dose 3–4 weeks before kidding. There is no meat or milk withdrawal period.

Blue tongue

Goats are definitely affected by this disease, which can be fatal, but there are many strains. Clinicians should carry out a risk analysis and use the appropriate strains. Polyvalent vaccines do not seem to be effective and therefore single-strain vaccines should be used. The vaccination regime recommended for cattle should be used, not that recommended for sheep.

Botulism

Two vaccines for botulism are approved for vets to import into the UK under special licence. One, Ultravac Botulinum is from Pfizer Animal Health, and the other is Botulism Vaccine from Onderstepoort Biological Products.

Brucella melitensis

There is no live vaccine licensed in the UK, although live vaccines are available elsewhere. A single injection of 1 ml needs to be given to 4–6-month old kids. It is not a marker vaccine and therefore vaccinated animals cannot be differentiated from animals that have sero-converted from the live bacterial infection.

Caseous lymphadenitis

Vaccination is available for this disease but it is not licensed in the UK. When the disease is endemic a combination of vaccination and clinical examination reduces the prevalence of infection more quickly than just treating or culling diseased animals alone.

Clostridial disease vaccination

This vaccination is vital for all goats. Vaccines containing ten different toxoids are now available against ten diseases: *Clostridium perfringens* types A, B, C and D; *Cl. chauvoei*; *Cl. novyi*; *Cl. septicum*; *Cl. tetani*; *Cl. sordellii*; and *Cl. haemolyticum*. Goats are not susceptible to all these conditions. However they are definitely susceptible to *Cl. perfringens* types C and D, *Cl. chauvoei*, *Cl. tetani* and *Cl. sordellii*. Clinicians must advise their clients carefully after balancing out the risks of each condition. Goats require two subcutaneous injections of the dead vaccine separated by 4–6 weeks. As the vaccine is not made specifically for goats it is advisable to vaccinate goats twice yearly. Ideally the vaccination of does should be given in the last third of pregnancy to boost the passive immunity for the kids. If this has not been carried out it is advisable to vaccinate the kids between 2 and 4 weeks of age.

Contagious agalactia

The live vaccine for this condition requires only a single 1-ml subcutaneous injection. It needs to be given under very strict circumstances to goats and must not be given to any goat which has active infection or which is incubating the disease. It must not be given in the last 2 months of pregnancy or in the first 2 months of lactation.

Escherichia coli

This organism can cause problems in young kids. Some protection can be afforded to kids by transfer of passive immunity via the colostrum. Does should receive 2 doses of the vaccine 4–6 weeks apart, with the second dose being given at least 4 weeks before kidding. In does which have received these 2 doses in a previous pregnancy only a single dose of vaccine needs to be given, at least 4 weeks before kidding.

Johne's disease

There is an oil-based, inactivated vaccine for this condition, which after a single dose produces a long-lasting cellular immunity. It should be administered early in life, or in the face of an outbreak to the whole goat herd. Vaccinated animals subsequently exposed to *Mycobacterium paratuberculosis* will create an immune response, preventing the bacteria from establishing in the small intestine. In animals that may already be infected, vaccination will delay the onset of clinical signs, thereby reducing mortality and morbidity rates. Faecal shedding is greatly reduced. This helps to stop the source of infection, as the bacteria will survive for over 1 year in the environment, withstanding extreme natural conditions. The disease is commonly transmitted by ingestion of feed, soil and water.

Orf

Vaccines to treat orf should not be used in goats as there is no evidence of protection, due to the incomplete immune response elicited.

Ovine enzootic abortion

Ovine enzootic abortion (OAE) will affect goats, and sheep vaccines against strains of *Chlamydophila abortus* can be used in goats. There are two vaccines licensed in the UK to control OEA in sheep and both are based on the 1B strain, which differs slightly from the wild-type strains but which gives a strong protective immunity.

The vaccine should never be given to pregnant goats. It is likely that goats will obtain a life-long immunity from a single dose. However company data only guarantee immunity for 3 years in sheep. Ideally they should not be given within 4 weeks of any other live vaccine. Animals may not be slaughtered for human consumption within 7 days of vaccination. There is an inactivated *Chlamydophila* vaccine licensed for sheep, which is in a water-in-oil adjuvant that can be given to pregnant sheep. However it would be unwise to give it to pregnant goats. Proven immunity for this vaccine only lasts for 18 months in sheep. It should be assumed that it will be similar in goats.

Q fever

A killed vaccine for this condition has recently been prepared in the Netherlands. It reduces the number of abortions and reduces the excretion of *Coxiella burnetii* organisms in the fluids and therefore the risks to humans (see Chapter 19).

Pasteurellosis

The *Pasteurella* vaccines prepared for sheep do not confer any immunity to goats and therefore should not be used, but there is a specific vaccine made for goats. It should be used according to the manufacturer's instructions and given to animals at risk. It is not available in the UK.

Peste des petits ruminants

There is a live, single injection vaccine available for PPR; 1 ml should be given subcutaneously to kids between 4 and 6 months of age and then repeated in another 3–6 months. After that an annual vaccination is recommended.

Rabies

There is a vaccine available for rabies, but it is relatively expensive and therefore unless there is a grave risk its use is probably not justified.

Rift Valley fever

The live attenuated vaccine available to treat RVF sheep is very effective in goats but must not be given to pregnant does. The inactivated vaccine available for pregnant sheep is not very effective in does. Vaccination with the live vaccine is highly recommended before service in does.

Salmonellosis

Several species of *Salmonella* can infect goats, but there is no good evidence that vaccines prepared for other species will confer immunity. Clinicians should advise against their use in goats.

Sheep pox

There is a live vaccine available for sheep that can safely be given to goats to treat this disease. Great care needs to be taken with the use of this vaccine, as kids require only 0.2 ml between the ages of 6 and 12 weeks. Older goats require 0.5 ml, and booster doses are required every second year. The injections should be given subcutaneously.

Toxoplasmosis

A live vaccine containing the S48 strain of *Toxoplasma gondii* is available to treat this disease, and is suitable for goats. Vaccination should be carried out with a single dose given at least 3 weeks before putting the doe to the buck. Goatlings may be vaccinated from 5 months of age. The vaccine lasts 2 years and so needs to be carried out every other year. This vaccine may be given at the same time as certain enzootic abortion vaccines.

8

Sedation, Anaesthesia, Surgical Conditions and Euthanasia

General Pre-operative Considerations

Tetanus cover

Sheep and goats are very prone to getting tetanus, and it is vital that every effort is made to cover all animals in the case of an urgent surgical procedure. An elective procedure should be delayed until full vaccination has been carried out, although the elective procedure of disbudding of kids should not be delayed. Full vaccination involves a double dose of vaccine separated by 4 weeks. For sheep an annual booster vaccination is sufficient, but in goats the boosters should be given at 6-monthly intervals.

If the procedure is urgent and the animal has had an initial course of two doses of vaccine some time ago, a single booster dose will be sufficient. However if this has not been carried out it is suggested that the patient should receive its primary dose of tetanus vaccine and 3000 IU of tetanus anti-toxin (TAT). This could be reduced to 1500 IU in very young animals. Cover with antibiotics is also important. If tetanus is a consideration, the antibiotic of choice is penicillin.

Analgesia

This is very important. The drug of choice with both sedation and anaesthesia is butorphanol. This can be given post-operatively as well as pre-operatively at 0.1 mg/kg every 6 h either intramuscularly, subcutaneously or intravenously. NSAIDs can be given at the same time, but it should be remembered that they nephrotoxic, so should be avoided if there is likely to be any kidney damage. The practitioner can use his judgement on which NSAID to use (see Chapter 6).

NSAIDs are very good pre-operative analgesics, but it must be remembered that steroids are more potent anti-inflammatory drugs than non-steroidals. As inflammation causes pain there may be good reason to use steroids for some analgesia, for example when flushing joints in lambs. Steroids and penicillin are the medicines of choice.

Antibiosis

Antibiosis drugs should be given as soon as possible in urgent cases. In elective procedures they should be given before surgery is planned, to allow for good tissue levels. Unless there are special considerations a combination of penicillin and streptomycin is the antibiotic of choice.

Gut fill

Ideally the gastroenteric organs should be as empty as possible, although practitioners should beware of withholding fluids from the young and from debilitated animals. Care should also be taken in hot climates. In some ways starving the patients is more important when heavy sedation or field anaesthesia is used, as there is no cuffed endotracheal tube in place to prevent rumen contents being inhaled. A protocol suggested by Mueller (2009) is to withhold concentrates for 24h preoperatively, forage for 12h and water for 8h. Young animals under 4 weeks of age should be treated as normal, except they should not be allowed to suckle for 2h before sedation or anaesthesia.

Fly control

This is important in all animals, particularly those producing fibre. A cream containing acriflavin and benzene hexachloride (BHC) should be applied to all wounds. The whole animal should be protected by synthetic pyrethrum compounds.

Sedation for Sheep

The fact that sheep are very tolerant of restraint and painful procedures should not be abused, and the safety of the animal is also important. Sheep are very sensitive to xylazine although this is the sedative of choice, so the practitioner has a dilemma. If sedation can be avoided with good restraint and accurate local nerve blocks that will be useful. Analgesia is important and should be used as much as possible. Butorphanol is a good analgesic and can be given at 0.1 mg/kg. Longer term analgesia can be maintained with NSAID (see Chapter 6). Caesarean sections are certainly best performed without sedation. Vasectomies, except in extremely wild rams, do not require sedation if the local infiltration is good. Castration and tail docking also do not require sedation if local anaesthesia is good. Although very young lambs legally do not require local anaesthesia in the UK, Australian workers (Lomax *et al.*, 2010) have shown the value of regional anaesthesia.

Sedation for Goats

If the practitioner has a choice, a GA is preferable to sedation and local infiltration in goats as they do not tolerate sedation and physical restraint as well as sheep (Mueller, 2009). However, for a caesarean section the method of choice is right lateral recumbency without sedation, but with very careful local anaesthesia.

Xylazine is the sedative of choice at 0.1 mg/kg given i/v. Up to 0.2 mg/kg of xylazine can be given i/m, but it should be avoided in the last month of gestation as it can cause abortions. It should also be avoided in cases of blocked urethra as it increases urine flow. In theory goats are less sensitive to detomidine and so these side-effects are avoided. On the other hand the sedative effects are less, even up to 0.04 mg/kg i/v. Lower doses of xylazine will give the same sedative effects as these higher doses of detomidine and may give fewer problems with abortions and increased urine output. The doses of both xylazine and detomidine can be halved if butorphanol is given at 0.1 mg/kg to achieve the same depth of sedation.

Goats are very sensitive to lidocaine hydrochloride, normally in a 2% solution. The maximum dose of 6 mg/kg should not be exceeded (i.e. 30 ml for a 100 kg goat). It should be noted that this is much less than in sheep. Great care should be taken with placement of the local block to give local anaesthesia without overdosing.

General Anaesthesia for Sheep

General anaesthesia in adult sheep is not a safe procedure. There are dangers of regurgitation of rumen contents and resulting inhalation. There is also a risk of bloat, either during anaesthesia or during recovery. The safest method is to premedicate with 0.1 mg/kg of xylazine intramuscularly. After 10 min ketamine can be given at 0.2 mg/kg intravenously. This will give approximately 20 min of anaesthesia.

The sheep should be kept in sternal recumbency. If longer anaesthesia is required intubation can be attempted, but this is difficult. A laryngoscope with an extra-long blade is required. A 10-mm endotracheal tube should be passed into the trachea and inflated. It is useful to pass a slightly bigger endotracheal tube (12mm) into the oesophagus, so that rumen reflux is cleared out of the pharynx. Isoflurane can then be given to effect. Recovery must be constantly monitored. The sheep must be kept in sternal recumbency. The endotracheal tubes should only be removed when a definite swallowing reflex is present.

One worldwide authority (Scott, 2007) has had considerable experience with the use of pentobarbital in emergency field situations. He states that it gives acceptable levels of surgical analgesia but recovery is extended for up to 2h, during which time bloat may occur, especially if the sheep becomes cast following attempts to stand. He states that it has obvious advantages in being very inexpensive and requiring no incremental doses during an average surgery time of 20–40min. His dose rate of pentobarbital is 20mg/kg injected intravenously. Approximately two-thirds of the calculated dose is given intravenously over 20–30s. The depth of anaesthesia is then determined after approximately 1min and the remaining one-third given if necessary. He states that there is little effect of incremental doses given after this induction period, and stresses the importance of a fully supervised recovery.

Alfaxalone is a useful anaesthetic for lambs. The preparation licensed for dogs and cats in the UK contains 10mg/ml. It should be given to lambs at 3mg/kg slowly intravenously and may be topped up by a further 2mg/kg if longer or deeper anaesthesia is required. Although in theory premedication with alpha-2-adrenoceptor agonists would lower the dose of alfaxalone, lambs are very sensitive to alpha-2-adrenoceptor agonists and so clinicians are not advised to use them unless they have prior experience.

General Anaesthesia for Goats

The simplest method is to premedicate with a combination of 0.1mg/kg of xylazine and 0.1mg/kg of butorphanol intravenously. This is followed in 5min by intravenous ketamine at 0.2mg/kg. This can be topped up by more ketamine up to three times. However for longer anaesthesia (e.g. 1h) a drip of xylazine and ketamine should be used. To prepare the drip, 50mg of xylazine and 200mg of ketamine should be added to 100ml of normal saline. Anaesthesia will be achieved in a 60kg goat by an infusion rate of 1ml/min.

All these methods should be restricted to adult goats. In young goats, particularly very young kids requiring disbudding, injectable anaesthesia should be avoided, in the author's experience. However some authorities recommend alfaxalone at 3mg/kg. The method of choice for kids is gaseous anaesthesia with a mask. Either halothane or isoflurane can be given to effect. It should be remembered that such mixtures can cause an explosion with oxygen, and the flow must be turned off if there is a naked flame. Halothane is preferred by the author as a longer effect is obtained from the inhalation of halothane compared to isoflurane, but supplies of halothane may cease.

Gaseous anaesthesia can be used in adult goats after premedication with a combination of 0.1mg/kg of xylazine and 0.1mg/kg of butorphanol intravenously. The goat should be kept in sternal recumbency with the head held straight and a mask held in place. Passing an endotracheal tube is difficult, and an assistant should hold the mouth open with a gag. With the use of a laryngoscope with an extra-long blade an 11-mm cuffed endotracheal tube can be placed in most adult goats. However regurgitation of rumen contents is always a danger on intubation and an even greater danger on recovery. The goat must be kept in sternal recumbency with its head up. The tube may be removed when reflexes are present but the head must be kept up until the goat is able to hold its own head up. In unweaned kids it is safe for them to be left in lateral recumbency.

Working in South Africa and the Netherlands, Dzikiti *et al.* (2011) have found that co-administration of isoflurane with an opioid analgesic drug such as fentanyl potentially reduces the dose of isoflurane required for general anaesthesia, and consequently may reduce the occurrence of adverse dose-dependent cardiopulmonary effects associated with isoflurane anaesthesia. The dose of anaesthesia can be tested by evaluating the purposeful movement in response to a noxious stimulus by clamping a claw with a pair of vulsellum forceps.

With all ages of goat, practitioners should be aware of the danger of hypothermia in anaesthetized goats. This is a particular danger in outside sheds in cold weather, and an assistant should constantly monitor rectal temperature. The safest method to warm a goat is by the use of hot water bottles under dry blankets.

Regional Anaesthesia in Sheep

Epidural anaesthesia

The normal site used by practitioners is the sacrococcygeal space. A 2.5-cm (1-inch) 20G needle should be used at a very shallow angle. This anaesthetic is very useful for replacing uterine or cervical prolapses. Lumbosacral epidural anaesthesia should only be attempted after suitable training. It gives sufficient anaesthesia for a variety of surgical procedures, such as caesarean sections (it is particularly useful if there are uterine adhesions from a previous caesarean section), vasectomies, fracture repair of the hind limbs and joint flushing. The downside of lumbosacral epidural anaesthesia is that hind limb paralysis may last for 4h.

Lower limb

Apply a tourniquet immediately above the carpal or tarsal joint. Two small rolls of bandage should be inserted either side of the Achilles tendon when applying the tourniquet to the hind leg. The mid area of the metacarpus or metatarsus should be clipped and surgically cleaned. A suitable superficial vein should be selected. Using a 2.5-cm (1-inch) 21G needle, 5–10ml (depending on the size of the animal) of 2% lignocaine should be injected extremely slowly into the vein. Within 5min full regional anaesthesia will be achieved. This will last for over 1h. Anaesthesia will cease as soon as the tourniquet is removed.

Regional Anaesthesia in Goats

Epidural anaesthesia

The normal site used by practitioners is the sacrococcygeal space. A 2.5-cm (1-inch) 20G needle should be used at a very shallow angle using 1ml of 2% lignocaine. This anaesthetic is very useful for replacing uterine or cervical prolapses.

Lower limb

This is can be carried out in a similar manner to that described for sheep.

Common Surgical Conditions in Sheep

Castration of adult rams

This can be carried out surgically or with the bloodless burdizzos. The latter are preferable if it is the fly season. It must never be carried out with a ligature or rubber ring. Sedation is rarely required but local anaesthesia is mandatory. In both methods 5ml of local anaesthetic should be injected into the neck of the scrotum on both sides, after suitable cleansing of the area. If a surgical approach is required a further 5ml should be injected into the caudal end of each scrotum. An open method of castration should be carried out unless there is evidence of an inguinal hernia.

With the ram standing and an assistant holding the tail, an incision is made at the caudal end of the scrotum containing the testicle, which is kept under pressure. The incision should be made through the skin and the tunics so that the testicle pops out. This is then grasped and pulled, ideally being twisted at the same time. There is no requirement for the use of an emasculator. The testicle and the spermatic cord should be removed and the area sprayed with an antibiotic spray. This should be repeated on the other side. Appropriate tetanus and fly protection should be given.

With the animal standing and restrained, the jaws of the burdizzo are applied to one side of the cranial neck of the scrotum making sure that the spermatic cord is included in the jaws. After 1 min the jaws are released slightly and moved 0.5 cm in a caudal direction and reapplied for 1 min longer. The procedure is repeated on the other side, making sure that none of the compression lines meet straight across the neck.

Burdizzos need to be oiled regularly and kept in a suitable **dry** place. Their action can be tested by applying them to two pieces of thick paper containing a piece of household string. The string should be severed after application of the burdizzo, but the paper should remain intact.

Castration and tail docking of young lambs

Castration and tail docking can be accomplished simply by applying a rubber elastrator ring to the tail and the neck of the scrotum within 48 h of birth. It is important that lambs receive colostrum, so these procedures should be delayed until this has been accomplished. Sufficient tail should be left on the lamb to cover the vulva in females and a similar length should be left in males. It is extremely important that **both** testicles are **distal** to the rubber band. If either one or both testicles are not felt then the lamb must be carefully marked. It is important that such an animal is sent for slaughter before reaching maturity. These animals are called 'rigs' and can be castrated in exceptional circumstances. In Australia and New Zealand a technique termed 'short scrotum' has been used. A ring is placed at the neck of the scrotum with both testicles proximal to it. The lambs will fatten more quickly than castrated animals but are also sterile. From a welfare point of view this procedure can be recommended if there is likely to be a delay in reaching slaughter weight, as the lamb experiences less pain than with conventional castration.

A recent small survey in Scotland has indicated that 100% of farms examined which have ceased both the practices have had some substantial improvements. These farms have been breeding from their own ram lambs and have been getting better performance from them compared to bought-in animals. They report that none of the stock had dirty back ends and that fly strike was not a problem. By careful management using dedicated grazing areas, crops, and supplementation all of the lambs are fattened before 1 December.

Coenurosis

Surgery for this condition is described in older textbooks in an extremely cavalier manner, and this type of surgery should not be carried out. The condition called gid is rare and requires careful diagnosis. Ideally a radiograph of the skull should be taken to visualize the fluid-filled cyst. The skull over the cyst will sometimes be thinner as the pressure has eroded the bone. However, in these cases there are likely to be severe neurological signs. Once a diagnosis has been made, the affected area of the skull should be surgically prepared. A 14 G needle should be pushed through the weakened skull into the cyst, and as much of the fluid as possible should be withdrawn. The sheep should be given antibiotics, NSAID and the tetanus status should be checked. Hopefully the animal will make a good recovery.

Dehorning of adult sheep

This procedure should not be undertaken lightly. There is no call for it to be performed for safety reasons in the uninjured sheep, as the lack of horns rarely makes the sheep any less dangerous to other sheep or to shepherds; however it has to be carried out under certain circumstances. If the horn is deformed and is growing into the head, sometimes the nonvascular tip – which has no nerve supply – can be removed with embryotomy wire. However normally the whole horn is pressing into the head and so has to be removed. If the sheep has damaged its horn it will need to be removed on welfare grounds, as well as to prevent further haemorrhage.

The operation can be performed under GA or under heavy sedation with a local regional block. After surgically preparing around the horn, the whole circumference of the horn needs to be infiltrated with local anaesthetic, with particular attention paid to the area (looking from above the horn) between 4 and 8 o'clock. With an assistant holding the horn a cut is made with an embryotomy wire saw in the skin 0.25 cm (one-tenth of an inch) below the horn. The direction of the cut needs to be approximately 15° below the horizontal line. There will be considerable haemorrhage. This can be controlled with a very hot dehorning iron if a small horn is being removed, but is unlikely to be successful if a large horn has been amputated. In this case individual vessels should be grasped with artery forceps and ligated. If the vessels are coming directly out of the bone tissue they can be blocked with small pieces of matchstick. The whole wound is then dressed with a cream containing acriflavin and BHC. A thick cotton wool pad is bandaged in place, taking care that it is not too tight nor restricting the trachea. The animal should be hospitalized if possible, or at least kept under careful observation for a minimum of 6 h. On no account should it be returned to other sheep as the lack of horns or horn will change its position in the pecking order and fighting will occur. The bandage will need to be changed at 48-h intervals. Antibiotic and NSAID cover should be continued for 10 days after the surgery, as secondary infection could lead to secondary haemorrhage with fatal results. Fly control is paramount as complete healing will take some weeks.

Digital amputation

This procedure is not commonly carried out. However it should be considered by clinicians if there is chronic septic arthritis in one intraphalangeal joint. The operation is welfare-friendly, particularly in lowland sheep which do not need to be too athletic. It is best to carry out the surgery under light sedation and a regional block. A tourniquet is required for both the regional block and for the operation. The animal is given preoperative antibiotics and NSAID.

The foot is trimmed to remove any overgrown horn, then the whole leg below the middle of the metacarpus or metatarsus is clipped and surgically prepared. A length of embryotomy wire is positioned between the cleats. With an assistant holding the affected cleat with a pair of vulsellum forceps, the cleat is sawn off with the wire at a 45° upwards angle. This cut will be made in the middle of the second phalange. The stump is then dressed with a suitable antibiotic cream and covered with a suitable dressing. The whole foot and leg to mid carpus/tarsus is bandaged with thin strips of cotton wool and standard bandages, which are then covered by gaffer tape, taking care that this does not actually touch the skin. The animal is kept under antibiotic and NSAID cover for a minimum of 10 days, and the dressing should be changed twice in this period. If a good healthy bed of granulation tissue has been formed a light protective bandage can be applied.

Entropian

Surgical correction is described in Chapter 14.

Enucleation of the eye

A surgical method is described in Chapter 14.

Repairing an inguinal hernia

Inguinal hernias are rare in rams. They are a genetic recessive disorder, so should only be repaired after castration. The left side is more commonly affected. If there is strangulation, then the animal will show colic-type pain. Because of the stoical nature of sheep these affected rams are often found dead. If the ram is alive and otherwise healthy, then normal slaughter for human consumption is the practical way forward. If the animal is a pet the hernia can be repaired after a closed castration. After sedation with xylazine the hindquarters of the ram are raised and the area is surgically cleansed in the normal manner. A skin bleb of 5 ml of 2% lidocaine is placed over each testicle and an instillation of 2 ml of lidocaine is put into each spermatic cord. A careful scrotal incision is made over the testicle, taking care not to incise the tunics. The testicle is drawn through the skin incision, milking any abdominal contents back into the abdomen. When the surgeon is perfectly certain that this has been accomplished, two large pairs of haemostats are placed over the cord. The proximal pair is removed and a transfixing ligature is tied in the groove left by the haemostats. If this surgery is being performed on a large mature ram then a pair of emasculators should replace the distal pair of haemostats. When the testicle has been removed the skin should be sutured with horizontal mattress sutures. Similar surgery should be carried out on the other side. The ram should be given antibiotics, NSAID and TAT by injection.

Repairing an umbilical hernia

Umbilical hernias are extremely rare in sheep. They have a high heritability and so repair should not be carried out in rams, which should be castrated and fattened. It is reasonable to repair an umbilical hernia in a pet ewe that is being kept for breeding, on the understanding that her progeny will not be kept for breeding.

Repair of umbilical hernias should be delayed until the lamb is at least 2 months of age, as often with age there is little reason to repair them as the abdominal opening is relatively small. If no more than three fingers can be inserted into the abdominal opening then the hernia can be closed with an elastrator ring. The lamb should be given antibiotic and NSAID cover and its tetanus status checked. It is then placed in dorsal recumbency. Raising the hernia sack to ensure there are no bowel contents, a rubber ring is placed as near to the abdominal wall as possible. Antibiotic cover and fly control should be maintained for a minimum of 10 days.

Replacing a prolapsed rectum

The causes of this very rare condition are obscure. It has been suggested that homosexual behaviour might be a cause, and it does appear to be more prevalent in rams. Severe coughing caused by lung worm or pneumonia has also been postulated as a cause. The sheep should be given antibiotic and NSAID cover. The tetanus status should be checked and fly control implemented. With the sheep in the standing position an epidural regional anaesthetic should be given, and the perineal area should be cleaned before a purse-string suture is put in place. It is important that this is placed before replacement of the rectum, otherwise the rectum will prolapse again while the suture is being placed. After replacement of the rectum, using plenty of obstetrical lubricant, the purse-string should be drawn tight to allow only one finger in the orifice. The animal should be kept on a laxative diet and checked regularly. The suture should be removed in 10 days. In the majority of cases it will remain *in situ*. However if it prolapses again, euthanasia is indicated.

Rig operation in rams

Retained testicles are very rare in sheep. If they are found when castrating young ram lambs, the lambs should be marked and recorded but no further action should be taken except to make sure that they are fattened quickly so that there is no ram taint to the meat.

A ram that has only one descended testicle will definitely be fertile; in fact, in the author's experience they have more libido and therefore cover more ewes. In some breeds, such as the Scottish Blackface, it is not even considered a fault. Occasionally practitioners will be asked to castrate a rig if it is required to be exported to certain countries such as the Republic of Ireland. Such an operation should not be undertaken lightly, as some retained testicles may be up near to the kidney. In these instances the best method is to carry out the removal laparoscopically in the standing ram. However if the testicle lies just inside the inner inguinal ring, normal surgical procedure can be carried out under heavy sedation. After sedation the scrotum and surrounding area should be clipped and surgically cleaned. A line block of local anaesthetic should be placed over the scrotum with more anaesthetic injected deeper into the inguinal area. After further surgical preparation an incision can be made over the scrotum cranially as far as the external inguinal ring. The tunics covering the retained testicle will be found by blunt dissection over the inguinal ring. These should be grasped by a large pair of artery forceps and the testicle drawn to the exterior. A transfixing ligature of absorbable suture material should be placed around the tunics dorsal to a second pair of artery forceps. The testicle should then be removed and the subcuticular tissues closed with a continuous row of sutures in absorbable material. The skin should then be closed with single horizontal mattress sutures of monofilament nylon. The ram should be given antibiotics and NSAID. The tetanus status should be checked.

Tail docking of an adult sheep

This is only required when a tail has been injured. Repair is fairly straightforward provided suitable aftercare is carried out. The sheep should be given preoperative antibiotic and NSAID cover and the tetanus status should be checked. The tail should be anaesthetized in the standing sheep with an epidural anaesthetic. The tail should be clipped out and surgically prepared. The surgeon should aim to remove at least one coccygeal vertebra above the injured section. Some skin needs to be left to effect a good closure so that the actual bony tissue should be removed by blunt dissection and the connective tissue of the tail cut through in-between vertebrae. The skin should be closed with several individual vertical mattress sutures of monofilament nylon. The tail must then be protected by bandaging and kept in place by securing it to a single piece of bandage around the circumference of the sheep in front of the udder or scrotum. The bandage should be replaced at regular intervals for at least 1 week after suture removal.

Vasectomy

From a disease control point of view the best candidates for this surgery are homebred lambs that are not fit to be kept as rams. It is best to allow them to mature to shearlings as the surgery is slightly more exacting in lambs and there is a danger in lambs that a spermatocele will be formed. This will cause pain and therefore should be avoided from a welfare standpoint. The pain will reduce the libido of the vasectomized ram (teaser) and therefore he will be less efficient in getting the ewes to cycle. The surgery should be carried out at least 2 months before the teaser is required. As the teaser is going to run with the entire rams, when not in use it is vital that really careful identification is carried out. Some practitioners prefer to remove one testicle at the time of vasectomy to ensure no mistakes are made between entire rams and vasectomized rams.

Excellent analgesia can be obtained by lumbosacral extradural lidocaine injection without the need for sedation, which is hazardous in sheep. However, this peripheral nerve block is not easy and requires precise needle placement and may result in a long period of hind limb paralysis. With adequate restraint the operation can be accomplished with just a skin bleb of 5 ml of 2% lidocaine on each side and instillation of 2 ml of lidocaine into each spermatic cord.

The ideal method of restraint is to have the shepherd sitting on a small bale of straw with his back to a wall. The ram is then sat on its hindquarters with its dorsal surface adjacent to the bale between the shepherd's legs. The wool is clipped off the scrotum and from the inner thighs. It is also helpful to clip off some of the hair from the belly, making a sterile preparation easier. There is a slight danger of long-term infection in the form of granulomatous tissue if sterility is not maintained. After surgical preparation the lidocaine is instilled. The area is again prepared for surgery.

A 5-cm (2-inch) incision is made in the neck of the scrotum over the spermatic cord but slightly medial to the cord. The spermatic cord is then exteriorized by blunt dissection. A pair of artery forceps is positioned between the skin and the cord. The shiny vas deferens will be seen on the medial aspect of the spermatic cord. It can be grasped with a pair of rat-toothed dressing forceps. Having ligatured either end with absorbable suture material, a 5-cm (2-inch) length is removed. The skin is closed with two horizontal mattress sutures of similar absorbable material. The process is repeated on the other side.

If the surgeon is confident that both of the vas deferens have been removed, these can be labelled and retained in formol saline in case of future litigation. If the surgeon has any doubts the cords should be submitted for histology before any harm can occur from a teaser being fertile.

Common Surgical Conditions for Goats

General

On the whole, surgical operations in goats are very similar to those carried out in sheep. Castration in young lambs is normally carried out using an elastrator rubber ring, and goats can be castrated in this manner. However they are often disbudded at an early age (see Chapter 16). It is very humane to castrate with an open surgical method at this time when they are already anaesthetized. Loop ear goats commonly injure their ears, and these are best stapled and then bandaged to protect them.

Atresia ani

This congenital condition may be inherited but this has not been proved; however it is prudent not to breed from these animals. Normally the condition is not seen until some time after birth. The place where the anus ought to be located is bulging out, full of meconium. This area should be cleaned, a skin bleep of local anaesthetic injected, and a small cruciate incision made with a scalpel. No suturing is required. The tetanus status of the kid should be checked and the animal examined in 48h to check that patency has been maintained.

Atresia recti

Unlike atresia ani, this condition is not often seen and its correction surgically is extremely difficult. Euthanasia is likely to be the kindest and most economical course of action.

Castration of adult bucks

This can be carried out surgically or with the bloodless burdizzo, and the latter is preferable if it is the fly season. It must never be carried out with a ligature or rubber ring. In both methods light sedation is recommended with the buck remaining standing. This can be achieved with 0.05mg/kg of xylazine given intramuscularly, and 5ml of local anaesthetic should be injected into the neck of the scrotum on both sides after suitable cleansing of the area. If a surgical approach is required, a further 5ml should be injected into the caudal end of each scrotum. An open method of castration should be carried out unless there is evidence of an inguinal hernia.

With the buck standing and an assistant holding the tail, an incision is made at the caudal end of the scrotum containing the testicle, which is kept under pressure. The incision should be made through the skin and the tunics so that the testicle pops out. This is then grasped and pulled, ideally being twisted at the same time. There is no requirement for the use of an emasculator. The testicle and the spermatic cord should be removed and the area sprayed with an antibiotic spray. This should be repeated on the other side. Appropriate tetanus and fly protection should be given.

With the animal standing and restrained, the jaws of the burdizzo are applied to one side of the cranial neck of the scrotum, making sure that the spermatic cord is included in the jaws. After 1min the jaws are released slightly and moved 0.5cm in a caudal direction and reapplied for a further 1min. The procedure is repeated on the other side, making sure that none of the compression lines meet straight across the neck.

Burdizzos need to be oiled regularly and kept in a suitable **dry** place. Their action can be tested by applying them to two pieces of thick paper containing a piece of household string. The string should be severed after application of the burdizzo but the paper should remain intact.

Castration of young kids

This can be carried out with an elastrator ring as in lambs, but this not the normal practice in the UK, where male kids are usually castrated by an open method. This is ideally performed at the same time as disbudding when the kids have been given a GA. However it can be performed under a local anaesthetic block, when 2 ml of 2% lignocaine is injected into each spermatic cord and a further 1 ml into the skin of the scrotum. A single incision is made into the scrotum on each side through the skin and the tunics. The testicle together with the spermatic cord is carefully drawn out and removed, and the wound is sprayed with antibiotic. The kid is given tetanus antitoxin, antibiotics and NSAID.

Castration can be carried out with a very small pair of burdizzos. A local block in the spermatic cord should be given but there is no need for local anaesthetic into the scrotum. Equally, there is no need for parenteral antibiotics, but NSAID and TAT should be given. The actual procedure is similar to that carried out in adult bucks.

Dehorning of adult goats

This procedure should not be undertaken lightly. There is no reason for it to be performed for safety reasons in the uninjured goat, as the lack of horns rarely make the buck any less dangerous to other goats or to goatherds. However it has to be carried out under certain circumstances. If the horn is deformed and is growing into the head sometimes the non-vascular tip, which has no nerve supply, can be removed with embryotomy wire. However normally the whole horn is pressing into the head and so the horn has to be removed. If the goat has damaged its horn it will need to be removed on welfare grounds as well as to prevent further haemorrhage.

The operation can be performed under GA or under heavy sedation with a local regional block. After surgically preparing around the horn, the whole circumference of the horn needs to be infiltrated with local anaesthetic, with particular attention paid to the area (looking from above the horn) between 4 and 8 o'clock. With an assistant holding the horn a cut is made with an embryotomy wire saw in the skin 0.25 cm (one-tenth of an inch) below the horn. The direction of the cut needs to be approximately 15° below the horizontal line. There will be considerable haemorrhage, which can be controlled with a very hot dehorning iron if a small horn is being removed. It is unlikely to be successful if a large horn has been amputated. In this case individual vessels should be grasped with artery forceps and ligated. If the vessels are coming directly out of the bone tissue they can be blocked with small pieces of matchstick. The whole wound is then dressed with a cream containing acriflavin and BHC. A thick cotton wool pad is bandaged in place, taking care that it is not too tight or restricting the trachea. The animal should be hospitalized if possible, or at least kept under careful observation for a minimum of 6 h. On no account should it be returned to other bucks as the lack of horns or horn will change its position in the pecking order and fighting will occur. The bandage will need to be changed at 48-h intervals. Antibiotic and NSAID cover should be continued for 10 days after the surgery, as secondary infection could lead to secondary haemorrhage with fatal results. Fly control is paramount as complete healing will take some weeks.

Enucleation of the eye

A surgical method is described in Chapter 14.

Repairing an inguinal hernia

Inguinal hernias are extremely rare in bucks and are a genetic recessive disorder, so they should only be repaired after castration. The left side is more commonly affected. If there is strangulation, then the animal will show colic-type pain. If veterinary assistance is sought within 2 h the small intestine can normally be replaced manually into the abdomen and castration can then be carried in the following manner.

After sedation with xylazine the hindquarters of the ram are raised and the area is surgically cleansed in the normal manner. A skin bleb of 5 ml of 2% lidocaine is placed over each testicle and an instillation of 2 ml of lidocaine is put into each spermatic cord. A careful scrotal incision is made over the testicle, taking care not to incise the tunics. The testicle is drawn through the skin incision, milking any abdominal contents back into the abdomen. When the surgeon is perfectly certain that this has been accomplished, two large pairs of haemostats are placed over the cord. The proximal pair is removed and a transfixing ligature is tied in the groove left by the haemostats. If this surgery is being performed on a large mature buck then a pair of emasculators should replace the distal pair of haemostats. When the testicle has been removed, the skin should be sutured with horizontal mattress sutures. Similar surgery should be carried out on the other side. The buck should be given antibiotics, NSAID and TAT by injection.

If an otherwise healthy buck is found on inspection to have an inguinal hernia, then normal slaughter for human consumption is the practical way forward. If the animal is a pet the hernia can be repaired after a closed castration as described above.

Repairing an umbilical hernia

Umbilical hernias are extremely rare in goats. They have a high heritability and so repair should not be carried out in bucks, which should be castrated and fattened. It is reasonable to repair an umbilical hernia in a milking or pet goat which is being kept for breeding, on the understanding that her progeny will not be kept for breeding.

Repair of umbilical hernias should be delayed until the kid is at least 2 months of age; often with age there is little reason to repair them as the abdominal opening is relatively small. If the abdominal opening is large, a full surgical operation will need to be carried out under GA. The kid should be given a GA and the area should be clipped and surgically prepared. An elliptical skin incision is made around the hernia sack. The skin is removed with blunt dissection. With great care, and also with blunt dissection, the hernia sac is undermined from the abdominal wall without entering the abdomen so that there is a rim of 1 cm around the orifice. Sterile nylon mesh is then sutured to the abdominal ring over the orifice with continuous stitches in monofilament nylon. After closing the wound with a continuous layer of subcuticular sutures of absorbable material, the skin is closed with single horizontal mattress sutures of monofilament nylon. The wound is covered with antibiotic spray. The lamb should be confined for a minimum of 10 days and receive antibiotics and NSAID cover. Obviously fly control and tetanus cover is vital.

Replacing a prolapsed uterus

The cause of uterine prolapse may be related to the birth of an oversized kid, but the most common cause is acute hypocalcaemia (see Chapter 9) at parturition. It is vital that the condition of hypocalcaemia is treated first as death may occur while the uterus is being replaced. The whole scenario should be treated with some urgency. However it is equally important that owners are educated so that they will be able to differentiate a prolapsed uterus from a retained placenta. Replacement should be carried out in a similar manner as described in the sheep (see Chapter 13). The owners should be counselled that the condition might reoccur at the next kidding but that this is not definite.

Replacing a prolapsed vagina

This is a very rare condition in does. Inexperienced owners should be instructed to differentiate this condition (which occurs prior to kidding) from a prolapsed uterus (which occurs after kidding). Replacement is straightforward and should be carried out in a similar manner to that described in sheep (see Chapter 13). The owners should be counselled that not only will this condition invariably reoccur at the next kidding, but also that it will be more severe, so that it is vital that the doe is not bred from again.

Replacing a prolapsed rectum

The causes of this very rare condition are obscure, but it has been suggested that homosexual behaviour might be a cause. It does appear to be more prevalent in bucks. Severe coughing caused by lung worm or pneumonia has also been postulated as a cause. The goat should be given antibiotic and NSAID cover, the tetanus status should be checked and fly control implemented. With the goat in the standing position an epidural regional anaesthetic should be given and the perineal area cleaned before a purse-string suture is put in place. It is important that this is placed before replacement of the rectum, otherwise the rectum will prolapse again while the suture is being placed. After replacement of the rectum, using plenty of obstetrical lubricant, the purse-string should be drawn tight to allow only one finger in the orifice. The animal should be kept on a laxative diet and checked regularly. The suture should be removed in 10 days. In the majority of cases it will remain *in situ*, but if it prolapses again euthanasia is indicated.

Vasectomy

This operation is rarely required in goats but can be performed in a similar manner to that carried out in rams. As goats are rarely as stoical as sheep and will not sit at ease on their hindquarters, sedation with xylazine is advisable at 0.1 mg/kg, given intravenously.

Euthanasia for Sheep

Use of a firearm with a free bullet

This is a very satisfactory method of euthanasia in adult sheep. However, in the UK the operator must either be a veterinary surgeon with a current firearms licence for the weapon concerned, or a licensed slaughterman with a similar firearms licence. The only exception to this is for the veterinary surgeon or the licensed slaughterman to use a shotgun with permission of the owner of the shotgun. There is no hard and fast rule on the size of the bullet or the bore of the shotgun, and operators should use their own judgement. With a large old horned ram a .310 or .320 calibre would be suitable; with a ewe or a younger sheep a .22 calibre would be adequate and safer. Equally, a 12-bore shotgun would be suitable for a ram, whereas a 4.10 shotgun should be used for a ewe or younger sheep. It must be remembered when using a shotgun that the end of the barrel needs to be no closer than 15 cm (6 inches) from the skull and can be up to 1 m (3 feet) away. The location of the target is the same for a firearm or for a shotgun. It is a point in the middle of a cross made between the ears and the eyes on the opposite side of the face. The position of any horns should be disregarded. It should be stressed that the sheep's head should be adequately restrained and no personnel should be behind the animal. With either of these methods the sheep should die instantaneously and there is no need to sever the carotids. It is not appropriate to use firearms for young lambs.

Use of a captive bolt pistol

This used to be the standard method of euthanasia in slaughterhouses. A .22 pistol with a captive bolt was fired into the brain by directing the shot in the middle of a cross made by two lines from the sheep's ears to its eyes. The animal was immediately bled out by severing all the major vessels in the neck. This method can be used for adult sheep and for fat lambs but should not be used for young lambs. No firearms licence is required. Farmers and shepherds should be given a short training course if this method is to be used on the farm.

Electrocution

This is the more modern method of euthanasia used in abattoirs. It is very important that the animals are bled out immediately after they are stunned. Guidelines are laid down for the strength and length of application of the current.

Chemical euthanasia

This is likely to be the method of choice for pet sheep. Veterinarians must obviously be not only totally welfare conscious but also mindful of the owners' concerns. For chemical euthanasia, good advice would be to use sedation first using intramuscular xylazine with a 4-cm (1½-inch) needle (2 ml of a 2% solution for an adult animal). The client should be warned that the animal might make a moaning noise. This is not from pain but from the effect of the drug. When the animal is in lateral recumbency, completion of euthanasia can be carried out by injecting 20 ml of triple-strength barbiturate into the jugular vein. The reasoning for this approach is first because larger doses of triple-strength barbiturate will be required without prior sedation, and second because it is not easy to inject large volumes intravenously into a standing sheep. It might be argued that a small dose of a solution containing 400 mg/ml quinalbarbitone and 25 mg/ml cinchocaine hydrochloride would be adequate. However the fluid is very viscous, and a large-gauge needle will be required. Also, the practitioner will be left with a part-used bottle of a solution containing 400 mg/ml quinalbarbitone and 25 mg/ml cinchocaine hydrochloride, as the smallest bottles of this solution available are 25 ml. Care is also required for sheep with long horns, for when they are in lateral recumbency the jugular is not particularly easy to visualize. The use of a small pillow under the neck will be helpful. Chemical euthanasia is the method of choice for small lambs. They should be held across the handler's chest, with the head restrained. The veterinarian can then raise the jugular and inject 5 ml of a triple-strength barbiturate solution with a 1-inch 21 G needle. If very large numbers of small lambs need to be destroyed, for example when affected or at risk from a highly contagious notifiable disease, then the triple-strength barbiturate solution can be injected with a 1-inch 19 G needle directly into the heart. The lamb should be held in a similar manner across the handler's chest.

Euthanasia for Goats

Use of a firearm with a free bullet

This is a totally acceptable method of euthanasia in adult goats. It should not be used in young kids. The position is in the centre of a cross made by two lines running from the eye to the opposite ear. The position of the horns is not relevant.

Use of a captive bolt pistol

This method as described for sheep is not normally used in goats, but is satisfactory. The position is the same for that used with a free bullet. The goat must be bled out immediately after stunning. There are extra-charged blank cartridges for use in captive bolt pistols for large-horned billy goats. Captive bolts should not be used in young kids.

Electrocution

This method is used in commercial goat herds. It could be used by the veterinary surgeon, but the author has not seen it carried out.

Chemical euthanasia

This is the normal method of euthanasia in pet goats and also in small goat herds in the UK. The same constraints apply to both goats and sheep, and are explained in the notes for sheep. Veterinary surgeons are urged to give a sedative first for euthanasia of most adult goats, unless they are moribund. The sedative of choice is 2% xylazine. Veterinary surgeons should realise that injecting large volumes of fluids into the jugular of adult goats is fraught with difficulties. On the other hand, it is relatively simple in well-restrained kids.

Euthanasia in General

It must be stressed that veterinarians must always check that whatever method has been used has been successful. They themselves must certify that death has occurred, and not rely on any helpers. In the normal circumstances euthanasia of any animal by a veterinarian using blunt trauma is **totally unacceptable**. However every veterinary surgeon is an individual and is legally and morally in charge in euthanasia situations, and must use her judgement. For example, there may be a fire in a lambing shed. The veterinarian happens to be passing in her car. She is off duty and has no firearm or lethal injection available for a small, very badly burned lamb. Is it better to administer one sharp blow with a hammer to the lamb's head or to wait for another veterinarian to arrive?

Certain religions demand that animals slaughtered for human consumption are killed in a specific manner. This mainly entails cutting the animal's neck vessels with a very sharp knife, without stunning the animal first. The legality of such methods varies from country to country, and their morality is outside the scope of this book. Veterinarians are urged to study the laws of the country in which they are working and should not condone any illegal methods of slaughter, however devout the owner.

9

Nutrition and Metabolic Conditions

Introduction

To satisfy the five freedoms – the ethical framework around which the codes of recommendation for the welfare of farmed livestock are presently crafted in the UK – all farm animals, including sheep and goats, must be given access to proper nutrition. This means not just that forage and water must be offered at all times, but that the nutrient balance is such that the animals do not suffer from hunger, thirst or malnutrition. In the UK and in the EU there are strict rules regarding the feeding and watering of animals in transit.

The diet of animals must be suitable to their production needs and must overcome any potential dietary shortcomings such as mineral deficiencies, energy shortfall or constituent imbalance. Herds and flocks should have an effective management plan (see Chapter 20). Feeding practice in particular must be good to optimize the health, welfare and productivity of the animals whether they are kept for meat, milk, fibre or even as lawn mowers (i.e. as pets). Judicious use of grazing can be used to satisfy the nutrient demands for a large part of the year for sheep and goats in the UK. The grazing has to be managed to maintain sward height and ensure that fresh grazing is available to the animals as needed, or the animals must be allow to roam to find new pasture. The roaming may be timed to make best use of the grazing to fit in with the weather, altitude, harvesting of crops or even the use of the garden.

In an intensive situation attention to stocking rates and the monitoring of sward height will allow the best use of grazing, with optimal swards of 4–6 cm, which can be maintained. Properly managed grazing patterns coupled with good forage preservation are the goal. Complications to diets start as soon as supplements are introduced. Balanced diets do not need mineral blocks or powder supplements *ad lib.*, and indeed some of these act to cause dietary imbalance, either by competing with nutrients in the diet, or by indirect competition. An example is the rich red mineral supplement that is often supplied by farm wholesalers. This contains high levels of iron and will effectively lower the adsorption of copper from the gut, perhaps even leading to marginal or deficient status. Similarly, imbalances of calcium, magnesium and phosphates can be precipitated by injudicious use of mineral supplements.

Measuring Feed Efficiency

Traditionally, nutritional performance is measured and shown as either feed conversion ratio (FCR), which is calculated by dividing the weight of food by the weight of gain, or as feed conversion efficiency (FCE), which is calculated by dividing the weight of gain by the weight of food. Another useful measurement is residual feed intake (RFI). This is a measure of the efficiency with which animals use their feed. It is calculated by subtracting the predicted food intake from the actual food intake.

RFI is therefore feed intake that cannot be accounted for by maintenance and production. Animals with a positive RFI are less efficient than average, whereas those with a negative RFI are more efficient than average. These differences in RFI arise from a number of sources including body composition, activity, ability to digest and metabolize feed, stress and feeding behaviour. Some of these are due to non-genetic factors such as heat stress, pathogens or metabolic disease (e.g. acidosis) but there is also a genetic component, and selection for animals on the basis of a negative RFI is worthwhile.

Poor Foodstuffs

Feeding mouldy forage is usually unintentional and occasionally unavoidable. However, the potential disease impact and reduced palatability of spoilt feed mean that this should be avoided if at all possible. Incorrect storage of forage intended for later feeding can result in the ideal conditions for growth of various organisms capable of causing disease in sheep and goats. These include:

- *Listeria monocytogenes* – an organism associated with various neurological diseases (see Chapter 14).
- Fungal organisms – diseases caused by fungi include placentitis and abortion, so particular care should be taken to ensure pregnant animals are kept away from spoilt feed. These fungi are not zoonotic diseases per se, but man can be directly infected by the spores. The fungi cause an extrinsic allergic alveolitis, otherwise known as 'farmer's lung'. Sheep and goats can develop a similar condition.
- *Bacillus licheniformis* – an organism that can cause abortions and stillbirths in sheep and goats.

It is therefore important that feedstuffs are stored correctly. Where areas of mould are seen then these should be removed and destroyed carefully. This care should also be exercised with mouldy bedding material.

Nutrition of Sheep

Nutrition in sheep, except on large integrated farms, is rarely very scientific. Equally, veterinary practitioners are rarely consulted. However, although a nutritionist will be the key person in helping farmers make decisions, it is important that practitioners are involved in any major changes. Nutrition will be an important part of preparing a flock health plan (see Chapter 20). One of the main problems to be addressed by farmers and their practitioners is weight loss in ewes. This is extremely common. Often it has a very insidious onset and is only recognized by an outsider such as the practitioner. It can be a result of poor shepherding, and the shepherd may be aware of this or in a state of denial. Great tact and communication skills need to be exercised by the clinician, who must always have welfare at the forefront of any agenda. The evidence should not be subjective but objective. Ewes should be weighed and, more importantly, be scored for condition.

Condition scores of ewes at tupping will have a direct bearing on lambing rates in fecund lowland sheep. A group of mules with a condition score of 2 at tupping will have a likely lambing percentage of 150%. This may easily rise to 200% if the condition score is 4. However the husbandry of the holding may not be able to cope with that higher lambing percentage. A more modest yet sustainable 175% could be achieved by having a condition score of 3.

However, the bottom line is that in a temperate climate at the end of summer, an overall condition score of 2 at tupping is too low. Many farmers regularly weigh their lambs but rarely weigh their ewes. They should be encouraged to carry out the simple exercise. On a well-managed holding a flock plan will be prepared and this will have targets for weights and condition scores at tupping, as well as lambing percentages. A target weight for a mule at tupping might be 75 kg.

A Texel ewe with a similar condition score would weigh 80kg and a Suffolk 90kg. If ewes are healthy, a daily weight gain of 250g is quite achievable, provided there is no undercurrent disease.

Often the problem of weight loss is overlooked on account of the weight of fleece. Condition scoring is vital. Visible emaciation will be seen at normal shearing time but may be glossed over as the ewes are rearing lambs. At this time they may have energy requirements of three times that at tupping and so it will be virtually impossible to raise either their weights or their condition scores, but every effort should be made. In winter-shorn flocks this window of visibility will not occur at this time and so really dangerous emaciation may occur and severe welfare conditions will prevail.

A general flock problem of low condition scores and weights may not be just due to suboptimum nutrition. Clinicians should keep an open mind and look for other causes such as parasitism, concurrent disease, lameness and dental problems. In flock problems, as with the individual thin ewe, a full clinical examination should be carried out in addition to other diagnostic tests.

Flocks that are kept truly extensively throughout the year face a variety of problems such as adverse weather conditions, for example sudden snowfalls with drifting in winter, wind and rain or snow around lambing time, lack of grazing during winter and predators (Winter, 1995). They require careful management to make sure the welfare of the animals is not compromised. Arrangements must be made so that the sheep can have unbroken access to fodder, and so that sufficient concentrates are readily available. Sheep are not wild animals and they must be regularly inspected. Winter housing may be the way forward to solve most of these problems. Such systems are becoming the 'norm' in the Scottish highlands, the mountains of Wales, the Lake District, the Pennines and the moors of Devon and Cornwall. Winter housing has been carried out for hundreds of years in the Alps and other high areas of Europe and Asia.

Traditionally, a younger age structure has usually been maintained in hill and mountain flocks, with ewes being drafted to less harsh conditions after three to five pregnancies. Careful management needs to be carried out with the use of breeds (see Chapter 1) so that hardier breeds are used in the worst conditions and those preferred by butchers are used in better conditions. Careful attention to fecundity needs to be considered. There is no value in having high lambing percentages at birth, only to have mortality rates of 30 or 40% within a few days.

Governments should be aware that large areas are maintained as attractive visas for the general public by extensive sheep farming. These environments will not be maintained if the sheep are removed, and so grants must be continue to be paid.

The first trimester of a ewe's pregnancy lasts for 45 days and is termed the time of implantation. In the UK, dietary energy supply for this period is likely to be adequate because autumn grass is still available after flushing ewes and there is very little energy demand from the developing fetus. The second trimester is termed the time of placental development. It lasts for 45 days from day 45 to day 90. Poor nutrition at this stage – which in the UK is during the winter, when weather conditions may be very bad – will impair placental development. In turn this will decrease lamb birth weights. Obviously it is not only the weather that will affect the nutrients available for placental development. Undercurrent disease such as chronic liver fluke infestation will have a marked effect. Apart from a decrease in the weight of lambs born, poor placental development will affect the actual birth weights of individual lambs. For example, one placenta will develop normally with a lamb at birth weighing <5 kg, but the other will be poorly developed, giving a twin of >3.5kg. The third or final trimester is when real fetal growth and development occur. It lasts for just over 50 days. Good nutrition in ewes carrying more than one lamb is vital during this period. Ewes carrying singles, unless they are radically underfed, can normally cope with the added nutritional requirements.

To summarize, in order to feed sheep sensibly and for the best production values, these simple rules need to be followed:

1. Plan your production targets.
2. Match your flock's body condition score to the stage of production.

3. Know your flock's metabolic and trace element status.
4. Plan your grazing and conservation pattern to maximize forage use.
5. Target concentrate delivery to the categories of sheep that need it.
6. Monitor your progress by judicious use of laboratory samples.
7. Review your progress from year to year.

Trace element deficiencies in sheep

Cobalt

Cobalt deficiency is called 'pine' and is mainly a condition of weaned lambs on pastures deficient in cobalt. The condition has a slow, insidious onset with multiple clinical signs. Lack of cobalt, which causes a deficiency in vitamin B12, leads to a decreased resistance to other common diseases such as parasites. It also reduces the lamb's immune response, so vaccination against clostridial diseases will be ineffective. There are two ways to confirm the condition: blood testing a sample for plasma B12 levels, or a trial of cobalt supplementation. Treatment is easy, with an intramuscular injection followed by cobalt supplementation by mouth of cobalt sulfate at 1 mg/kg. This will need to be continued at monthly intervals until the animals are fed on concentrates. In future years, lambs and even ewes should be drenched at regular intervals while on the deficient pastures, or given specifically prepared cobalt boluses, which lodge in the reticulum.

Copper

Copper is rarely deficient per se, but normally occurs when sheep graze pastures high in molybdenum. It can also occur when pastures are high in sulfur and iron. The normal manifestation in the UK is the condition of swayback (see Chapter 14), but in other countries the signs are more variable. In Australia low copper will cause anaemia and poor wool quality – 'steely wool' – which may be confused with haemonchosis (see Chapter 10). In New Zealand low copper will cause lambs to have poor bone mineralization, which may be confused with rickets. Throughout the world low copper will cause poor growth rates and an increase susceptibility to disease. Copper is stored in the liver so the ultimate diagnosis is copper level estimations. However, plasma copper levels will drop as soon as the liver is depleted. Care needs to be exercised as copper is toxic to sheep and its excess must be avoided (see Chapter 17). When copper levels are known to be a problem the safest method of supplementation is copper oxide needles given orally in a gelatine capsule. Copper can be given by injection as copper heptonate. However there are no longer any injectable licensed preparations available in the UK.

Selenium

Selenium deficiency is usually considered with vitamin E deficiency, as deficiency of either will give the same clinical manifestation. The condition is called 'white muscle disease' or 'stiff lamb disease', and the correct name is nutritional muscular dystrophy. In the UK it is principally seen in areas with low soil selenium when sheep are fed on home grown cereals and root crops, but it is not common. It can also be seen when there is poor mixing of mineral additives. It is a condition of worldwide occurrence in selenium-deficient areas. Green forage crops normally have good levels of vitamin E but this is not the case in dry or drought conditions. In the UK young lambs less than 6 weeks of age are mainly affected. Initially they are stiff and then become recumbent. Diagnosis on clinical signs is possible after a full examination but should be confirmed with blood samples tested for glutathione peroxidise as an indicator of selenium. Vitamin E levels can also be measured.

Older lambs may just present with poor growth rates. After a blood test has confirmed the diagnosis, lame lambs will respond rapidly to selenium/vitamin E supplementation by injection, and growth rates will improve in older lambs. Infertility has been seen in low selenium areas. Fertility in these areas can be improved by selenium/vitamin supplementation in the ration, and this type of supplementation will prevent the disease in future years.

Body condition scoring in sheep

Although the ultimate measure is body weight, average weights for varying stages of pregnancy and for various breeds are available, and body condition score is extremely useful in giving an objective assessment of a ewe's condition. It depends on feeling the amount of muscle and fat deposition over and around the vertebrae in the loin region between the vertebral process and the transverse process and the skin. When assessing body condition score it is important that the ewe is relaxed and standing in a race, and not crushed up in a pen. The score is from 1 to 5:

1. The animal is extremely thin. The vertebral process can easily be felt and the transverse processes are very obvious.
2. The vertebral process are more rounded and there is a reasonable eye muscle. The transverse processes are easy to feel but are covered with flesh.
3. The vertebral process can be felt as a rounded bone but it is not possible to feel between the vertebral processes.
4. The backbone is a smooth, slightly raised ridge.
5. The spine can only be felt by pressing down firmly between the fat-covered eye muscles.

Nutrition of Goats

There is very little research in goat nutrition published in English, and most values of requirements are extrapolated from dairy cows or sheep. One of the main problems in feeding goats is the limited numbers in a herd and the wide range of milk yields, from 600 to 1500 l per lactation. Often goats have long lactations when they fail to get in kid but are run with the higher-milking animals in the milking herd. Such goats require much lower energy density diets. They are thus overfed and get fat. Goats have a very short pregnancy compared to cows. Metabolic problems tend to happen at the end of pregnancy. It is very difficult to manage kidding dates. This is even worse if the does are allowed to run with the buck. A useful figure is that a goat's dry matter intake will be 2.8% of its body weight. This will decrease to 2.7% in early lactation.

Trace element deficiencies in goats

Cobalt

This is extremely rare in goats as their browsing will provide sufficient cobalt.

Copper

This may occur in goats and the causality is very similar to that of sheep.

Selenium

This condition is more common in the USA than in the UK, as goats in the former are fed lucerne (alfalfa) hay. Legumes may take up insufficient selenium in areas where that element is deficient. The signs in goats are very similar to those in sheep.

Metabolic Diseases in Sheep

Hypocalcaemia

In sheep, even in dairy sheep, this is a disease of late pregnancy prior to parturition. The condition can occur in all breeds and seems to follow within a few hours of a stressful experience. The stress may be a change of feed or weather, or even just a gathering and handling session. The ewes tend to be in the last third of pregnancy, and the number of lambs *in utero* does not seem to be a factor. The ewes will be anorexic, ataxic or recumbent. Heart rates will not be raised; rectal temperatures will be below normal; rumen movement will be reduced, and by definition the blood calcium levels will be low. Obviously, samples should be taken before treatment. However treatment should not be delayed waiting for results, as a positive response to treatment with calcium borogluconate is diagnostic. Ideally a 50-kg ewe should receive 3 g intravenously, accomplished by injecting 75 ml of a 20% solution. The effect will be rapid, with the ewe returning to normality within 2 h.

Treatment by subcutaneous injection will be effective but will take longer, around 12h or overnight. With help, intravenous injections are easily accomplished into the jugular vein. However, if practitioners are alone, and the ewe is near to parturition, a good site for intravenous injection is the mammary vein. With the ewe resting on her rump and with her back to the practitioner, the vein can be easily injected by leaning over her shoulder. A 19G needle should be used and the solution should be given slowly. Ideally the bottle should be warmed to blood heat and not taken straight out of a cold vehicle. Care should be taken with all calcium borogluconate injections that cleanliness is observed. The solution per se is an irritant and so any bacterial infection will cause an unpleasant abscess. There is no need to use 40% solutions subcutaneously; they are more irritant than 20% solutions when injected subcutaneously, and when injected intravenously they are more likely to adversely affect the heart.

Hypocalcaemia can occur in sheep from the ingestion of certain plants (see Chapter 17). These contain oxalates, which rapidly bind up the blood calcium and cause hypocalcaemia with the normal signs as described earlier. Plants found in the UK that come to mind are fat hen (*Chenopodium album*), rhubarb (*Rheum rhaponticum*) and sugarbeet tops (*Beta vulgaris*). Plants to be aware of in other areas include buffelgrass (*Cenchrus ciliaris*) in the tropics, greasewood (*Sarcobatus vermiculatus*) in North America and Mexico and soft roly-poly (*Salsola kali*) in Australia. All will cause hypocalcaemia and show similar signs.

Hypomagnesaemia

This condition is rare in sheep. Magnesium, which is readily available in most feeds, needs to be ingested and absorbed daily. If the transit time through the bowel is too rapid then insufficient magnesium will be absorbed. Although lush green grass is a very good source of magnesium, it causes a rapid transit time of ingesta through the bowel and so can provoke the condition. If blood levels of magnesium are low then any stress will cause the signs, which are neurological. Sternal recumbency is rapidly followed by lateral recumbency and convulsions. The heart rate and rectal temperature are raised. There is frothing at the mouth and rapid eye movement. The legs will paddle. The sex of the animal is not relevant, although it is possible that the condition is more common in entire adult males. Certainly the condition can occur in pregnant and lactating animals. In temperate climates it is a condition of the spring and autumn. This is due to the likelihood of lush grass at these times and the very changeable weather, which may act as a trigger. The classic situation for hypomagnesaemia in sheep is animals grazing lush pasture under fruit trees. The ground will have received large quantities of nitrogen either as inorganic nitrogen or as organic nitrogen in muck. Treatment in sheep is rarely successful if they are convulsing. Although blood magnesium levels can be restored to normal, there is usually irreparable brain damage. Treatment can be attempted: it should consist of a **subcutaneous** injection of 50ml of a 25% magnesium sulfate (up to 100ml can be given to a large ram). It is important that this drug is given subcutaneously, as it will cause death if given intravenously. It is prudent to give other supportive treatment such as a mixture of 20% calcium borogluconate, 5% magnesium hypophosphite and 20% glucose given subcutaneously, coupled with NSAID. Historically the mixture of calcium called PMD (phosphorus magnesium dextrose) was given intravenously. However deaths in sheep have been reported and so clinicians are now advised to stick to the subcutaneous route. It should be remembered that these cases are on a knife edge and so any treatment by any route may well cause death. Shepherds should be advised accordingly; this is particularly important with pet sheep.

Hypophosphatemia

This condition, which causes recumbency in cows, does not seem to affect sheep. A deficiency in phosphorus may cause other signs, for instance a generalized lack of calcification of bones and a pica for anything containing phosphorus, such as bones. This is well documented in other countries, for example South Africa, Australia and New Zealand. However it is not likely to occur in the UK, where real deficiency of phosphorus has not been recorded.

Ketosis

In sheep this occurs during the last weeks of pregnancy, as the name 'pregnancy toxaemia' suggests. It is the most important metabolic disease in sheep. The condition is also called 'twin lamb disease' as it is often associated with multiple pregnancies, but it can occur in ewes carrying only one lamb. The trouble actually starts prior to tupping. Ewes in the UK are given access to good grass after weaning and become too fat. At tupping ewes should be 'fit, not fat'. The ewe needs to put on weight slowly during pregnancy, on good forage. During the last 6 weeks of pregnancy regularly increasing amounts of concentrates need to be included in the diet or, in later lambing flocks, the ewes need to receive more and better quality grass. If the ewes are too fat during the later stages of pregnancy they will be unable to use this fat. It will be deposited in the liver and cause ketosis, when a raised level of ketones will be found in the serum. If the ewes receive a stress – even just having multiple lambs *in utero* may be sufficient stress – they will develop pregnancy toxaemia. They will be anorexic and depressed, and this will quickly lead to recumbency, bruxism and the classic stargazing carriage of the head. Treatment is often unrewarding unless instituted immediately the first signs are seen. It should consist of intravenous injections of 50 ml of 40% glucose solutions three times daily, and oral high-energy drenches. Some recommend giving an injection of dexamethasone. This will initiate parturition if that is imminent, and may solve the problem. However if parturition is not yet near it will result in an abortion, from which the ewes rarely recover. Therefore if there is any doubt about how close to term the ewe may be, intravenous injections of NSAID are safer and more beneficial.

Metabolic Diseases in Goats

Hypocalcaemia

In goats the condition is mainly seen post parturition, normally within 48 h. The signs of the condition are the same as for sheep, but the timing is different. The condition is not only seen in high milk-yielding goats but also in relatively low milk-yielding animals. Unlike sheep, goats will shake prior to ataxia and recumbency. Observant goat keepers will recognize the disease in this early stage. Another early indication is a slow parturition. Normality will be restored promptly with treatment. Hypocalcaemia is sometimes listed as a cause of 'sudden death' in goats, but I think this is extremely unlikely. It could occur in parturient animals that are unsupervised, in other words it is a condition of 'found dead' rather than peracute mortality. Treatment is exactly the same as for sheep. As this is a condition of the individual animal rather than a flock problem, the intravenous route of administration of the calcium borogluconate should be followed. The use of the mammary vein is not appropriate in goats. The condition is normally cured with one intravenous injection. There is no rationale for giving subcutaneous calcium borogluconate to 'last longer'. Calcium borogluconate is an irritant and goats will vocalize loudly. Clinicians should reflect that it is just as painful in sheep but they are more stoical. I think we all should be more conscious of welfare in sheep. The use of NSAID may well be beneficial in post-parturient goats. Clinicians should always check the mammary glands of goats for signs of mastitis. This condition can occur at the same time as hypocalcaemia and should be treated accordingly. In a straightforward case of hypocalcaemia the rectal temperature will be lowered and the faeces firm. In some cases of mastitis, particularly early in the course of the disease, the temperature will be raised and there will be diarrhoea. Later on in cases of toxic mastitis, as in cows, there will be collapse, very watery diarrhoea and a subnormal temperature. These animals will require fluids as well as the calcium borogluconate. It can be argued that it is too late for antibiotic treatment as the toxin is causing the signs; however it is prudent to give intravenous and intramammary antibiotics in these cases. Unlike in sheep this condition is likely to reoccur at subsequent parturitions and so goat keepers should be prepared. Equally, they should adjust the feeding of their pregnant females as the condition can be prevented by careful nutrition. On very rare occasions hypocalcaemia will occur in goats when they come into oestrus. The signs are the same, and the disease can be confirmed with serum calcium levels. Equally rapid recovery will be accomplished with treatment.

As in sheep, hypocalcaemia can be caused by the ingestion of certain plants containing oxalates (see Chapter 17).

Hypomagnesaemia

This is a rare condition in browsing goats as they obtain adequate amounts of magnesium daily, but it will occur in herds of goats fed on lush pastures. These are usually high-producing dairy herds. It can readily be prevented by small amounts of concentrate supplementation. The clinical signs are straightforward and progressive. The goat will be inappetent and will shake. This should not be confused with oestrus, as these mild signs are often shown by certain individuals. However, in cases of hypomagnesaemia the neurological signs will rapidly become more severe, leading to recumbency and opisthotonous. Then there will be convulsions and salivation. Sometimes the rectal temperature will be raised. The pulse will be rapid and shallow, and all gut sounds will cease. Death will occur in a few hours. Treatment with 50 ml of 25% magnesium sulfate subcutaneously, followed by 50 ml of a solution containing 20% calcium borogluconate and 5% magnesium phosphate intravenously will raise blood magnesium levels. However the outcome may not be good if there has been irreparable brain damage. Diagnosis can be made on clinical signs and confirmed by low magnesium blood levels. In the dead animal a presumptive diagnosis can be made by low magnesium levels in the aqueous humour.

Ketosis

The condition known as pregnancy toxaemia is rare in pregnant goats, unlike sheep, but it will occur in very heavily pregnant goats with multiple fetuses. The signs will be anorexia and lethargy. Rectal temperature will be normal but the pulse rate will be raised and rumen movement will be absent. Treatment is only successful if promptly delivered before recumbency. It consists of 100 ml of a 40% glucose solution given intravenously. Often practitioners give a mixture of glucose, calcium borogluconate and magnesium phosphate as well. A concentrated electrolyte solution should be given by mouth, and this can be given as a drench. Great care needs to be taken to avoid inhalation pneumonia. A safer method is to use a calf feeding bag. The use of corticosteroids is controversial. They will improve the liver metabolism but will also initiate kidding within 48 h. If the kids are not too premature, this may be successful, with the doe improving and the kids viable. However if the kids are premature they will die and the resulting metritis will kill the doe. The condition can be prevented by not allowing does to be too fat at service and putting them on a slowly increasing concentrate diet towards the end of pregnancy. In large herds, does may be scanned and those with multiple fetuses can be separated and fed more.

The more common form of ketosis is seen in goats 2 or 3 weeks after kidding. This is equivalent to acetonaemia in dairy cows and is more common in dairy goats. If ketone levels are high the condition can be called nervous acetonaemia. The goats will show neurological signs. These are relatively mild, with the goat walking with its head excessively raised, with starry eyes. They rarely become recumbent but will certainly be hyperaesthetic. Treatment is straightforward, as dexamethazone can be given at 1 mg/kg as the doe is not pregnant. High percentage glucose drinks will also be helpful. The condition can be prevented by paying attention to the post-kidding diet. The animals need highly digestible fibre and good carbohydrates.

Fatty liver syndrome

This syndrome occurs in does that are overfat at the time of kidding. Normally they have only one or two very small kids; otherwise they would have developed ketosis before parturition. The name of the condition says it all: the liver is too full of fat. The goats have a reduced food intake. The body fat is then mobilized, and this stresses the already-compromised liver. Dexamethazone and high doses of vitamin B are helpful, and antibiotics will aid recovery even though there is no infection. Prevention can be carried out by not allowing goats to get too fat at any time, particularly before pregnancy or in the early weeks of pregnancy.

Acidosis

This is really a poisoning. It occurs by a sudden rise in high-energy feed or by the goats getting access to a food store. Rumen fermentation leads to an increase production of lactic acid, resulting in ruminal and systemic acidosis. Signs include lethargy, anorexia, abdominal pain, rumen stasis, diarrhoea and death. Aggressive treatment is required. Calcium borogluconate and glucose should be giving by intravenous injection. A drip line will need to be set up with Hartmann's solution to which can be added high doses of vitamin B. Bicarbonate and kaolin will be helpful by mouth.

Chronic Wasting Disease in Sheep

The thin ewe is a very common sight in sheep flocks and presents a difficult challenge to the clinician. A careful history should be taken to assess onset and progression of clinical signs. It is important to ascertain if this is an individual problem or a flock problem. A full clinical examination should be carried out on all the affected animals and the findings should be recorded. Problems with nutrition should be considered first. It may be that there are fundamental problems with nutrition. If the ewes are at grass it may be that the stocking rate is too high or that the pasture is too poor. This may be a particular problem in times of drought or snowy/ frosty weather. The forage should be examined carefully to check not only on nutritional value but also palatability, availability and of course quantity. Lastly, the weight of concentrates being fed needs to be recorded.

It may not just be poor nutrition which is causing the wasting and low body condition score. The age of the flock is very relevant particularly when oral problems are considered. Incisors and cheek teeth should be examined. An orf problem will be obvious and will affect body condition scores.

The legs and feet of the sheep should also be examined. These may have multiple problems, including foot rot, interdigital dermatitis, scald, foot abscesses, strawberry foot rot, foot trauma, arthritis and fractures.

If there is a whole-flock problem it is valuable to carry out a metabolic profile by taking blood samples. The number needs to be representative not only of the very poor ewes, but also of the more normal ewes. This will indicate any metabolic problems such as trace element deficiencies (cobalt, copper, selenium and zinc). Liver enzymes will give an indication of liver fluke infection. However faeces samples will have to be taken to provide evidence of other endoparasites, protozoal parasites and some chronic infections, for example Johne's disease. Fleeces should be examined for evidence of ectoparasites including lice, mange mites and ticks. Fly strike will be obvious, but it is conceivable that fly worry from horn flies could affect general health.

Chronic Wasting Disease in Goats

This condition is very common in goat practice and presents a difficult challenge to the clinician. A careful history should be taken to assess onset and progression of clinical signs. It is important to ascertain if this is an individual problem or is occurring regularly, or is even occurring in a group of goats. A full clinical examination should be carried out on all the affected animals and the findings should be recorded. Problems with nutrition should be considered. It may be that the plane of nutrition is too low for the whole group, or that too high a stocking rate is creating bullying. This may be a particular problem in rapidly expanding herds, when goats from a large number of small herds are bought. Animals suffering from chronic wasting need to be identified by careful observation; they can then be fed individually. It goes without saying that there should always be sufficient trough space and rack space to allow all the goats in a group to eat at the same time. Obviously the fodder must be of good quality. The conditions that cause chronic wasting in sheep will also affect goats. They may be oral (e.g. orf) or locomotory, with arthritis being the most common. Because goats are browsing animals, trace element deficiencies (e.g. cobalt, copper, selenium and zinc) are very rare. On the other hand the chronic infections of Johne's disease and tuberculosis are more likely. Endoparasites should not be forgotten, with liver fluke being top of the list, followed by intestinal nematodes. Respiratory nematodes are rare. The chronic irritation and blood loss of ectoparasites should not be underestimated. These include lice, mange, fly worry and ticks. Neoplasia may affect old goats. The diagnosis of chronic wasting from all causes will be challenging and is likely to be made at post-mortem.

10

Gastroenteric System

Anatomy of Ovine and Caprine Teeth

Sheep and goats have 32 permanent teeth. Incisors and canines are absent on the maxilla. On the mandible the single canine on each side has migrated forward to join the three incisors. This gives the impression that there are four incisors on each side. These are present at birth. The central incisor is replaced at 1 year and 3 months, the next at 1 year and 9 months, the third at 2 years 3 months and the final incisor at 2 years 9 months. Obviously there is individual variation. A lamb or kid has all 12 of its deciduous premolars at birth or soon afterwards. After approximately 4 months the first molar erupts. Between 9 and 12 months the second molar erupts. Between 1 and 1.5 years of age all 12 deciduous premolars are replaced by permanent premolars. Also at this time the third and final molar erupts. Therefore a sheep and a goat have a full mouth of permanent teeth at 3 years of age.

Mouth and Dental Problems in Sheep and Goats

Introduction

If this is a general flock or herd problem of excess salivation it is vital that FMD is considered. If there is any doubt the appropriate authorities should be contacted. Several systemic diseases can also cause excess salivation, including blue tongue, Nairobi sheep disease, orf, PPR, sheep pox and vesicular stomatitis. The difficulty in diagnosing FMD arises from the fact that often only mild disease is seen in sheep, and also because lesions associated with common endemic diseases of sheep, such as interdigital dermatitis (see Chapter 15) and orf (see Chapter 16) are similar in appearance (Watson, 2004). There are other causes of ulceration in the mouths of sheep that mirror FMD lesions, yet they are not FMD. These have been termed ovine mucosal and gum obscure disease (OMAGOD). These ulcers occur in the buccal or inner lip mucosa below the incisors. They are caused by trauma associated with grazing bare or rough pastures or by the use of mineral and feed blocks (Fig. 10.1), and may be encountered in up to 25% of the flock. They will only be seen on careful clinical examination and do not cause excess salivation.

Mouth Problems in Individual Neonatal Lambs

There may be excess salivation, and the clinician should always check for systemic disease. If the lamb or kid is normal in other respects but not sucking, then mouth problems should

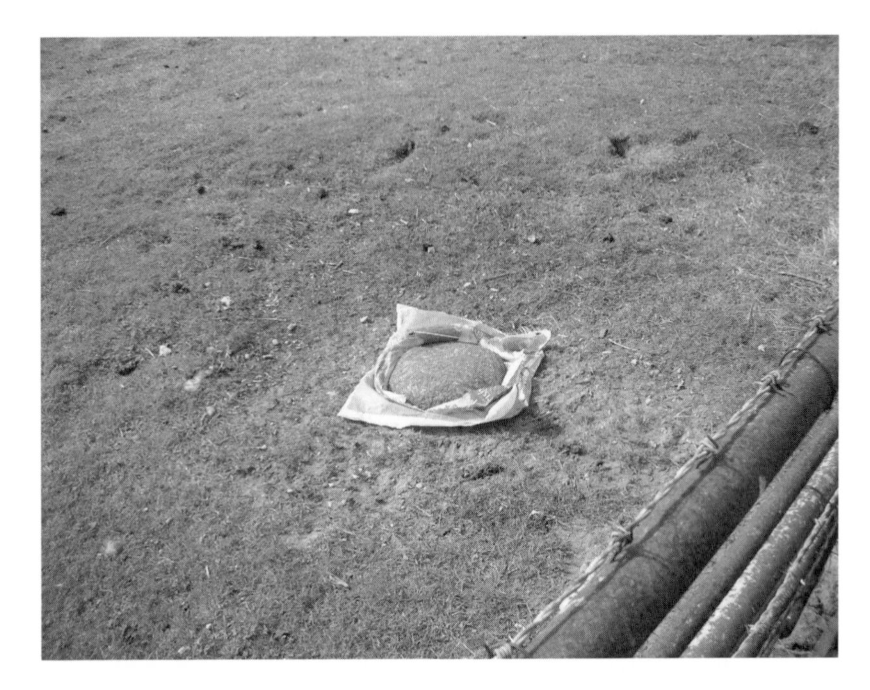

Fig. 10.1. Mineral block.

be suspected whether or not salivation is excessive. Damage to the mandibular symphysis is common after poor parturition technique. Often the tongue is swollen from a prolonged lambing or kidding. Tongue damage may occur as a result of predator or dog attacks. Clinicians should check for congenital problems, the most common of which is cleft palate. This will normally cause milk to come down the nose as the neonate sucks.

Neonatal lambs will get periodontal orf lesions soon after birth, which will not necessarily be visible externally. The lesions will be eruptions on the mucosa. This may be a flock problem rather than just an individual affected lamb. Periodontal orf is common in artificially reared lambs.

Mouth Problems in Growing Adult Sheep and Goats

Obviously if several animals are affected, the differential list will be different from a single sheep or goat being infected. However in either case individual animals have to be examined. First the clinician needs to decide what signs are being shown. There is likely to be excess salivation. This may be coupled with cud spilling, which is normally manifest as a green discolouration around the mouth. The whole head should be examined before the lips are peeled back to examine the incisors and the mucosa. Then, with the use of a gag and a good light source (preferably a head torch), the inside of the mouth and the teeth can be examined (Fig. 10.2). It is very important that clinicians examine the outside of the mouth carefully first. Squamous cell carcinomas may be found in the oropharynx of old small ruminants. Tumours of the salivary glands may be seen but these seldom metastasize to the local lymph nodes. If there is a fracture of one or both mandibles, the gag should not be used, and if there is any doubt, a radiograph should be taken. This should be a lateral oblique with the side of the jaw most likely to be affected nearest to the plate. The x-ray machine should be placed lower than the head and point up at an angle of 30°. The whole mandible should be radiographed, so a

6 days post infection. The clinical signs are associated with virus replication in endothelial cells, which results in haemorrhage, ischaemia, inflammation and oedema. The lesions are common in areas subject to mechanical trauma and abrasion, such as the feet, mouth and eyes. Fever, with temperatures up to 42°C, may occur. In milking sheep and goats there is reduced milk yield. There are respiratory signs and abortion in sheep and goats. BTV causes not only gross abnormalities to the central nervous system (CNS) of the fetus, but also generalized growth retardation and fetal lymphoreticular hyperplasia (Richardson *et al.*, 1985). There is conjunctivitis, mucosal inflammation and oedema. Petechiae, ecchymoses and cracked lips will be seen, leading to excess salivation. There is coronitis causing lameness.

The diagnosis is confirmed by PCR for viral RNA. This can detect all 24 serotypes. The virus can be sequenced and isolated. If serology is required, ELISA and serum neutralization test (SNT) may be carried out.

When treating affected animals all handling should be gentle, with as little movement as possible.

The differential diagnosis for sheep and goats must include FMD and vesicular stomatitis. PPR, sheep pox, orf and facial eczema must be considered in sheep and goats. On the whole there is a much lower mortality in FMD than in BTV. Facial swelling is much more marked in BVT compared with FMD. On the other hand vesicles and ulcers are characteristic of FMD but are less common in BTV. Clinicians should remember that FMD is highly infectious but BTV requires a vector.

There is no specific treatment for BTV. Antibiotics and NSAID are helpful, and nursing is vital. This should include offering water and mushy food, and providing deep bedding out of the sun and heat. Affected animals will never return to full production. There will be a lasting milk drop in milking goats and sheep, with an increase in mastitis. There is an increased incidence of lameness in all species. There will be long-term fertility problems including abortions, stillbirths, weak lambs and kids and early embryonic deaths. In fibre animals there will be wool loss and staple breaks. There is an increase in pneumonia cases and long-term 'poor doers'.

Since 1998 there have been 12 different invasions of BTV into Europe with 12 different vaccines required to help control them. The vaccines available are inactivated (dead) vaccines against specific serotypes. The most up-to-date are highly purified by liquid chromatography (see Chapter 7).

Foot and mouth disease

The clinical examination of sheep was among the many practical problems encountered during the 2001 pan-Asia type O FMD outbreak in the UK and was a cause for concern for many veterinary surgeons (Watson, 2004). The severity of FMD will vary markedly with the strain of virus, the breed of animal and the type of husbandry. The disease spectrum will range from unapparent infection detected only by subsequent flock serosurveillance through to high morbidity outbreaks with very noticeable diseased sheep and goats.

The main signs are lameness and reluctance to move. Excess salivation is rarely seen in sheep but is commonly seen in goats. A thorough examination of the whole flock will reveal the typical erosions and ulcers on the mouths and feet of a considerable number of animals. There will be a radical drop in milk yield in milking sheep and goats. Lambs and kids suckling their mothers will be crying and hungry. Several animals will be acutely ill with pyrexia. Recovery in sheep is quick, with the disease passing through the flock in a few days. Recovery is not quite so quick in goats. The earliest signs are vesicles – fluid-filled sacs within the epithelium. The fluid is clear, slightly yellow and slightly viscous. The vesicles are thin walled and therefore very transitory. Often the whole infection will only last 2 days in an individual sheep. Over 90% of sheep will have foot lesions and sudden severe lameness will be very evident. This is the commonest clinical sign associated with FMD in sheep and goats. Whole groups will frequently lie down and be very unwilling to rise. Diagnosis may be confused in young lambs which are showing the genetic condition of red foot, which is only seen in Blackface and Welsh Mountain sheep. These affected lambs will show mouth ulcers as well as the severe foot disease resulting in horn shedding. OMAGOD will also cause diagnostic problems later on in an outbreak. Serum will need to be tested for antibodies to confirm FMD. It is possible that FMD may be confused with BTV but careful assessment of clinical signs will clarify the diagnosis.

Sheep in particular are very important for disseminating the virus to other species, usually because there are delays in recognizing the clinical signs, which are often apparently mild. Continued close vigilance by flock owners and veterinary surgeons is therefore of the utmost importance in an outbreak.

The spread of FMD virus can occur in a number of ways. The most important is by direct contact between infected and susceptible livestock. However it can also occur with feeding infected milk, or using infected semen or embryos. The virus can be airborne or carried by people or species of animal not susceptible to the virus (e.g. sheep dogs), and can be carried by vehicles and any other fomites.

Virus production in infected animals remains high until antibodies develop at approximately 4–5 days post infection. Some animals will remain as carriers.

Malignant catarrhal fever

Malignant catarrhal fever (MCF) is a disease of cattle caused by a group of herpes viruses, including alcelaphine herpes virus 1 and ovine herpes virus 2. The most important is alcelaphine herpes virus 1. The normal host of this virus is the wildebeest (gnu), in which it is asymptomatic. The disease in cattle appears in the Masai cattle in Kenya and northern Tanzania at the time of the wildebeest calving season from the end of January to the beginning of March. Goats are not affected, but occasionally Masai sheep will show symptoms of lethargy and pyrexia. There is inflammation of the mucosal surfaces, mainly mouth necrosis and keratitis with conjunctivitis. Sheep are likely to recover unless they are suffering from malnutrition or some other disease. However, the UK sheep, in common with the wildebeest in Africa, are normally asymptomatic carriers. Cattle are the main host, and their prognosis is grave. Diagnosis is either with an ELISA or a PCR but there is no treatment or vaccine available.

Nairobi sheep disease

Nairobi sheep disease (NSD), which occurs in sheep and goats, is caused by a nairovirus. It is spread by ticks, mainly the brown ear tick, *Rhipicephalus appendiculatus*, and is mainly seen in areas in east Africa where this tick occurs. However, it has been reported in Botswana and the Congo, where it is spread by *Amblyomma variegatum*. Although the virus can be found in the urine and faeces it is not spread in these, but transovarially and trans-stadially by the brown ear tick. It can stay alive in the tick for more than 2 years.

It is a particularly deadly disease in sheep with up to 90% mortality in exotic breeds, and over 30% mortality in local breeds. Goats normally have a lower mortality.

The disease is acute, with illness shown within 5 days of being bitten by an infected tick. There is acute depression, high fever, mucopurulent haemorrhagic nasal discharge and haemorrhagic diarrhoea. Pregnant animals will abort. Petechiae and ecchymotic haemorrhages will be seen in the mucosa of the mouth. These same haemorrhages will be seen throughout the gastrointestinal tract on post-mortem. The lymph nodes throughout the body are swollen and oedematous.

Diagnosis can be made on clinical grounds and confirmed by blood samples for an ELISA test. There is no treatment. Prevention can be carried out by very strict twice-weekly dipping in a suitable acaricide or regular use of pour-on cypermethrin products. It is hoped that a vaccine will be prepared in the near future.

Peste des petits ruminants

PPR is caused by a *Morbillivirus* and is related to rinderpest, although unlike rinderpest it is not contagious to cattle. On the other hand rinderpest can affect goats but appears to be less virulent as the mortality rate may be as low as 50%, whereas the disease in cattle, in the author's experience, causes 100% mortality. However, rinderpest has now been totally eradicated. PPR is often termed goat plague. It is a disease with a high morbidity and mortality in goats, and affects sheep in the same way. It is seen in Africa, the Middle East, Central Asia and the Indian subcontinent. At the end of 2010 the Food and Agriculture Organization (FAO) was concerned about an outbreak in Tanzania that threatened over 13.5 million goats and 3.5 million sheep in that country. The FAO advised an emergency vaccination campaign around the disease outbreak, with further vaccination campaigns in the bordering areas of Malawi, Mozambique and Zambia. Sheep and goats are critical to food and income security for pastoral communities in sub-Saharan Africa. Clinicians should not be concerned that they will miss this disease as the signs are very obvious. There is high fever with erosions on the mucous membranes of the mouth and eyes, acute bloody diarrhoea and also signs of pneumonia. Whole herds will quickly become infected and the majority will die. There is no specific treatment, but oxytetracycline injections seem to reduce the number of deaths and NSAID may be useful. A vaccine is available for use in sheep and goats (see Chapter 7).

Rotavirus

Rotavirus spp. have been found in most farm animals in many countries, and seven serotypes are recognized. However, their pathogenicity in lambs and kids is not clear cut. They will definitely cause diarrhoea but often there is another pathogen isolated at the same time. This may be a bacteria, e.g. *E. coli*, or a protozoa such as coccidia. Clinicians cannot treat the virus so attention should be drawn to the other pathogen.

Bacterial Diseases Affecting the Gastroenteric Tract

General

Physiological diarrhoea is seen in lambs and kids, particularly in bottle-fed animals. The signs are normally self-limiting.

Clostridial disease

Clostridial diseases are important in all mammals but are particularly important in sheep. They are also are important in goats but there are some differences. There has been less research carried out in goats.

Bacillary haemoglobinuria

This has been reported in sheep in the UK but it is rare. Actually it is primarily a disease of cattle in central Ireland and is sometimes called bacterial redwater; it is caused by *Clostridium haemolyticum*. This is a disease of older sheep, which may be found dead or severely ill. The disease occurs in areas of high rainfall, particularly when summers are wet. Haemoglobinuria is the main sign in sheep. Aggressive treatment with penicillin and fluid therapy, particularly whole blood, may be successful in pet sheep and goats. On post-mortem anaemic liver infarcts are pathognomic for the condition in both sheep and goats.

Blackleg

Caused by *Clostridium chauvoei*, this is primarily a disease of cattle. The disease in sheep is extremely rare in the UK; this may be because immunization against the disease is usually included in a multivalent vaccine. The disease in sheep may follow shearing wounds and dog bites. The disease is much more common in Africa, where it is found in hair sheep and goats. The organism is common in the soil. The first sign shown in sheep and goats is lameness, and on careful examination the animal will show a very swollen painful area over a wound.

Treatment with high doses of penicillin and NSAID is rarely successful.

Black's disease

The correct name for this condition is infectious necrotic hepatitis. It is caused by *Clostridium novyi* type B. It is relatively common in sheep and is also seen in goats. The trigger factor is acute fluke, that is, the migration of immature flukes through the liver. Acute fluke occurs in sheep in the autumn. In theory acute fluke could occur in goats but they tend to get the chronic form. Control can easily be carried out by vaccinating all animals against *Cl. novyi* type B. Fluke control is vital not only to prevent Black's disease but also to prevent the damage caused by the flukes in the liver.

Botulism

Unlike the previous two conditions, the organism *Clostridium botulinum* multiplies in the soil and in silage, and not in the sheep or in the goat. The organism produces toxin outside the body, so the severity of the disease will relate to the amount of toxin ingested. Sheep are more resistant to the toxin than are goats; they are more fastidious than goats and do not eat silage contaminated with soil. The author has seen a flock of sheep affected with botulism in Western Australia that had a mortality of over 50%. The animals had been in drought conditions and there was no association with silage feeding. Diagnosis is not difficult if the pathognomic sign of a flaccid anus is seen when you take the rectal temperature. There is no specific treatment, but animals will recover if they can be kept alive with oral fluids.

Braxy

This disease, caused by *Clostridium septicum*, only occurs in sheep. It appears to be a 'British disease', as the author has discussed it with European colleagues and they are unfamiliar with the condition. Australian, New Zealand and South African veterinarians have not recorded the disease either. The trigger factor is thought to be eating frosted root crops. In the UK, these are classically fed in Norfolk throughout the winter, and include stubble turnips and sugarbeet tops. When they are consumed in a frosted condition they cause an abomasitis, which is thought to allow entry of *Cl. septicum*. *Cl. septicum* is included in several polyvalent vaccines. This disease has not been recorded in goats.

Enterotoxaemia

Enterotoxaemia is more commonly called pulpy kidney and is caused by *Clostridium perfringens* type D. It is a sheep disease, but it is also a very common disease in goats. It is the most common clostridial disease in the UK, and can be found in growing lambs in commercial flocks that have not been vaccinated adequately. The toxoid is included in **all** the vaccines and so there is little excuse for vaccination failure. However, these are the main reasons for lack of or inadequate vaccination:

- The sheep keeper erroneously assumes that lambs from vaccinated mothers will be covered until they reach slaughter weight. This is not the case, and lambs from vaccinated mothers should have their first dose of vaccine by 10 weeks of age followed by a second dose 4–6 weeks later.
- Lambs from unvaccinated mothers should be vaccinated as early as 4 weeks of age, with a second dose 4–6 weeks later. Where the risk is very high (e.g. in the orchards in Kent) a dose of vaccine should be given within the first 2 days of life.
- Lambs are often sold at weaning and given the first dose of vaccine. They are then said to be 'vaccinated', which is not the case because the second dose is required. If the administration of the second dose is unduly delayed the whole vaccination should be started again.

Some hobby farmers have a complete mental block with vaccination, and this ignorance is not acceptable from a welfare stance. Enterotoxaemia can actually occur in any aged, unvaccinated sheep. It is associated with growing sheep but in pet sheep the disease can occur at any time.

The disease is normally manifest by sudden death, although observant keepers will see sick, cold, moribund animals. There is no treatment. Diagnosis will not pose a problem on post-mortem. The abdomen, pleural cavity and pericardium will be filled with fluid, usually bloody. The kidneys will be friable as the common name suggests. There is a high level of sugar in the urine, which can be tested by a small animal dipstick.

Lamb dysentery

This is a rare condition in commercial flocks because of vaccination. It does not seem to occur in hobby flocks. It is caused by *Cl. perfringens* type B. It is a disease of young lambs, which often die before they develop dysentery. The only method of control is to have lambs born from fully vaccinated ewes. The ewes need to have received a booster injection 4–6 weeks prior to lambing. Obviously the lamb needs to have received adequate colostrum in the first 12 h of life to achieve passive immunity. It is not seen in goats.

Malignant oedema

This disease, found in goats as well as sheep, is caused by several clostridial organisms: *Cl. septicum*, *Cl. chauvoei*, *Cl. perfringens* and *Cl. novyi*. Animals can be found dead or *in extremis*. They show swellings, which are often gaseous. The disease may follow wounds obtained by rams fighting, when it is often called 'big head disease'. In goats the organism may gain entrance at parturition and cause massive swelling of the hindquarters. Aggressive treatment with penicillin and NSAID may be successful if started promptly.

Sordellii abomasitis

Clostridium sordellii causes disease in sheep and goats. It produces two toxins; one is haemolytic and the other is lethal. It attacks the abomasums of sheep and has different manifestations in the various age groups. In young lambs over 3 weeks of age it will cause acute abomasitis, and in older lambs it will cause sudden death from abomasitis. In adults it will cause sudden death or abomasitis that leads to death, often from ulceration and peritonitis. This manifestation is seen in goats. A vaccine is now available that is recommended in sheep and goats. As the same vaccine is prepared for cattle, it should be pointed out that there are two different dosages: 2 ml per dose for cattle, and 1 ml for sheep. Goats should receive the sheep dose.

Struck

This disease is common in Kent but very rare elsewhere in the UK. It is caused by *Cl. perfringens* type C. As the name suggests, it causes sudden death. There is no standard trigger factor. However, I think it is likely that the very heavily fertilized grass under fruit trees is the culprit. *Cl. perfringens* type C has been recorded in goats.

Tetanus

The causative organism, *Clostridium tetani*, is well known, as is its pathogenesis. In the author's experience it is now very rare in sheep, mainly owing to vaccination. It can occur following castration and tail docking in pet sheep, which are often unvaccinated. It is common in goats. All young disbudded kids should receive tetanus antitoxin. Stiffness and rigor will be seen before the jaws become clamped together. Initial treatment should be large doses of TAT and also large doses of penicillin. Animals may recover if they are given adequate nursing.

***Escherichia coli* O157**

This is not a pathogen in sheep or goats, but is carried by them and therefore poses a danger to man. The commensal bacterium of concern is VTEC O157:H7. It causes no clinical signs in small ruminants but precautions must be taken by farmers, particularly those with farms open to the general public. In the UK routine testing found it to be present in the faeces samples of approximately 3% of small ruminants (see Chapter 19).

Escherichia coli pathogenic to neonates

Historically this disease was rare in lambs because of their extensive husbandry and the relatively rare birth of triplets. That is not the case today, when the majority of lambs are born inside or in lambing pens in polythene tunnels. Triplets are common. Lambs are often not just hand reared but are batch suckled on plastic feeders. Coupled to this, shepherding is not so traditional, so that sheep keepers – particularly hobby farmers and non-commercial owners – may have less experience. Pathogenic *E. coli* will also occur in kids.

Basically, *E. coli* infection is largely about poor management rather than virulent pathogens. The old adage 'a lamb that has had adequate colostrum is hard to kill and a lamb that has not is hard to save', still holds good. *E. coli* are the normal inhabitants of a lamb's intestine. In the second day of life a healthy lamb will have 10^{10} *E. coli* bacteria/g of its faeces.

Lambs will harbour the *E. coli* bacteria with the K99 antigen, but these enterotoxigenic *E. coli* are rare. However, they may be found in 2% of flocks and in these flocks lamb mortality as high as 75% has been recorded. With this disease there is nearly always a septicaemia. The condition may be peracute so that death may occur before the lamb is seen to scour. Isolation of the organism from heart blood is diagnostic. Often colostrum will be seen in the stomach but will be unclotted. Forty per cent of these strains of *E. coli* are resistant to ampicillin. Amoxicillin with clavulonic acid is likely to be the antibiotic of choice; in the author's experience oral combinations of neomycin and streptomycin are not effective. There is no licensed *E. coli* vaccine available in the UK.

Having said that, colibacillosis caused by pathogenic organisms is rare in lambs. There is a much more common condition in which *E. coli* plays a role: 'watery mouth'.

This condition is much more common in triplets than in singles or twins. It is also more common in male lambs. The main cause is likely to be a lack of sufficiently good quality colostrum within the first 6h of life. The weakest triplet, or a ram lamb that has had a rubber ring put on too soon, is obviously at risk. Interestingly, lambs born to ewes that are penned up separately straight after birth are more at risk. This does not seem logical, as one would assume such lambs would be more likely to get adequate colostrum. The reason is therefore unclear. Obviously there is likely to be a build-up of *E. coli* in the pens, and watery mouth cases increase later in the lambing season. Colostrum certainly has a protective effect, not only physically as it has a laxative property, but also by giving immunity to strains of *E. coli*. Watery mouth outbreaks can be controlled by giving antibiotics by mouth or by injection soon after birth as a prophylactic. However the best advice would be to avoid such a regime as it will increase antibiotic-resistant strains of *E. coli*. It may also increase the number of strains with the K99 antigen. A better method of control would be to change the husbandry practices as follows:

- Rubber rings should not be put either on the tail or the scrotum until the lambs have received sufficient colostrum. Triplets are most at risk. There are many proprietary brands of colostrum available if the ewe does not have sufficient. This should be administered by stomach tube if the lamb does not have a good sucking reflex. (The use of cow colostrum is too hazardous and the method of freezing yoghurt pots of the colostrum from ewes with singles too labour-intensive except in the smallest of flocks.)
- If ewes are being lambed under cover it is vital that there is sufficient space for them. It is vital that there is a good **dry** bed (*E. coli* delights in wet straw) fully refreshed in each lambing pen after each ewe moves out. Ewes and lambs if possible should be turned out within 48h.
- Ewes with their lambs must be checked several times a day to see that all the lambs are feeding.

To sum up, *E. coli* is not a major pathogen in lambs but its importance should not be discounted. Good management is vital. Antibiotics should not be used to supplement bad management.

Similar advice should be given to large goat herds if *E. coli* infection becomes a problem.

Johne's disease

Johne's disease occurs throughout the world. It has actually only been recorded in a relatively few countries in sheep and in a much larger number of countries in goats, wherever they are kept. It is reasonable to conclude that it is a danger to sheep and goats everywhere. Johne's disease primarily is a pathogen of cattle but the strains affecting small ruminants tend to be fairly species specific, but clinicians should not be complacent and should always beware of the dangers. Milk or colostrum from infected cows, for example, should not be fed to small ruminants, and colostrum from one species of small ruminant should not be fed to another species. In cattle the main sign is diarrhoea. This is not the case in small ruminants, which tend to suffer ill thrift. In all animals, the disease is always fatal once clinical signs develop. On very rare occasions certain animals will show signs of remission, but these will be short lived and deterioration will soon set in. Euthanasia is the only option. It should be remembered that there is thought to be a link between Johne's disease in animals and Crohn's disease in man, and therefore the carcasses from animals affected with Johne's disease should not go for human consumption. Normally the small ruminant has become so emaciated that the carcass is not worthwhile anyway. It should also be remembered that the bacteria will survive pasteurization for 15 s and so the holding time for pasteurization for milk has to be increased to 25 s.

The normal method of transmission is from dam to offspring soon after birth through colostrum, milk and faeces. Transplacental infection can also occur, particularly in animals showing advanced signs of ill thrift.

Johne's disease can be diagnosed by an ELISA blood test, which is fairly sensitive once the animal shows signs of the disease. However it is too insensitive to be used as a screening test in clinically normal animals. Faecal smears stained with Ziehl–Neelsen have a high specificity but a sensitivity of only 30%, as shedding of the organism is very intermittent in small ruminants. The strains found in small ruminants are very difficult to grow on culture. They are particularly slow growing and can take over 3 months to grow. The use of liquid cultures may speed up a positive diagnosis but 3 months is required for a negative result, which may not be particularly sensitive.

Clinicians might think that a post-mortem examination would be definitive, but gross pathology is not very reliable. There may be granulomatous lesions in the intestines and local lymph nodes but these may not be obvious. Histology from multiple sites is vital. The key point about this disease in sheep and goats is that it is difficult to diagnose and is **not** manifest as diarrhoea as in cattle. However, as in cattle, the disease is likely to be present in many more situations than would be imagined, and it may not be clinically apparent until the animal is not only an adult but has had several offspring.

Control of Johne's disease in goats is possible using the Weybridge vaccine. Kids should be given half the cattle dose into the brisket at less than 4 weeks of age. Owners should be warned of the unsightly lumps that may occur at the site of injection. Snatching kids at birth to ensure adequate colostral intake from known negative dams and rearing them artificially away from the dam's environment is worthwhile. It is vital to maintain clean rearing environments for kids. The infection may be spread congenitally as well as via infected milk and colostrum, and so family line culling may be worth considering. All floor feeding should be stopped and all the water troughs should be raised.

Protozoal Diseases Affecting the Gastroenteric Tract

Coccidiosis in sheep

Coccidiosis is confusing in lambs as they become more susceptible to coccidiosis just at the stage when their protective immunity to cryptosporidiosis has developed. There are 11 species of *Eimeria* that are thought to be pathogenic in lambs. The most serious are *E. crandallis* and *E. ovinoidalis*. Their primary site of infection is the ileum but they also cause damage to the colon and the caecum, and the resultant oedema damages the gut wall. Haemorrhage and villus atrophy occur, reducing fluid absorption and causing diarrhoea. *E. crandallis* causes grey mucoid faeces and *E. ovinoidalis* causes more haemorrhage. Nodular lesions are often seen; these are of doubtful significance but are thought to be formed by *Eimeria bakuensis*. This species is not thought to be very pathogenic in the UK but causes problems in Central Asia. All these species of *Eimeria* that are pathogenic in sheep have oocysts that are relatively small, no larger than 30 µm. This contrasts with coccidia in goats.

There is a complex clinical picture with all species of coccidia. Several species may be involved, and there may be other pathogens such as *Rotavirus*. The nutritional status of the lamb is critical and of course there are stress factors such as transport, muddy conditions (particularly around the water supply) and a sudden change of diet, usually a flush of grass (Fig. 10.4).

Lambs become infected with oocysts early in life, but as they have a long prepatent period, often in excess of 28 days, clinical signs appear much later after the infection has built up. It is important for the clinician to be aware of this as the cause for the outbreak may well be historical and not apparent to the shepherd. Clinicians also ought to judge high oocyst counts with caution, as they may be boosted by non-pathogenic species. At the other end of the spectrum, acute or even fatal disease may occur before significant numbers of oocysts of pathogenic species appear in the faeces. Laboratory findings must be linked with clinical findings. Sadly, a firm diagnosis may require a post-mortem with a mucosal scraping. Control of coccidiosis must be a balance: animals need sufficient infection to produce immunity, but not enough to cause clinical disease. Low stocking densities and good hygiene with dry bedding are all required for lambs indoors. Outside, it is vital to avoid muddy areas around the water supply and creep feeders.

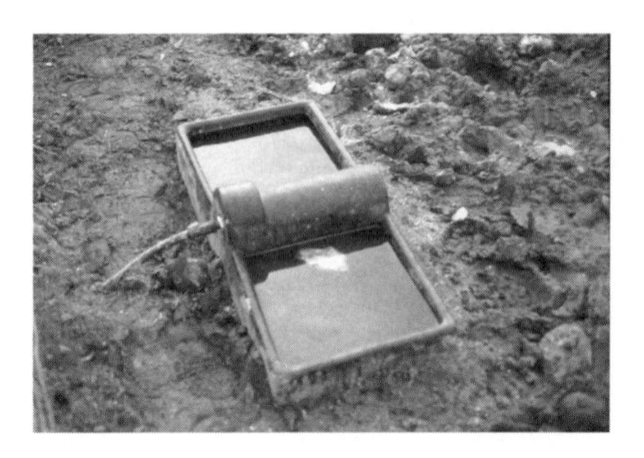

Fig. 10.4. Muddy water trough.

The numbers of oocysts excreted into the environment by the ewes can be controlled around lambing time by a prophylactic dose of decoquinate in their feed. It is possible that this will reduce the passive immunity passed on to the lambs with their colostrum, so timing is important. It needs to be fed exactly at lambing and not too early. Of course decoquinate can be fed to the lambs in their creep continuously over the 28 days when they are most at risk. Once again, this may delay the build-up of the lambs' own premunity, so that an outbreak of coccidiosis may occur 10 days after the decoquinate is withdrawn. Ideally the lambs should be moved onto fresh, clean grazing on the day the decoquinate is withdrawn.

Decoquinate is not the only medicine available. Diclazuril and toltrazuril, together with the more old-fashioned sulfadimidine, can be used. Diclazuril is given orally and can be used not only to prevent coccidiosis but also to treat the disease. On the whole it is best to treat the whole group rather than just the clinically affected lambs. Clinicians should warn shepherds that initially the diarrhoea may get worse straight after treatment, as the drugs acts on multiple stages of the life cycle. There is a rapid release of antigen leading to good development of immunity. Whole-group therapy is also advised for toltrazuril treatment. This oral treatment can be used to reduce oocyte production and clinical signs. Naturally the availability of both of these drugs should not be an excuse for poor hygiene. Treatment with sulfadimidine by injection is considerably cheaper, but requires daily injections for 3 days (see Chapter 6).

Whatever treatment is given to kill the coccidia it must be a recommendation that oral rehydration therapy is carried out at the same time for the badly affected animals.

Coccidiosis in goats

Coccidia are host specific, unlike coccidiasina. It is therefore sensible to discuss each of the infections in small ruminates separately. There does not appear to be any crossover between lambs and kids.

Numerous *Eimeria* species are found in goats worldwide. They have very variable pathogenicity. The picture is complex as often there are mixed infections of coccidia and/or mixed infections with other pathogens. The clinician needs to be careful that the diagnosis of coccidiosis is correct. When there are large faecal oocyst counts it is easy to assume that coccidia are the cause of the diarrhoea, only to find that these are a relatively non-pathogenic strain and the real cause is an enteric virus. Equally, only a relatively modest oocyst count of a highly pathogenic strain such as *Eimeria ninakohlakimovae*, which is found worldwide and is equivalent to the sheep pathogen *E. ovinoidalis*, would be highly significant. Clinicians are faced with another problem. A relatively mild pathogenic strain (e.g. *Eimeria kocharli*) may actually cause severe disease when the challenge is overwhelming and the affected animals have a very low premunity. The author has experience of a large outbreak in pedigree goats that had been brought down to the coast of Kenya from up-country. They had been severely stressed by a horrendous journey of over 400 miles that took over a week on account of 35.5cm (14 inches) of rain falling in 24h. They had been mixed with local goats, and mortality was over 95%. Only a single species of pathogen was ever isolated. In Central Asia, in contrast, workers in Iran (Razavi and Hassanvand, 2007) found that 84.5% of goats in an outbreak were infected with several species of *Eimeria*. Pathogenic strains of coccidia and non-pathogenic strains of coccidia tend to have oocysts that are relatively small, like oocysts found in sheep. They are rarely larger than 30μm, except *E. kocharli*, which is nearly 50μm. The very common *Eimeria christenseni* is nearly 40μm. *E. christenseni* is found world-wide but *E. kocharli* is restricted to Africa and Central Asia.

In general coccidiosis in kids causes relatively mild signs of diarrhoea, or pasty faeces, loss of condition or failure to thrive and grow. The signs tend to become more severe as more kids are brought through the system and the environment becomes more contaminated. The signs may also be severe when there is very poor hygiene or in artificially reared animals. In the latter case it is vital that hygiene is of a very high standard.

Several studies have suggested that coccidiosis is one of the most important diseases of kids, especially in their first 3 months of life. However it is important for clinicians to differentiate between infection and disease. All kids become infected with coccidia but their presence does not necessarily lead to the development of clinical signs of disease and, in many situations, low levels of challenge can actually be beneficial by stimulating protective immune responses in the kid. Development is particularly dependent on husbandry and management.

As with lambs, the most pathogenic species of coccidia are those that infect and destroy the crypt cells of the large intestinal mucosa. Coccidia that invade the large intestine are more likely to cause pathological changes, particularly if large numbers of oocysts are ingested over a short period of time. The rate of cellular turnover is slower in the large intestine and there is no further intestine caudally to compensate. In heavily infected kids, the mucosa becomes completely denuded of cells, resulting in severe haemorrhage and impaired water resorption, leading to diarrhoea, dehydration and death.

To control the disease kids should be in small groups and age matched. If possible they should also be size matched. Regularly moved, portable pens are ideal. Eradication is not possible and coccidiostats such as decoquinate should not be used as a substitute for good management. The dose of decoquinate is 0.5mg/kg/day for up to 28 days. Monensin is another useful drug as a preventative in goats. It should be given at a dose rate of 1mg/kg/day. It is **not** licensed in the UK and should not be used as the cascade principle would be broken. However, elsewhere it can be used daily for 1 month. Strategic dosing can be carried out for 5-day periods with amprolium at a dose rate of 50 mg/kg. Once again this is **not** licensed for use in the UK. There is a risk of kids developing cerebrocortico necrosis (CCN) (see Chapter 14) with this treatment for coccidiosis.

The clinical picture is confusing as a neurological type of coccidiosis has been described in kids. The author has had personal experience with this condition in east Africa. The kids develop severe diarrhoea, which develops into tenesmus and dysentery. If the kids are chilled they become extremely depressed, and become incoordinate with muscle tremors. They will appear to be blind. Finally they develop convulsions and die.

Cryptosporidiosis

In 2010 the incidence of this disease in lambs was found to be rising in the UK, having dropped in 2007 and 2008. The morbidity in many outbreaks has been as high as 10%, and some farms have recorded morbidity rates of 50%. The reason for this increase is likely to be the poor wet weather in the spring delaying turn-out of ewes with lambs at foot.

Cryptosporidiosis is the result of an infection caused by a protozoan of the genus *Cryptosporidium*. There are as many as 16 species. However few of them are pathogenic to domestic animals and small ruminants in particular. The most important species is *Cryptosporidium parvum*. This will cause diarrhoea in lambs and will also affect humans, although the most important species in humans is *Cryptosporidium hominis* (see Chapter 19). *C. parvum* has a direct life cycle with infection occurring by the faecal–oral route. Normally the infection in lambs and kids is not a monoinfection but more commonly a mixed infection with other pathogens. The highest mortality rates in lambs occur between 4 and 10 days. Kids are infected a little later and the highest mortality rates occur between 5 and 21 days. Obviously it is impossible to ascertain whether the deaths are due to the *Cryptosporidium* or to another pathogen. The oocysts are fully sporulated and infective when they are excreted in the faeces. Very large numbers are excreted during the prepatent period, resulting in heavy environmental contamination. Transmission can occur directly from lamb to lamb or indirectly via a fomite, which may be a human. Infection can result from faecal contamination of food or water. For bottle-fed lambs or kids, infection can be via contaminated milk. For suckling lambs or kids, infection can occur from dirty contaminated teats. Ewes and does can contaminate the environment, because if they are harbouring *C. parvum* they will show a periparturient rise in oocyst excretion. Oocysts are resistant to most disinfectants and can survive for several months in cool and moist conditions. Their infectivity can be destroyed by ammonia, formalin, freeze-drying and exposure to temperatures below freezing and above 65°C. The contamination of the environment rises sharply as the lambing continues. Lambs born later in the season are more at risk, particularly if colostrum intake is low. Age-related resistance unrelated to prior exposure is observed in lambs. This does not occur in kids. Case fatality rates in cryptosporidiosis are generally very low unless another pathogen such as a *Rotavirus* is also involved. The possibility of auto-infection should not be ruled out in lambs or kids, nor should an infection from calves either nearby or when they have been housed in the shed earlier in the year. The infectious dose of *C. parvum* oocysts for a neonate is very low.

In clinical cases in all small ruminant neonates, the faeces tend to be pale and liquid. Fresh blood may be seen but tenesmus is not a feature. In severe cases the animal will be depressed and dehydrated. Lambs may show abdominal pain but this is rare, and it is much more common in kids. The condition is easy to diagnose as large numbers of oocysts will be seen in the infected faeces. Ziehl–Neelsen is a useful stain as the oocysts are small and relatively nonrefractile.

Control of the condition requires attention to detail in all aspects of hygiene to lessen cross contamination and auto-infection. Halofuginone lactate can be used for prophylaxis and treatment. It is licensed for use in cattle in the UK. It is available as an oral solution containing 0.5 mg/ml of halofuginone lactate. The dose is 2 ml/kg/day for 7 days.

At the end of the lambing season it is vital to steam clean the building. This should also be carried out in goat houses.

Cryptosporidiosis does not seem to be a problem in adult sheep or goats, only in young animals.

In conclusion it should be stressed that cryptosporidiosis is a zoonotic disease. Naturally shepherds and goat keepers must be warned. However, what is more important is that members of the public – particularly children – must adopt strict hygiene measures. These must be prepared and displayed in writing on farms that are opened to the public commercially.

Giardia

This is a zoonotic pathogenic protozoan that is transmitted by the faecal–oral route. It can affect sheep and goats, but only in young animals, where it is associated with diarrhoea. It does not affect adults. However it can affect adult humans as well as children (see Chapter 19). It has a long maturation period of 2 or more weeks so it is not found in lambs or kids under 4 weeks of age. It is rare that it actually causes disease in animals unless there is massive environmental contamination. This usually occurs when wildlife contaminates the drinking pond. The organism has a predilection for the small intestine. Treatment should be either with fenbendazole at 10 mg/kg orally for 3 days, or metronidizole at 25 mg/kg given either orally or as an enema for 3 days.

Sarcocystis

This parasite is seen all over the USA and in South America. It has only been seen in imported animals in the UK. It is spread by dogs and wild carnivores and so safe carcass disposal is vital to prevent the spread of the organism. Small ruminants are the intermediate hosts. They may exhibit a variety of signs, such as anaemia, fever, vasculitis, myositis, abortion, chronic wasting and sudden death. However these signs are so diverse that the disease is rarely diagnosed in life.

Parasitic Diseases of the Gastroenteric Tract

Intestinal cestodes

Adult tapeworms such as *Moniezia expansa* occur in sheep and goats, and can be found in the latter if they are running with sheep. This species is found throughout the world. *Moniezia benedeni* and *Thysaniesia giardi* are found in sheep and goats in Peru. The secondary host is an oribatid mite found on the pasture. The prepatent period is 40 days. Some authorities suggest that they are of no clinical significance, but in large numbers they may cause ill thrift, and intussusceptions have been reported on post-mortem. They are well controlled with albendazole. Other species found in sheep and goats in the semitropical areas of Africa and Asia are of the genus *Avitellina*. In the tropical areas of these continents there are no oribatid mites, but psocid mites are found. The latter act as secondary hosts to *Stilesia globipuncta*. These tapeworms are also controlled by albendazole and are rarely associated with clinical disease. Two further tapeworms can be considered here. They do not actually live in the intestines but in the bile ducts and the pancreatic ducts. They are considerably smaller and their presence often goes unnoticed. These are *Stilesia hepatica* and *Thysanosoma actinioides*. They occur in tropical areas of Asia and Africa. The latter species is also found in the Rocky Mountains in North America. Control is not easy, and weekly dosing with double-strength albendazole for three treatments is recommended. Both these species cause clinical signs which vary from mild diarrhoea to violent diarrhoea and liver failure signs. Liver enzymes will be raised in serum samples.

Those tapeworms that have sheep and goats as secondary hosts form metacestodes (see Table 10.1). It should be remembered that the metacestode stages of *Taenia multiceps*, referred to as *Coenurus cerebralis*, cause 'gid' in sheep and goats (see Chapter 14). They are also found in the muscles and subcutaneous tissues, as well as the brain. The metacestode stages of *Taenia hydatigena*, referred to as *Cysticercus tenuicollis*, occur in sheep and

Table 10.1. Metacestodes found in sheep and goats.

Cestode species	Primary host	Metacestode species name	Where found in the secondary host	Comment
Echinococcus granulosus	Small carnivores	Hydatid	Abdomen and pleural cavity	Very common worldwide with a high zoonotic risk
Taenia hydatigena	Small carnivores	*Cysticercus tenuicollis*	Travel through the liver to end in the mesentery	Deaths have been reported in goats from damage due to migration through the liver
Taenia multiceps	Small carnivores	*Coenurus cerebralis*	Brain, muscles and subcutaneous tissue	Will cause gid (neurological condition; see Chapter 14)
Taenia ovis	Small carnivores	*Cysticercus ovis*	Heart and skeletal muscles	Asymptomatic

rarely in goats. In very rare cases these may result in acute manifestation and death. Hydatid disease or echinococcosis due to *Echinococcus granulosus* occurs frequently in sheep in the UK, but only rarely in goats. This is not the pattern elsewhere in the world, where *E. granulosus* is very common in goats.

Cysticercosis was seen in 7% of 9000 lambs reared in Somerset on a single holding in 2009 (Eichenberger *et al.*, 2011). The infection was linked to footpath contamination by dogs.

Intestinal nematodes

Many nematodes are found in sheep and goats, and the principal species are shown in Table 10.2. Practitioners, like the owners of small ruminants, need to radically change their thinking on the control of intestinal nematodes. The old instructions about regular use of anthelmintics should be totally discarded. Animals should only be treated if they need to be treated. The difficulty for practitioners and farmers is the problem of knowing when they need to be treated. The overuse of anthelmintics has brought on universal resistance to the three standard types of anthelmintic. It is vital that the new class, which has recently been released, is not rendered useless by overuse and the build-up of resistance. One of the main new instructions is that no animal must be underdosed. So if animals are in a group, it is important that the dose is worked out for the largest animal in the group and that is the dose used for the whole group. Certain anthelmintics have a narrow safety range (e.g. levamisole in goats), so it is important that accurate weighing and dosing is carried out. This will not be a problem in small herds where each animal can be treated as an individual. However in larger herds, if there is a marked difference in size then it is important that the dosing groups can be small enough to accommodate the variations. In Africa and Central Asia sheep and goats are run in large groups of mixed species. In many ways this is ideal as helminths are not a problem in large tracts of Africa where there are a large number of different species grazing the same land. However when dosing animals with anthelmintics, it is important that the species are separated and the correct weights for the two groups are estimated accurately. When decisions have to be made regarding the need for worming, it is also important that the two species groups are treated separately. Equally, it must be remembered that there is a close crossover of helminth species between sheep and goats and therefore there will be a crossover of resistant species of worms between sheep and goats.

In both sheep and goats it is vital to separate animals into age groups, as the need for dosing will be different for most situations. However, clinicians should remember that

Table 10.2. Intestinal nematodes in sheep and goats.

Where found in the animal	Helminth species	Comments
Abomasum	*Haemonchus contortus*	Causes life-threatening anaemia
Abomasum	*Ostertagia circumcincta*	Common, causing clinical disease of diarrhoea and weight loss
Abomasum	*Ostertagia leptospicularis*	Infections caught from deer
Abomasum	*Ostertagia trifurcata*	Common, causing clinical disease of diarrhoea and weight loss
Abomasum	*Skrjabinagia kolchida*	Infections caught from deer
Abomasum	*Teladorsagia davtiani*	Common, causing clinical disease of diarrhoea and weight loss
Abomasum	*Trichostrongylus axei*	Very common; also seen in equids
Small intestine	*Bunostomum trigonocephalum*	Uncommon, but will cause serious disease
Small intestine	*Capillaria longipes*	Often seen but rarely of clinical significance in sheep or goats
Small intestine	*Cooperia curticei*	Common, often causing clinical signs of diarrhoea
Small intestine	*Cooperia onocophora*	Caught from cattle and may cause clinical signs
Small intestine	*Moniezia expansa*	Very common in sheep and goats. Only significant in high numbers
Small intestine	*Nematodirus battus*	A life-threatening disease of lambs and kids
Small intestine	*Nematodirus filicollis*	Common, and may well cause clinical disease
Small intestine	*Nematodirus spathiger*	Common, and may well cause clinical disease
Small intestine	*Strongyloides papillous*	Will cause clinical disease in young kids
Small intestine	*Trichostrongylus colubriformis*	Common cause of clinical disease
Small intestine	*Trichostrongylus vitrinus*	Common cause of clinical disease
Large intestine	*Oesophagostomum venulosum*	Common, but causes little disease
Large intestine	*Trichuris ovis*	Common, but of no clinical significance
Large intestine	*Chabertia ovis*	Uncommon; of no clinical significance
Large intestine	*Skrjabinema ovis*	Very common oxyurid parasite

where *Haemonchus contortus* is involved it is likely that all the animals are to be treated, regardless of age and, indeed, of species. To complicate the situation further, the hormonal state of the females must be considered. Historically it was thought that there was a rise in faecal egg output by ewes in the spring. This was called the 'spring rise'. It is now known that parturition, not spring, was the trigger. This position is the same with goats. Ewes and does have a post-parturient rise, which is not related to the season of the year, the coming of the rains, nor the hemisphere where the small ruminants are kept.

In sheep and goats it is important to remember that helminths should not be considered in isolation. The clinician has a goal of maintaining the status quo; this means that each animal has a relatively small worm burden so that it maintains some immunity to a large worm burden, but does not suffer disease or subclinical disease. This balance is much easier to attain if the nutritional status of the grazing, particularly the amount of protein available to the animal, is adequate. The provision of sufficient minerals and trace elements will also help to maintain the status quo.

The aim of the practitioner and the small ruminant keeper must be to minimize the use of anthelmintic treatment. Anthelmintics should **only** be used when it is necessary to prevent clinical disease. In this way the rate of selection for resistance will be reduced and drug efficacy will be preserved for as long as possible. To do this it is important that the number of worms in **refugia** is increased. Worms that are not selected by anthelmintic treatment are said to be in refugia. This refers to those worms whose larvae are on the pasture, or are at stages in animals not affected by treatment, or worms in untreated animals. The larger the population of worms in refugia, compared with the population of worms exposed to treatment, the slower resistance will develop. After treatment there are always some worms that survive in the host; these are resistant worms. If the offspring of these worms are in the majority, resistance to the anthelmintic will develop rapidly. To prevent resistance developing, a substantial number of worms need to be left untreated each time anthelmintics are used, so that essentially these non-resistant worms provide the subsequent generations of worms. It is now considered that where sheep and goats are continually exposed to worms it is a good idea to have a few worms inside the animal. These not only help develop a form of immunity, but also prolong the effectiveness of the available anthelmintics. The selective treatment of animals significantly increases the percentage of the worms in refugia.

Every holding and every group of animals must be considered separately; there should be no blanket treatments. In fact effective worm control prevents unnecessary dosing, which is also good economically. However it is vital to prevent resistant worms being brought on to a holding. Therefore in a closed or semi-closed situation the aim with any new animals is total deworming. This may involve a combination of the 'old' three wormers given at the correct dosage or the 'new' wormer recently available. Drugs may be given at the same time but should not be actually mixed. After drenching the animals should be housed, or at least kept off the pasture for 48h to allow any eggs that are still viable to be shed. The new animals can then be introduced onto the pasture grazed originally to pick up the 'non-resistant' worms and thus dilute any resistant worms.

Controlled grazing methods will help to avoid infection. Grazing animals on corn aftermath as practised in Central Asia is an excellent method of avoiding infection. Any method of allowing pastures to rest will be beneficial, as soil organisms such as earthworms, dung beetles and nematophagous fungi will reduce pasture burdens. Mixed species (e.g. rabbits and horses) will also be helpful. Cattle grazing will also help, but some species of helminth cross between cattle and sheep, or between cattle and goats, so practitioners should not give blanket advice but continue to monitor the situation. Preventing close cropping of grass is good, as rarely do worms climb more than 3cm up the stems. The ideal control of pastures is to plough and have a break crop such as lucerne or kale. Making hay also helps pasture contamination considerably but, like resting a pasture for a year, is not totally effective. Resting a pasture for only 3 years can be considered totally effective. Of course zero grazing is the ultimate method of control and may be considered in large milking herds of sheep or goats. Small young ruminants are most at risk, so it is important to protect them from contaminated pastures and also to remember that their mothers will be contaminating the pasture on account of the 'post-parturient rise phenomenon'. Each flock or herd has different problems, but various ideas can be put forward to the owner. The time of parturition can be altered. This is relatively easy in sheep and goats, with their 5-month gestation period. Parturition can be carried out indoors and turn-out delayed until their mothers' faecal egg output is lower and the over-wintered larvae have died on the pasture.

The minimum frequency of dosing should be used, and as stated earlier the correct dose must be used to avoid underdosing. The dose of the anthelmintic has been tested in sheep so that is not a problem provided the sheep are weighed. It should be stressed that **only anthelmintics licensed for sheep should be used** (not products licensed for cattle or horses). The problem lies with goats, which have no licensed products. General advice for goats would be to use twice the sheep dose with benzamidazoles and avermectins, which have a wide safety margin. As stated earlier, levamisole does not have a wide safety margin and so the dose can be increased to 1.5 times the sheep dose but no higher than this. Deciding when to change anthelmintics is problematic. The most up-to-date advice must be only to rotate drugs when resistance is suspected, not on an annual basis. Faecal egg outputs should be monitored. It is important to sample individuals and not a bulked-up sample, or the egg count will be diluted. The number of samples is difficult to decide upon. In very small flocks or herds each animal can be treated as an individual. In larger flocks or herds 10% can be used as a yardstick. In very large groups a compromise has to be reached. Testing before treatment will provide information about the worm status of the group and whether anthelmintic use is necessary. Testing after treatment will show the efficacy or otherwise of treatment. It takes 3 days for all the eggs in the gastrointestinal tract to pass out, so if treatment is 100% effective there will be virtually no eggs present at that time. However there is a shock effect of the anthelmintic, which means it will stop egg production but not actually kill the mature worms. It is therefore prudent to wait for 2 weeks after treatment before sampling. Worms acquired after treatment will not normally produce eggs for 3 weeks. The practitioner can therefore advise the owner on the likelihood of anthelmintic resistance to the drug being used and the advisability of a change of drug. Practitioners must stress that if there is resistance to one drug in a group of drugs then there will be resistance to all the other members of that group of drugs. Owners can easily get confused by the different packaging of the products.

As yet no natural plant anthelmintics such as garlic are effective in controlling worms, although many owners are totally convinced of their efficacy.

Although goats are affected by the same nematodes as sheep, it is thought that they are more susceptible because they are principally browsing animals and their resistance to these endoparasites is less highly evolved (Taylor, 2002). However this is unlikely in a worldwide context, as goats have been grazing with sheep for many thousands of years. In Europe goats do seem to be more sensitive then sheep to endoparasites when kept on lush pastures with poor parasite control. They carry heavier nematode burdens, which are reflected in higher faecal egg counts. These can persist for long periods, especially in lactating goats. The periparturient rise can last for the whole of lactation, up to 18 months. Clinical disease is indicated by a count of 2000 eggs/g, and more than 500 eggs/g indicates subclinical disease. At a subclinical level there will be a reduced milk yield and lower weight gains.

It should be remembered that sheep and goats kept in dry semi-desert conditions or in mountainous areas do not suffer from the clinical effects of intestinal parasites.

In all small ruminants, intestinal nematodes will cause various signs and symptoms depending on the species of nematode, which determines the place where the adults are found. Probably the most serious is *Haemonchus contortus*, which is a blood-sucking parasite in the abomasum. It will cause severe, life-threatening anaemia in both species and at all ages. Diagnosis by faecal worm egg output is normally too late. Clinical diagnosis by assessing the pallor of the mucous membranes is vital so that prompt anthelmintic treatment can limit the number of deaths.

Ostertagian nematodes cause the gastric glands in the abomasum to become hyperplastic and cause an increase in pH, which leads to a leakage of pepsinogen into the plasma. This can be measured in a serum sample to aid diagnosis. On post-mortem following heavy infections the mucosa of the abomasum will show raised nodules giving the well-known 'Morocco leather' appearance. In all small ruminants heavy infections can lead to mucosal necrosis and sloughing. The sign in the living animal is violent blackish diarrhoea.

Intestinal nematodes produce villous atrophy and crypt hyperplasia. Diarrhoea is of a more chronic nature, and there will be a protein-losing enteropathy. This will cause setbacks in growth rates of young animals and weight loss in older animals. Diagnosis will be made by raised individual faecal worm egg counts. Individual counts are important to avoid dilution effects, which may give misleading results.

Infections of the nematode *Nematodirus battus* can lead to very serious problems; it causes scouring in lambs and may well be associated with viral, bacterial or coccidial infection. A heavy infection will cause profuse watery yellowy-green diarrhoea, leading to severe dehydration and death even before eggs are seen in the faeces. The eggs are roughly twice the size of other intestinal nematodes found in sheep and are easily recognized. Lower levels will cause ill thrift. Historically *N. battus* affected 4–8-week-old lambs that had been grazing on pastures grazed by young lambs in the previous summer. The eggs required a frost before they could become infective. However the pattern in the UK is now changing, with infections occurring in older lambs. Pastures which have been grazed by young cattle or ewes are no longer safe, and the species has now been found to be resistant to benzimidazole anthelmintics in the UK (Mitchell *et al.*, 2010). However at present the benzimidazole anthelmintics are still recommended for treatment of *N. battus*, as resistance at the time of writing was not widespread. Many of the other species of nematode worms are becoming resistant to the three standard wormer types, so treatment is difficult. It has been suggested that stock should receive a therapeutic dose of all three wormer types at 3-weekly intervals.

Trematodes

Liver fluke infection in sheep

In the UK there has been a massive increase in prevalence of fasciolosis (liver fluke infection). It is no longer commonest in the wetter, western areas of the UK and Ireland. However the distribution is dependent on the presence of the intermediate aquatic snail host, *Lymnea truncatula*, which is now more or less ubiquitous. The levels of infection and incidence of disease are linked to the rainfall from May to October. Adult flukes in the bile ducts of cattle and sheep are passed onto the faeces on the pasture, where they lay their eggs. The eggs hatch in the warmer months (>10°C) in water, releasing motile miracidia. These infect the snails in which the development continues through sporocyst and redia stages, releasing cercariae. In wetter summers there is a massive shedding of eggs on pastures during August–October. These encyst into metacercariae on the herbage and are ingested by the ruminant. The immature flukes migrate through the liver to the bile ducts. In cattle this is not as dangerous a stage but in sheep there is often massive damage to the liver resulting in death. These deaths will occur from September to December. More chronic infections, as seen in cattle with adult fluke in the bile ducts, occur in February and March. Sheep will be weak and anaemic. The classic sign is oedema in the mandibular space, a condition known as 'bottle jaw'. Mild winters increase the numbers of hibernating snails, which shed more cercariae in the following spring. Diagnostic signs in sheep are fairly straightforward, as seen in Table 10.3.

Control programmes must take into account topography, geographic location and prevailing weather conditions. Draining endemic areas will help to eliminate snail habitats. Fencing off wet areas in the autumn prevents access to these snail habitats. In average rainfall years all sheep should be dosed twice, in October and January, with a drug (e.g. triclabendazole) that is effective against immature stages. They will need to be dosed again in May, and at this time only this

Table 10.3. Diagnostic signs of fasciolosis in sheep.

Disease type	Peak incidence	Clinical signs	Fluke numbers	Eggs per g of faeces
Acute	October– January	**Sudden death** or dullness anaemia, dyspnoea, ascites and abdominal pain	1000+ mainly immature	0
Subacute	October–January	**Rapid weight loss, anaemia,** submandibular oedema and ascites in some cases	500–1000 adults and immature	<100
Chronic	January–April	**Progressive weight loss, anaemia,** submandibular oedema and ascites	200+ adults	100+

can be with a combination roundworm and fluke drench (see Chapter 6). In areas that have previously experienced high rainfall, sheep may require additional dosing in both the winter and the summer season.

There is strong evidence (Sargison and Scott, 2011) that there is resistance of *Fasciola hepatica* to triclabendazole. This has serious economic consequences. The population genetics of *F. hepatica* will inevitably prove to differ from those for parasitic nematodes, and therefore refugia-based strategies that have been developed to slow the emergence of resistance in parasitic nematodes cannot be extrapolated to *F. hepatica*. Farmers should attempt to develop evasive strategies, such as fencing off snail habitats; managing snail habitats and areas that are conductive to the survival of free-living stages of *F. hepatica*; and the strategic use of fasciolacidal anthelmintic treatments with the aim of reducing *F. hepatica* egg shedding and miracidial infection of snails.

Liver fluke infection in goats

Goats can become infected with *F. hepatica*. This may take the form of acute disease, as is common in sheep. There will be a massive rise in liver enzymes, diarrhoea, acute depression and death. In the UK this normally occurs in the autumn, as early as September. Any time during the winter goats may show a more chronic form with some anorexia, lethargy, weight loss and decreased milk production. The control and treatment of the disease is similar to that advised for sheep.

Conditions of the Stomach including Surgical Procedures

Gastric disorders of sheep

Acidosis

This condition occurs with grain overload. It can occur in a variety of situations, such as when sheep have broken into a feed store or when sheep are given cereals for the first time and several stronger animals eat more than their share. Signs will vary from mild abdominal discomfort and lethargy to acute collapse and death. In peracute cases the animals will be found dead and show no sign of violent watery diarrhoea, which is the main sign in slightly less acute situations. All affected animals will show a lowered rectal temperature and an increased pulse. They will have toxic-looking mucous membranes.

Bloat

In theory sheep could get bloat in a similar manner to cattle with an oesophageal foreign body such as a potato. This does not seem to occur, as sheep are careful with chewing and swallowing their food. They will get a frothy bloat from over-eating a legume (e.g. clover). They will then become recumbent and die unless treated fairly rapidly. Treatment is best accomplished by stomach tubing to relieve the gas if possible, and passing vegetable oil down the tube to flatten the gas. If that is not possible a trocar and cannula can be inserted into the left flank as described below for goats.

Gastritis

Severe pain and vomiting will be seen in affected sheep as a result of poisoning with certain plants (e.g. rhododendron) (see Chapter 17).

Rumen atony

In sheep this condition is secondary to a primary lesion affecting the vagus nerve, for example inflammation of the mesenteric lymph nodes from *Mannheimia haemolytica* infection. The sheep will be off-colour, with pyrexia. Prognosis is guarded. Aggressive treatment with antibiotics and NSAID is required.

Rumen impaction

This condition will be seen in sheep that have consumed a toxic dose of acorns (see Chapter 17). It is also seen in tumours affecting the stomach (see below). Finally it is also seen in *Actinomycosis bovis* granulomas on the caudal end of the oesophagus. The sheep will be slightly off-colour with some evidence of chronic bloat. They are not normally pyrexic.

Treatment is with daily doses of streptomycin, which should be repeated for 10 days.

Tumours affecting the stomach in sheep

All tumours in the gastroenteric system of sheep are rare. However, the most common are rumen papillomas, which will be found either on post-mortem or when examining the rumens of sheep slaughtered for meat. Very rarely will they be seen in younger animals, but the majority are seen in cull ewes. In contrast to cattle they are not found in the oesophagus. They are benign but may be as large as 2 cm in diameter. In exceptionally rare cases they may appear on histological sections to be squamous cell carcinomas, but these do not metastasize.

Adenomatous polyps are found in the abomasum, and on extremely rare occasions adenocarcinomas are seen. These will metastasize to the small intestine and pancreas. However they may stay static for months and only cause problems in advanced pregnancy.

It is believed that environmental carcinogens interact with genetic factors, because in New Zealand more cases occurred in British breeds than in fine wool breeds (Head, 1990). Bracken has been incriminated in the UK and Australasia, but the tumour also occurs on New Zealand farms without bracken. It occurs in Iceland where there is no bracken and a case has been seen in a sheep which has been known not to have had access to bracken (Head, 1990). The influence of a rumen papilloma virus is debatable. Certainly sheep with rumen papilloma do not always have intestinal adenocarcinomas, and not all guts with adenocarcinomas exhibit papilloma in the rumen.

Gastric disorders of goats

Acidosis

Normally this is a peracute condition in goats and requires aggressive fluid therapy with antibiotic and NSAID support. Injections of vitamin B may be helpful. Apart from grain overload this may occur after goats have eaten potatoes and pea straw at the same time.

Bloat

This is rare in goats as they are seldom given access to very rich clover pastures.

Rumen atony

This is a very rare condition. In the author's experience it tends to follow either acidosis or bloat.

Rumen impaction

This is a common condition in goats that have eaten something totally unsuitable, such as polythene string or cloth. A rumenotomy may be required.

Tumours affecting the stomach

These are extremely rare in goats. They are squamous cell carcinomas seen on post-mortem. Suspected tumours seen on ultrasound are likely to be phytobezoars.

Conditions of the Intestines including Surgical Procedures

Colic in sheep

General

This is extremely rare in adult sheep, but pain will be seen in bottle-fed lambs when there is too much gas in the abomasum. Treatment with a solution containing 4 mg butylscopolamine bromide and 500 mg metamizole/ml at a dose of 1 ml/20 kg intravenously is normally effective.

Intussusception

This can occur in any age of sheep or goats but is extremely rare. The author has only seen three cases, two in young lambs and one in a neonatal kid, and all were only seen on post-mortem. Another author (Scott, 2010) reports two cases in neonatal Texel lambs. The clinical signs started with depression, inappetance/reluctance to suck, abdominal discomfort manifest as an arched back, increasing abdominal distension with gas over several days, and tenesmus with passage of scant mucus containing fresh blood, which caused variable staining around the tail and perineum. Frequent painful vocalization alerted the shepherd to the illness and euthanasia was performed on welfare grounds. The diagnosis was obvious on post-mortem, but would have been very difficult in life, although ultrasonography might have been helpful. Surgery, although possible, would not have been an option economically.

Colic in goats

General

Abomasal bloat will occur in bottle-fed kids, which should receive the same treatment as bottle-fed lambs. Torsion of the bowel or intussusceptions can occur in adult goats, but are outside the author's experience. Ultrasonography might be helpful with diagnosis. An exploratory laparotomy is essential to diagnosis.

Tumours of the intestines

Adenocarcinomas of the intestine are one of the most common tumours seen in sheep and goats. The pathognomic sign is ascites. This is easier to recognize in sheep which have become extremely thin; goats may also become thin but have an abdomen full of fat. Palpation will aid the clinician with diagnosis. Surgery is not justified and euthanasia should be carried out.

Diseases of the Liver

General

Sheep and goats suffer to a large extent with the same diseases of the liver.

Abscesses

These may form in the livers of sheep and goats either by haematological spread or by local invasion from the rumen. They may be caused by a variety of organisms. The most common in sheep is *Fusobacterium necrophorum*, in goats *Corynebacterium pseudotuberculosis*. Clinically the animals will be ill with pyrexia, and jaundice may be a feature. There does not seem to be a chronic condition as seen in cattle. Diagnosis may be helped by raised liver enzymes, liver biopsy and transabdominal ultrasonography. Obviously aggressive antibiotic treatment is required.

Black's disease

This is caused by *Clostridium novyi*. It is mainly a sheep disease but is definitely seen in goats.

Fascioliasis

This is the most important liver disease in sheep and goats.

Plant toxicity

This can occur in sheep and goats (see Chapter 17).

Rift Valley fever

The viral RVF disease occurs in primarily in sheep and goats. It does affect man and so technically it is a zoonosis, but it is normally spread by insect vectors. An outbreak occurred in laboratory workers at Kabete in Kenya in the 1960s. It is possible that the laboratory technicians and vets had become infected while on safari in the Rift Valley. Equally, it was a strange coincidence that at the time they were all involved in investigating the disease in the laboratory. The disease in man is similar to very severe influenza (see Chapter 19).

The disease is caused by a *Bunyavirus*. Nairobi sheep disease (NSD) is another *Bunyavirus*. RVF virus affects sheep and goats but is also found in cattle, camels and game animals (buffalo and antelope). There is therefore always a reservoir of the virus. It also can survive in the eggs of the mosquito *Aedes mcintoshi*. The groups of RVF viruses are confusing. The east African strain has recently been found in Saudi Arabia and the Yemen. This strain is found throughout southern Africa including Swaziland and Madagascar. There is also a west African strain found mainly in Senegal and Mauritania, and a separate strain found in Egypt. The disease is spread by mosquitoes and perhaps by other insects. It is also possible that there is direct spread from viraemic sheep and goats.

In sheep and goats the disease is most severe in very young lambs and kids and there is an extremely high mortality. Mortality is fairly high in growing sheep and goatlings. Although it is normally mild in adults it always causes an abortion storm. Aborting animals may die from other infections brought on by the abortion. All surviving animals develop a lifelong immunity. The disease may be so peracute that the lambs and kids are found dead without showing any signs. Blood taken from a live animal and heart blood taken from a newly dead animal can be tested with an ELISA for confirmation of the diagnosis. The liver shows grey-yellow necrotic foci distributed throughout its parenchyma. Virus isolation will give a definitive diagnosis. There is no specific treatment, but administration of 30 ml of serum collected from convalescent animals given intravenously or intraperitoneally may reduce mortality rates.

Tumours of the liver

Tumours of the liver are found in sheep. They are nearly always formed from liver tissue except for very rare melanomas, which normally start in the lungs and spread through the diaphragm. Primary liver tumours are rarely malignant and do not cause emaciation. This is only seen in malignant tumours which grow large rapidly and invade the lymph nodes. Polycystic lesions are commonly seen in the liver of healthy animals and are not cancerous. Tumours of the liver are extremely rare in goats and are normally carcinomas found at post-mortem. In theory they could be seen on ultrasound or, by luck, picked up on liver biopsy.

Diseases of the Pancreas

Pancreatitis as a clinical entity on its own is not recorded in sheep and goats. However it may become an entity as a secondary complication to peritonitis or liver disease. The pancreas may also be infested with cysticerci from *Taenia* spp., whose primary host is a small carnivore.

11

Respiratory and Circulatory System

Non-infectious Conditions of the Upper Respiratory Tract in Sheep

Chondritis of the larynx

This condition is confined mainly to rams, particularly Texels. The animals will show respiratory distress and make a loud snoring noise. The rectal temperature will remain normal. The lungs are difficult to auscultate. However the animals remain quiet and apparently normal. Prompt treatment with antibiotics such as oxytetracyclines and dexamethazone will cure the disease. Ideally a long-acting preparation of oxytetracycline and dexamethazone should be injected every second day for five treatments. If treatment is delayed the inflammation of the larynx can be reduced but the noise will continue. The rams can still serve normally.

Nasal foreign bodies

These are extremely rare and are normally grass seeds. If they are in a rostral position they will cause a unilateral nasal discharge, but if they are in a more caudal position they will cause a bilateral nasal discharge. Removal is extremely difficult.

Nasal tumours

These are very rare but may occur more commonly in sheep kept as pets. The most common are polyps or adenopapillomas. These can be removed if large and near the nasal orifice. However if they cannot readily be visualized and cause a nasal discharge, that will cause a problem with diagnosis. A pragmatic approach would be to treat the sheep for nasal myiasis (see Chapter 6) and with antibiotics. If the tumour is a squamous cell carcinoma the condition will deteriorate rapidly and euthanasia will be the only option. Tumours may also be adenocarcinomas of the turbinates. These are normally sporadic, although clusters have been reported in North America and have been seen by the author in Kenya. It is thought there may be a genetic factor linked to a virus. They show clinically in old sheep as a reduction in the upper airways causing snoring. There is initial success following treatment with antibiotics and dexamethazone or NSAID, but the noise and distress return and euthanasia is indicated.

Non-infectious Conditions of the Upper Respiratory Tract in Goats

Collar trauma

This can be seen in tethered goats if they are attacked by carnivores. Normally the collar trauma is the least of the goat's problems. Clinicians should examine the neck carefully for bite wounds.

Nasal foreign bodies

In common with sheep, these are extremely rare. However, goats tend to be more inquisitive and so may sniff in powdery edible substances such as flour, which will cause very aggressive sneezing that is normally short lived.

Nasal tumours

These are even rarer in goats than in sheep. However polyps will be seen that are likely to be benign adenopapillomas.

Infectious Conditions of the Upper Respiratory Tract in Sheep

Enzootic nasal adenocarcinoma

This condition is caused by a retrovirus that causes tumours of the mucosa covering the turbinates. It is principally found in South Africa, but not in the UK, Australia or New Zealand. Diagnosis is mainly on clinical signs of a chronic seromucous nasal discharge. A PCR that can be used on this discharge, but not on serum, is available. This might be the same condition seen by the author in Kenya. Diagnosis can be confirmed on post-mortem. No treatment or vaccine is available.

Nasal myiasis

The adult fly *Oestrus ovis* deposits larvae around the nostrils. These invade the nasal cavity and develop into second-stage instars which invade the sinuses in the head. The mature larvae are sneezed out up to 1 year later. They are easily treated with ivermectins and rarely cause problems.

Rhinitis

This rare relatively mild condition, with a transitory nasal discharge, will occur in weaned lambs. The cause is *Salmonella arizonae*. The condition is self-limiting and it is probably better not to give antibiotics.

Infectious Conditions of the Upper Respiratory Tract in Goats

Enzootic nasal adenocarcinoma

This condition is caused by a retrovirus that causes tumours of the mucosa covering the turbinates in sheep. It can also affect goats if they are herded together. There is no treatment or vaccine available.

Nasal leech

The parasite involved is the leech *Dinobdella ferrox* and, when seen in a mixed flock of sheep and goats, the percentage of goats affected is higher than that of the sheep. This is the opposite effect to that caused by the nasal bot *O. ovis* (in a mixed flock, a higher percentage of sheep than goats will be affected by *O. ovis*). *D. ferrox* has attacked the legs of the author when trekking in the Himalayas. However in goats the leech invades the nostrils causing sneezing and a bloody nasal discharge. Systemic ivermectins are not effective. However, if instilled up the nose they are said to be effective and the leeches are expelled within a few hours.

Nasal myiasis

O. ovis is found in goats but is much less common than in sheep. This is very striking when a mixed flock of sheep and goats is examined. The morbidity in the sheep may be over 50% but that of the goats will be under 5%. Problems can be experienced in pygmy goats when the larvae are too large to be expelled. However, if the signs of sneezing can be controlled for a few days after ivermectin treatment, the larvae will macerate and then be expelled.

Retropharyngeal lymph node abscessation

These abscesses are caused by *Corynebacterium pseudotuberculosis*. Owing to the proximity to the carotid artery, euthanasia is advised.

Rhinitis

This condition can be caused by caprine herpes virus. There will be a purulent nasal discharge leading to more severe systemic signs. This is rare in North America and is not found in the UK. Bacterial rhinitis can occur but it is normally linked with *Pasteurella multocida* pneumonia.

Non-infectious Conditions of the Lower Respiratory Tract in Sheep

General

Diagnosis of lower respiratory disease in sheep is difficult in the live sheep. The respiratory rate may be high in perfectly healthy sheep. Factors outside the control of the sheep such as the ambient temperature and the humidity will affect the respiratory rate, which will vary between 20 and 200 breaths/min. Fleece cover and fat cover will both affect the respiratory rate, as will pregnancy. Any sheep with anaemia will have an increased respiratory rate.

Infectious conditions can be investigated by paired serology for Maedi–Visna, Jaagiekte, bovine respiratory viruses and *Mycoplasma* spp. There is a more invasive technique, bronchoalveolar lavage, via the trachea (see Chapter 4). However the welfare aspects of such a technique might be questioned as normally the diagnosis can be made on post-mortem, if a group of sheep is involved.

Because of their fleeces, sheep are very prone to drowning. However, when shorn they can swim, as can hair sheep.

Aspiration pneumonia

This may be seen in several animals in flocks drenched by an inexperienced shepherd (Fig. 11.1).

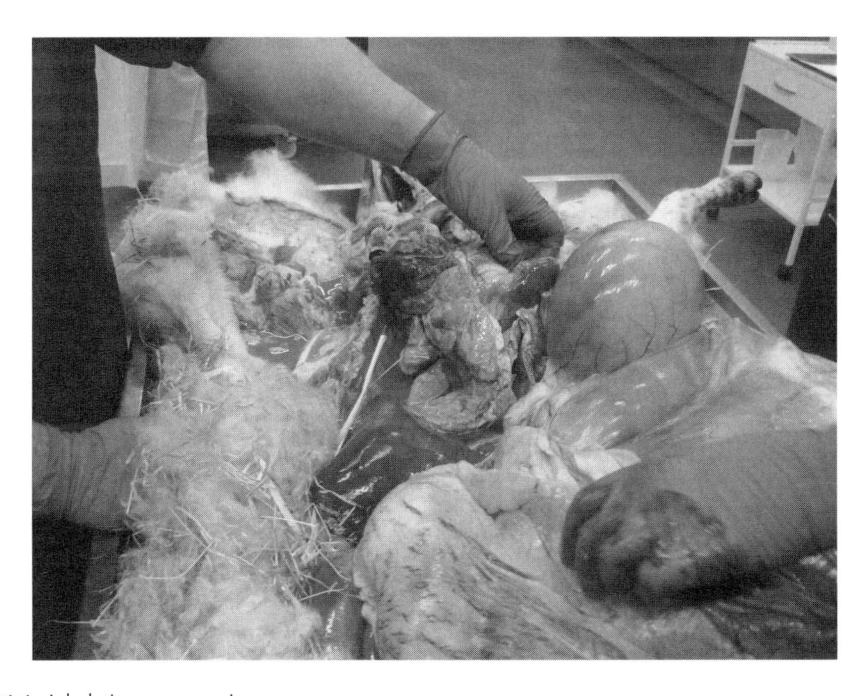

Fig. 11.1. Inhalation pneumonia.

Ruptured diaphragm

This is an exceptionally rare diagnosis but it can occur (Fig. 11.2). In theory a diagnosis could have been made in the live sheep with ultrasonography, and – also in theory – surgery could have been performed. No cause was known but trauma was assumed in this 5-year-old ewe.

Tumours

Respiratory tumours are normally contagious in sheep and are caused by one of the *Betaretrovirus* spp.

Non-infectious Conditions of the Lower Respiratory Tract in Goats

Aspiration pneumonia

As most goat keepers are caring individuals this condition is extremely rare except following a GA, which is a known hazardous procedure.

Drowning

This is rare as goats are good swimmers.

Tumours

There is a relatively high incidence of thymomas. The clinical signs are diverse and include respiratory distress, ventral oedema and a marked visible jugular pulse. In some animals the only sign will be wasting. Squamous cell carcinoma will be seen in goats as secondaries in the lungs. The clinical picture will be similar to tuberculosis. Euthanasia and a post-mortem examination should be carried out.

Winter cough

This is a rare condition caused by an allergic response to fungal spores in hay and straw. Post-mortem will reveal gross emphysematous areas of lung. An alveolitis is seen histologically. Treatment can be attempted with

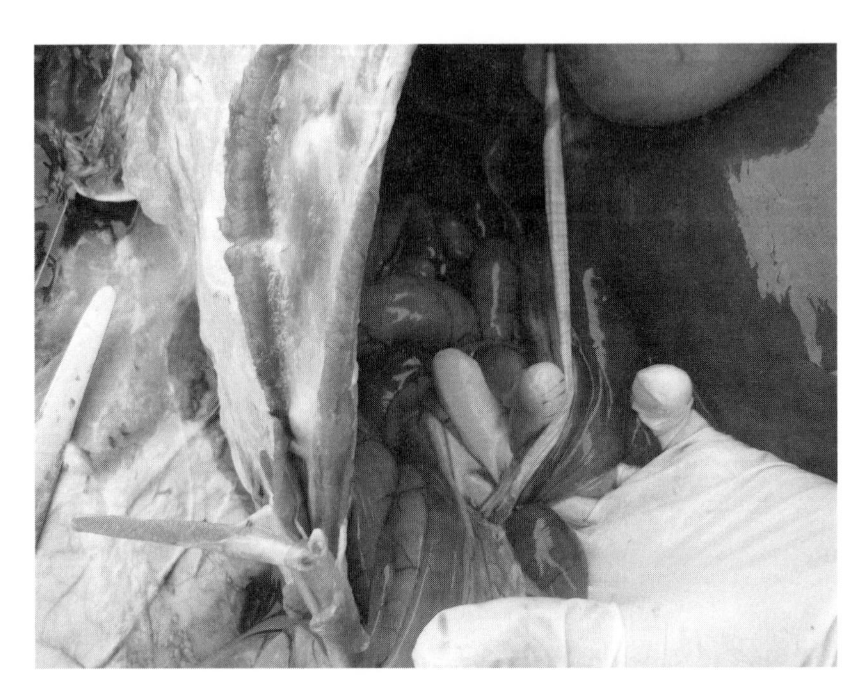

Fig. 11.2. Ruptured diaphragm.

clembutoral injections given intravenously in acute cases. Further treatment can be given orally at 0.5g/10kg. However the only real cure is for the goat to be kept outside permanently, and never given hay or straw. Inside, dust-free environments using shavings and silage might be successful with dedicated management.

Other causes of respiratory distress

The list of poisons that will cause respiratory distress is very long. Any poison that causes anaemia will cause respiratory signs. The most common is an excess of brassicas. They are fine for goats when fed in moderation, but if they are the only item in the diet, poisoning is inevitable. Not only will goats be anaemic but they will also have red urine.

Copper poisoning will cause respiratory signs in goats. There is rarely a problem with the diagnosis as the jaundice is very obvious. The affected goats invariably die and therefore euthanasia should be performed. Cases are now very rare in the UK because copper is no longer allowed to be used as a growth promoter in pig food, which was sometimes fed to goats. Molasses blocks containing high levels of urea should not be given to goats. If goats just licked as sheep and cattle do then there would be no problem, but they have a tendency to bite chunks off the block and get urea poisoning. This certainly causes respiratory distress. Nitrite/nitrate poisoning is also seen in goats but it is very rare. It will occur if goats are allowed access to broken bags of fertilizer, when they will show acute respiratory distress and die. Methylene blue is the specific intravenous antidote (see Chapter 17). In theory nitrate poisoning could occur after fertilizing a goat paddock with nitrate fertilizer, but such an event would be extremely rare.

Anaemia as a result of *H. contortus* infection, or infection with any blood parasite, will cause respiratory distress in goats. Clinicians should not be confused by the increase in respiratory rate shown by does in oestrus.

Infectious Conditions of the Lower Respiratory Tract in Sheep

Viral infections

There is no evidence that infectious bovine rhinotracheitis (IBR), parainfluenza III (PI3), respiratory syncytial virus (RSV) or bovine virus diarrhoea (BVD), which infect cattle, could cause respiratory disease in sheep. Ovine PI3 is distinct from both bovine and human PI3. Most clinical cases of ovine PI3 occur in 10–12-week-old lambs. The clinical signs are mild with a short duration of pyrexia and a serous nasal discharge. The ewes are normally asymptomatic but will show mild interstitial pneumonia.

It is not advisable to vaccinate sheep with cattle vaccines. The killed vaccines would be worthless and the live intranasal vaccines might be a disaster.

Blue tongue virus can be spread transplacentally. Virus serotype 8 was demonstrated to occur naturally by workers in Belgium (Saegerman *et al.*, 2011) (see Chapter 10).

Sheep pulmonary adenomatosis or Jaagsiekte is a bronchoalveolar carcinoma caused by a retrovirus, seen clinically in sheep from 2 years of age. Animals will appear not to thrive. They remain bright and continue feeding even though they become hyperpnoeic and lag behind the rest of the flock. This is how the disease first got its name in South Africa in 1825; it means 'driving sickness'. Fluid progressively accumulates in the lungs and can be heard on auscultation. There is often secondary *Mannheimia haemolytica* infection, which may well kill the animals. Diagnosis can be made earlier by the 'wheel barrow' test. The hind legs of the sheep are raised and then fluid will pour out of the sheep's nose. There is also a reliable PCR. Initial treatment with antibiotics and NSAID may appear to be helpful but the good effect will be short lasting. On post-mortem the ventral lobes of the lungs will be full of grey nodules up to 2cm across. There will also be nodules in the local lymph nodes. There is no treatment and animals should be culled as soon as a diagnosis is made. Care should be taken when buying replacements into a flock because of the insidious nature of the disease, which may take up to 3 years to appear.

Bacterial infections

M. haemolytica is a major cause of bacterial pneumonia, either as a primary or secondary infection. In the majority of combined infections it is presumed that the involvement of other respiratory pathogens will disrupt the lung's protective mechanisms and predispose the animals to a secondary *M. haemolytica* infection. The source of the infection is usually carrier adults, although the organism can survive in the environment, on grass or bedding, and in water. Outbreaks normally occur in fattening lambs but indoor-lambing ewes can be affected. Often the trigger factor can be difficult to pinpoint as it takes up to 1 month for an outbreak to occur. Housing is obviously one of the main predisposing causes, but movement from a hill environment to a fattening lowland situation can be the trigger. Often lambs will only have received the first of the two-dose vaccine at that time. Weather changes may play a part and the chill factor is very important. On the hill with rocks and deep heather the lambs can get shelter, but on arable land when fenced away from the hedgerows, there is a marked chill factor. This can easily be avoided by liaison between the farmer and the shepherd but this may be lacking if the sheep owner is only hiring the land.

Animals may be found dead, or vigilant shepherds may pick them out in the early stages of the disease with a high temperature and a nasal discharge. Coughing and an ocular discharge can also be a feature. The organism can be found in the blood as well as in the lung tissue in younger lambs.

Treatment with antibiotics, especially more modern ones developed for cattle, can be rewarding if the disease is caught early enough. Morbidity can reach 40% with a figure half that of mortality, so blanket antibiotic treatment should definitely be considered. NSAID will definitely help affected animals and will also decrease the number of chronically affected animals.

Vaccination with two doses of vaccine (see Chapter 7) must be carried out before possible outbreaks, but the logistics of this are difficult for shepherds with hill lambs.

M. haemolytica infection may occur secondarily to a *Mycoplasma* infection. Mycoplasmas are found in sheep throughout the world but they alone do not seem to be able to cause pneumonia. The most common is *Mycoplasma ovipneumoniae* but *Mycoplasma arginini* and even *Mycobacterium bovis* may also be found. They all appear to cause subclinical disease and require *Mannheimia haemolytica* to cause clinical disease. In turn a trigger factor such as transport, mixing and markets is required.

It should not be forgotten that mycoplasmas have a definite role in other syndromes, for example keratoconjunctivitis (see Chapter 14), polyarthritis (see Chapter 15) and mastitis (see Chapter 13). The mastitis maybe linked with 'contagious agalactia', which is a notifiable disease in the UK (see Chapter 13).

Other bacteria also have a role in some pneumonia outbreaks in sheep throughout the world. Specific pathogens include *Bibersteinia trehalosi* (formerly called *Pasteurella trehalosi*) and *Pasteurella multocida*, both of which can cause pneumonia in fattening lambs. *Bordetella parapertussis* will definitely cause a mild infection in young lambs in its own right with no other pathogen present. However deaths will only occur if another pathogen is present.

The role of *Histophilus somni* is confusing. This bacterium has had other names in the past, namely *Histophilus ovis*, *Haemophilus somnus* and *Haemophilus agni*. It can be found as a sole pathogen in sheep pneumonia and may also cause pneumonia in goats worldwide. However there does not seem to be a crossover with cattle. *H. somni* has been found to cause other problems in sheep, namely epididymo-orchitis, metritis, meningoencephalitis and mastitis.

Chest abscesses caused by a variety of organisms including *Streptococcus zooepidemicus* and *Erysipelothrix rhusiopathiae* will occur in ewes, but are really quite common in thin older rams. Auscultation is usually unrewarding. However the animals will have a constant raised rectal temperature and will cough on excursion. Treatment may be rewarding but is labour intensive. Animals should be given penicillin daily for at least 4 weeks.

Tuberculosis in sheep is rare and is usually an incidental finding at slaughter or at post-mortem examination. However an outbreak in the UK with clinical signs has been described by one author (van der Burgt, 2010). Chronic weight loss was seen in 10% of a flock of 220 Lleyn sheep, and *Mycobacterium bovis* was isolated from three carcasses. As a diagnosis of chronic wasting disease with possible respiratory signs, tuberculosis should not be overlooked.

Parasitic pneumonia

Dictyocaulus filaria will cause clinical signs in young sheep, normally in the autumn. Severe signs are rare, and deaths are very rare. Strong immunity is generated so *D. filaria* is rare in adult sheep. The worms are effectively killed by ivomectins. Two other lungworms, namely *Protostrongylus rufescens* and *Muellerius capillaries*, are seen in sheep normally as an incidental finding at slaughter or post-mortem. However they can cause respiratory distress and weight loss in lambs. They too are sensitive to ivomectins. Lungworm larvae may be seen using the Baermann technique (see Chapter 4).

The intermediate stages of the tapeworm *Echinococcus granulosus*, 'hydatid cysts', will occur in a sheep's lungs and are normally asymptomatic. They are a zoonosis (see Chapter 19).

Infectious Conditions of the Lower Respiratory Tract in Goats

Viral infections

There is no evidence that IBR, PI3, RSV or BVD, which infect cattle, could cause respiratory disease in goats. It is not advisable to vaccinate goats with cattle vaccines. The killed vaccines would be worthless and the live intranasal vaccines might be a disaster.

BTV that occurs in goats will cause respiratory signs. Goats should be vaccinated against the relevant serotypes of BTV in a similar manner to cattle, that is, a double initial dose (unlike sheep, which only require one dose).

Pulmonary adenomatosis, 'Jaagsiekte', will occur in goats but is rare.

Contagious caprine pleuropneumonia

Contagious caprine pleuropneumonia (CCPP) is still seen in Africa and the Middle East, so it certainly could reach Europe and even the UK; however it is unlikely that practitioners will miss it. It is a terrible disease, even in naive goats in Africa, causing 100% morbidity and often over 75% mortality. If it occurred in Europe or the UK there might be 100% mortality. However in a partially immune population it was not nearly so striking. There are other *Mycoplasma* spp., which may be differentials.

CCPP is a contagious disease of goats caused by *Mycoplasma mycoides* subsp. *capri*. It is now called *Mycoplasma capricolum* subsp. *capri-pneumoniae*. It is notifiable to the Office International des Epizooties (OIE). It is species specific and only occurs in goats, although there was a myth in Kenya (which had no foundation) that the disease was spread by impala. Historically goats were very important to the Masai, although their cattle were their pride and joy. They recognized CCPP and also realized that, although it looked similar to contagious bovine pleuropneumonia (CBPP), it was rarely seen in their cattle. They also realized that it was a different disease. In reality goats can get CBPP as kids if they are fed infected cows' milk, but cattle cannot get CCPP.

Practitioners in the field in the UK need not be alarmed by CCPP. However, for those working in laboratories, it is not a simple condition to study as there are other *Mycoplasma* species that infect goats. These can be isolated from healthy animals and do not normally cause disease, but others will actually cause pneumonia if inoculated into goats. Species isolated in the UK include *M. ovipneumoniae*, *M. conjunctivae*, *M. arginine* and *Acholeplasma oculi*. All of these may cause mild respiratory incidents, often called 'post-show flu'. They may affect the whole of the herd but are normally self-limiting.

However if treatment were required, oxytetracyclines and NSAID must be recommended. *M. ovipneumoniae,* however, has been associated with severe respiratory disease in a goat herd in Kosovo (Rifatbegovic *et al.*, 2011). Mortality was high due to the poor conditions on 200-head goat farm.

In most countries there is a compulsory slaughter policy for goats with CCPP. They should not be treated, as if they survive after treatment with oxytetracyclines and NSAID, they will remain as carriers.

Bacterial infections

These are the main cause of pneumonia in goats, and the two culprits are *Pasteurella multocida* and *Mannheimia haemolytica*. They can occur singly or in a mixed infection. Goats, particularly young animals, will show high temperatures and a markedly increased respiratory rate. They will even mouth breathe. Clinicians should not be tempted to use tilmicosin, which is very useful in sheep respiratory infections. This drug has a very narrow safety margin in goats. A mixture of penicillin and streptomycin are the antibiotics of choice, given daily at the sheep dose. There are no licensed products for goats. Oxytetracycline can be used, employing a long-acting dosage if revisiting is difficult. It should be remembered that goats are ruminants and must never be given antibiotics by mouth except in young kids. It is also very foolish to contemplate giving young kids suffering from pneumonia anything by mouth on account of the danger of inhalation pneumonia. There are very many modern antibiotics licensed for use in cattle, but there is little point in using them in goats, as resistant bacteria are very rare in goats. However, NSAID help in cases of goat pneumonia. To prevent the spread of the disease fresh air is important. Goats become infected when kept in places such as airless caravans, hot airless show tents and airless trailers. Good ventilation, free of draughts, is required. Do not vaccinate goats with sheep *Pasteurella* vaccines as they are worthless in goats. On the other hand vaccinating goats against clostridial diseases is very worthwhile. It is just the 'P' combinations that should be avoided. Angora goats seem particularly prone to *Pasteurella* pneumonia.

Actually, pneumonia in goats is relatively uncommon. However goats will often show signs that mimic pneumonia, such as respiratory distress, raised respiratory rate and mouth breathing. Their rectal temperature will also be raised to 40°C (103°F). Giving these goats antibiotics and NSAID may well be beneficial, and these drugs will certainly not do any harm. However clinicians should make the correct diagnosis, which will be much more rewarding for the goat, the owner, and themselves.

Goats will get tuberculosis (TB). The most common affected organs are the lungs and so goats will show respiratory signs. Normally these will be chronic, but there are many manifestations. The first signs will be a goat showing chronic weight loss. This may then turn into acute respiratory distress if a tubercle bursts in the lungs. Goats can be infected with cattle TB (*Mycobacterium bovis*) and human TB (*Mycobacterium tuberculosis*). Recently goats have been awarded their own TB, *Mycobacterium caprae*. This totally dispels the myth propagated by goat keepers selling goats' milk that goats are free from TB. It is a notifiable disease so if in doubt practitioners in the UK must inform the Department for Environment, Food and Rural Affairs (DEFRA).

M. bovis is very rare in wild Caprinae. There has only ever been one case reported in the Iberian ibex (*Capra pyrenaica*) (Cubero *et al.*, 2002). The Iberian ibex is a medium-sized mountain ungulate found throughout the Iberian Peninsula. The reason for its resistance to TB is unknown. However a native Portuguese breed, the Serrana, found in the north-east of Portugal, has been reported to have contracted the disease (Quintas *et al.*, 2010). The affected animals presented initially with dry coughing, progressive emaciation and occasional diarrhoea, and there were high mortality rates. Post-mortem examination revealed circumscribed, yellowish-white, caseous or caseocalcareous lesions of various sizes, often capsulated, especially in the lungs and mediastinal lymph nodes, or in the mesenteric lymph nodes. Ziehl–Neelsen stains showed acid-fast bacilli and *M. bovis* was grown on culture. The Portuguese authors concluded that TB may be more common than previously thought, and should be included in the differential diagnosis of any cases of chronic respiratory disease. There can be further confusion in the diagnosis of TB because goat herds can show concurrent caseous lymphadenitis (Sharpe *et al.*, 2010). The gross post-mortem findings, such as abscessation and lesion distribution, can be very similar. Both diseases may affect the lung, thoracic lymph nodes, and viscera. A definitive diagnosis can be made by culture but this can take months. Ziehl–Neelsen and Gram staining of histological sections can be very helpful.

Parasites affecting the respiratory system

The most common parasite to cause respiratory distress in of all ages of goats is *Haemonchus contortus*. It causes severe anaemia, which then results in respiratory distress. The mucous membranes will be totally white and rectal temperature will be normal. Acute *Fasciola hepatica* will give similar signs. In theory a massive infestation of sucking lice would cause anaemia and respiratory distress. *Oestrus ovis,* the sheep nasal bot, will infect goats. The goats will not be ill but will keep sneezing, and goat keepers may well see the large larvae. Ivomectin injection is very effective as a single treatment.

There are many protozoal parasites that will cause anaemia in goats worldwide. The respiratory signs are secondary to the anaemia.

Nematodes affecting the lungs

In general lungworms are of no real significance in sheep and goats, but there are some exceptions to that rule. When there is mixed grazing with cattle, *Dictyocaulus filarial* can cause real problems in younger animals, namely first-season lambs and kids. There is a vaccine available for cattle that uses live irradiated larvae. This has not been used in small ruminants and therefore cannot be recommended. Treatment with injectable ivomectins is very effective. *Protostrongylus rufescens* is often found on post-mortem in the small bronchi, but its presence is rarely related to disease. Mild coughing is often seen in small ruminants and is on the whole disregarded by owners. Nevertheless, *Cystocaulus* spp., *Muellerius capillaris* and *Neostrongylus linearis,* which are found as nodules in the lung parenchyma, may all cause significant bronchopneumonia with emphysema if present in large numbers. Animals should not only be treated with injectable ivomectins, but also with antibiotics and NSAID.

Diseases of the Cardiovascular System

Heart attacks

Heart attacks as described in man are very unlikely to occur in sheep and goats, so sudden death in these species cannot be attributed to this cause. However muscular dystrophy, 'white muscle disease', affects lambs and kids (see Chapter 9). It can occur in neonates and also in older animals; they will normally be found dead.

Heartwater

The rickettsia *Ehrlichia ruminantium* used to be called *Cowdria ruminantium*. It occurs in sheep and goats in Africa south of the Sahara and also in sheep and goats in the Caribbean, and the tropical areas of North and Central America. It is a tick-borne disease and so its distribution is linked to suitable *Amblyomma* spp. vectors. In the author's experience the principal tick in Africa and the Caribbean is the three-host tick *Amblyomma variegatum*. The organism passes trans-stadially through the tick and may event spread transovarially. The disease has various forms, which make diagnosis difficult. On the whole acute heartwater occurs 2–4 weeks after new sheep or goats move into a tick area. They will show high fever and acute respiratory signs, which may be due to the cardiac symptoms. Pericarditis may be heard on auscultation. Mortality rates can be as high as 90%, as once convulsions occur death is inevitable.

However there may be a less acute form with a fever but with animals recovering without developing neurological signs. Diagnosis is difficult in the living animal, and it is hoped that a PCR will be developed soon. Signs on post-mortem will include marked hydropericardium, hydrothorax and pulmonary oedema. The kidneys will be swollen but not soft as in enterotoxaemia. The organism will be found on histological samples stained with Giemsa. The most reliable site is the brain cortex.

Treatment is tetracyclines, ideally given intravenously initially, followed by intramuscular injections of 10 mg/kg. It is advisable to inject long-acting tetracycline preparations at 20 mg/kg to all the animals that have been exposed to the infected ticks. Naturally all the animals should be treated to remove the ticks and prevent reinfestation (see Chapter 6).

Iliac arterial thrombosis

This condition could occur in sheep and goats, but the author can find no references in the literature.

Poisonous plants

There are very few poisonous plants that actually stop the heart. Foxgloves and oleander (see Chapter 17) are the most common plants to cause cardiac signs.

Rupture of the aorta

This occurs in sheep and goats that harbour the nematode *Spirocerca lupi*, which occurs in tropical areas of Asia. The parasite lives in nodules in the aorta, and on rare occasions the blood vessel will be weakened and rupture. A similar parasite, *Onchocerca armillata*, has been found in India. This very rarely causes rupture but is often associated with chronic blood loss and anaemia. Injections of ivomectins are effective treatment.

Schistosomiasis

These trematode parasites live in blood vessels and can cause a variety of different signs and symptoms. They occur throughout the tropics but are also found in Central Asia, the Middle East and the Mediterranean. They are elongated trematodes that have separate sexes, unlike liver fluke. The male lives in a groove in the female. They are found in small ruminants as well as in a variety of other species, including man. They mainly live in the mesenteric and portal veins and so cause diarrhoea, dysentery, anaemia, emaciation and death. The pulmonary form causes respiratory signs. Oral praziquantel at 25 mg/kg is effective treatment if repeated at weekly intervals for a minimum of 5 weeks.

Vegetative endocarditis

This condition occurs in small ruminants. If the tricuspid valve is affected it is called right-sided heart failure, and there will be ascites, peripheral oedema and a marked jugular pulse. This will be seen in goats and hair sheep. It will not be seen in wool sheep unless they are recently shorn. If the bicuspid valve is affected it is called left-sided heart failure, and there will be oedema of the lungs. This may show as a dull area in the ventral thorax. The animal may well have a cough when it is exerted, and the resting pulse rate may well be raised. Clinicians should remember that dropped beats are normal in sheep and goats. It is possible to have vegetative lesions on both sides of the heart. The combination of signs will be confusing.

Diagnosis can be confirmed with a 5.0 MHz scanner. A variety of bacteria can cause the condition, and *Erysipelothrix rhusiopathiae* is a common cause. Animals should be treated with antibiotics for at least 2 weeks. The author normally uses a penicillin and streptomycin combination, but clinicians may prefer to use a longer-acting antibiotic if the owners are unable to inject the animals themselves. The condition may be incurable. However if the signs diminish that is excellent, but if the animal is pregnant the owner should be advised to give a 2-week course of antibiotics immediately after parturition in case the condition flares up.

Ventricular septal defects

Ventricular septal defects are extremely rare in lambs and very rare in kids.

Viral myocarditis

This condition is seen in small ruminants. It is associated with FMD infection and results in sudden death.

Diseases Affecting the Haemopoietic and Lymphatic Systems

Anaplasmosis

This is an arthropod-borne, rickettsial disease of ruminants. There is confusion as the main organism is *Anaplasma phagocytophilum*.

Babesiosis

Babesia spp. are tick-transmitted protozoan parasites of the red blood cells. In the UK sheep can be infected with *B. motasi*, a sheep parasite, and *B. capreoli*, a parasite of red deer. The parasites rarely cause problems on their own, but they exacerbate concurrent tick-borne fever. Ticks become infected when they ingest a blood meal from a parasitaemic host. Within the tick, the *Babesia* spp. probably reproduce sexually, and are transmitted between larval, nymph and adult stages, and transovarially, through infection of the eggs by a vermicule stage of the parasite. *Babesia* spp. enter the salivary glands of the ticks and are transmitted to the sheep. Rapid, asexual division of the parasite occurs within the host's red blood cells, leading to haemolysis. The severity of the disease depends on the pathogenicity of the *Babesia* spp., host immunity and the level of challenge. The diagnosis of babesiosis is based on knowledge of *Babesia* spp.-infected tick activity and can be confirmed by identification of the parasite in Giemsa-stained red blood smears. Babesiosis can occur in goats.

Theileriosis

This disease is often subclinical. It is caused by the tick-borne protozoa *Theileria ovis* and *Theileria recondite*, which are similar to *Babesia* spp. They initially infect the lymphocytes and then the erythrocytes of the sheep. They have been isolated worldwide and associated with disease, but in the UK have only been found in Wales, where they were subclinical.

Tick-borne fever

This disease in sheep is caused by infection of white blood cells with the rickettsial organism *Anaplasma phagocytophilum*. Goats can harbour the infection but very rarely show any signs. The ticks regurgitate their gut contents during blood feeding, and these transmit the disease. Often all the nymphs and adult ticks on a farm are infected. The infection of the white blood cells causes neutropenia, lymphopenia and thrombocytopenia. The sheep will show pyrexia and malaise within 24 h of infection. This will last for 3 weeks and make the sheep, particularly the lambs, more susceptible to concurrent secondary viral and bacterial infections. There are antigenic variations so often no immunity is established. Lambs cannot be protected by colostral antibodies and so they are most at risk to contracting louping ill and joint ill. Naive pregnant ewes moved into infected areas may abort, and rams may be infertile. The disease can be avoided by bringing the ewes out of the area to lamb. The ewes and lambs can be returned after being treated with an effective pour-on treatment to prevent tick infestation. Diagnosis can be made by seeing the *A. phagocytophilum* inclusion bodies in cytoplasmic vacuoles of monocytes and neutrophils in Giemsa-stained blood smears. Splenomegaly will be seen on post-mortem. PCR and ELISA tests will be available soon.

Trypanosomiasis

Trypanosomes are, other than a very few exceptions, spread by tsetse flies (*Glossina* spp.). These flies are found in Africa south of the Sahara and north of the Limpopo River. Trypanosomiasis is therefore mainly restricted to this very large belt across Africa. The tsetse cannot withstand low temperatures and so it is not found at altitudes of over 1500 m, altitudes below which wool sheep are not kept, so they are not affected by trypanosomiasis. However goats and hair sheep will contract the disease. If there are large numbers of tsetse flies the challenge to the animals and indeed the humans will be too great, and so only game animals will exist in these areas, many of which include the famous national game parks. Sheep and goats will contract trypanosomiasis in areas where there are not so many tsetse flies.

Trypanosomes are flagellate protozoa with an undulating membrane. The three main species that infect sheep and goats are, in order of size, *Trypanosoma brucei*, *Trypanosoma vivax* and *Trypanosoma congolense*. There is considerable debate as to how pathogenic these trypanosomes are to sheep and goats. They are definitely pathogenic, but whether they can cause disease in their own right is questioned. In the author's experience they will die of the disease if they are stressed in any way, for instance by starvation, intestinal parasites or being driven on foot over long distances. *T. vivax* and *T. congolense* can readily be seen in the bloodstream and are best found on a thick smear stained with Giemsa, but can also be found with more careful observation on a thin smear also stained with Giemsa. They primarily cause anaemia and pyrexia. *T. brucei* tends to invade the lymphatics so swollen peripheral lymph nodes will be seen. The trypanosomes may be seen in the blood but also may be found on a lymph node smear.

The perceived tolerance to trypanosomiasis shown by sheep and goats may be because tsetse flies would rather feed on other mammalian species. Certainly pregnant goats are bitten more frequently than non-pregnant females, and males are very rarely bitten. The author only has experience with *Glossina morsitans* and *Glossina pallidipes*. Other *Glossina* spp. may have different feeding habits. In the author's experience goats and sheep that are born and reared in a tsetse area seem considerably more tolerant than naive animals.

Diminazene aceturate can be used to cure all these infections. It is supplied in 1.05 g sachets for reconstitution in 12.5 ml of water to make a 12.5% solution. This will treat ten adult goats. It should be made up in as sterile a manner as possible to avoid causing abscesses. Isometamidium can be used to treat all three species but there is widespread resistance and so the author would not advise its use without careful follow-up.

Quinapyramine can be used as either the sulfate or the chloride preparation. There is also now very widespread resistance in infections of *T. brucei*, *T. congolense* and *T. vivax*, and so this drug, together with homidium either as the sulfate or chloride preparation, is probably best avoided.

Tumours of the Cardiovascular System

By far the most common tumours are haemangiomas. These may be found in the spleen, liver, intestine and subcutis. They are normally benign but will haemorrhage and cause anaemia. Clinically, this will resemble haemonchosis. Fibromas are very rarely seen in the heart muscle. These do not normally show clinically, only on post-mortem.

12

Urinary System

Introduction

Some urinary conditions are linked with the genital system (see Chapter 13). Sheep and goats suffer from similar urinary problems.

Congenital and Hereditary Conditions of the Urinary System

Renal agenesis

This condition may be hereditary. However it is normally seen as a terminal condition and so euthanasia is advised. It is often linked to gonadal agenesis. If it is unilateral, both renal agenesis and gonadal agenesis may well go unnoticed in females. In males there may be a misdiagnosis, considering them to be rigs. Hopefully surgery will not be attempted. In the author's experience ultrasonography is not helpful but perhaps with more sophisticated equipment and a more skilled operator, that may be the way forward. Equally, laparoscopy could make diagnosis clearer.

Persistent patent urachus

This is usually a congenital condition as the urachus fails to close at birth. However if it occurs a few days after birth it is likely to be as a result of a septic omphalophlebitis. Differentiation is important as treatment is likely to be different. If the urachus remains patent at birth, it can be ligated immediately and the animal should receive antibiotics for 10 days, after which the clinician should carry out a careful check. The tetanus status should be ascertained, and fly control is important.

In the event of the urachus not closing with this treatment or if it has become patent some days after birth as a result of infection, more aggressive surgery needs to be carried out. The neonate should be anaesthetized (see Chapter 8) and surgically prepared. The practitioner should perform a laparotomy so that the urachus can be traced back to the bladder. It should be sectioned and the bladder closed with a double layer of continuous Lembert sutures of an absorbable material. The umbilical vessels should be ligated proximally to any infected and diseased tissue. This tissue should then be totally removed. The abdomen should be closed with interrupted sutures of monofilament nylon. These all should be laid individually before any are tightened in a 'vest over pants' configuration. When the practitioner is satisfied that there are enough sutures to close the abdomen and that no small intestine is trapped, the sutures can be tightened. It is very important that no extra sutures are added after this on account of the danger of perforation of the small intestine. A subcuticular layer of continuous sutures of an absorbable material should be laid before the skin is closed with interrupted horizontal mattress sutures of monofilament nylon. It is important that the animal receives aggressive antibiotic treatment for 10 days, when the sutures – if clean and dry – can be removed. If there is any doubt, they should be left in place and further antibiotic treatment should be given.

Medical Conditions of the Urinary Tract

Nephritis and nephrosis occur in sheep and goats. The presenting sign will be general malaise and low-grade abdominal pain. It is rarely painful enough to be termed colic. Nephrosis is a distinct clinical entity in young lambs of between 2 and 4 weeks of age, which will stop sucking and yet appear to be thirsty, as they will stand over the water supply. The cause is unknown. Clinicians may be asked to examine these cases post-mortem. They may be mistaken for clostridial disease; indeed the condition may be as a result of an unknown toxin. There is no treatment.

Surgical Conditions of the Male Urinary Tract

General

The male urinary tract is similar in sheep and goats. The urethra is long and narrow, with a sigmoid flexure and a small urethral appendage. Gelded males appear to be more susceptible to obstruction than entire males. Obstruction is virtually unheard of when the animals are at grass, but is really quite common in animals fed dried food. The animals will be seen to strain. The urethra can be felt pulsating just below the anus. No urine will be passed and the hair near the tip of the prepuce will be dry.

The classes of sheep most at risk include: early-born, indoor-reared lambs; artificially reared lambs; ram lambs bred for showing or use in their first year; and store lambs on a finishing ration. Urethral obstruction may occur in up to 10% of affected male sheep whether castrated or entire. Surgical treatments have a good success rate and have welfare implications, so preventative measures are very important. These should focus on reducing calculus formation. The most common types of calculus seen in animals on a cereal-based ration are phosphates, usually calcium or magnesium salts. They form in the kidney medulla and are often found at slaughter or post-mortem as incidental findings. However as soon as they start to obstruct the flow of urine, the development of clinical signs will start. If they block a single ureter this will cause nephrosis, which will remain subclinical as the second kidney will compensate. There is a danger of pyelonephritis in this diseased kidney. The lamb then will become ill with a raised rectal temperature. However, if both become blocked the lamb will quickly be become clinically ill, anorexic, and have a hunched gait and painful kidneys. This condition is more common in ewe lambs but a blocked urethra is more common in males.

Urethral obstruction in male lambs has the signs described above. These will quickly turn to bladder or urethral rupture, renal failure and death. Early diagnosis is very important and can be aided by ultrasonography. An author (Scott, 2000) states that diagnostic quality images of the abdomen and bladder of sheep can be readily obtained using a 5-MHz sector transducer connected to a real-time, B-mode ultrasound machine. Scans can be recorded using a thermal printer or digital recording equipment. These scanners can be used to examine the abdomen in sheep, although the depth of field is limited to 10cm. The bladder of a normal male sheep is contained within the pelvis, and therefore cannot be visualized during ultrasonographic examination. A bladder that extends for up to 10cm or more over the brim is considered an abnormal finding. Every effort must be made to prevent the formation of calculi. One of the main problems is the excretion of phosphorus in the urine. Naturally there are differences between individuals, and there are also differences between breeds. Breed differences have been studied in the Netherlands. Most at risk are Texels followed by Blackface,

East Friesland, Finnish landrace and, lastly, Suffolks. Texels excrete four times more phosphorus in their urine compared to Suffolks.

Obviously the mineral content of the diet is important. Cereal diets are high in phosphorus and low in calcium, so additional phosphorus must not be fed. Lambs gaining 200 g/day should not receive more than 0.6% of phosphorus in their diet in their early life. This should be reduced to 0.4% of phosphorus in their diet in later life. Normally in ruminant diets a good regular supply of magnesium is very important. However in this instance the diet should not contain more than 0.2% of magnesium. Magnesium is absorbed more than twice as efficiently from a concentrate diet when compared to a roughage diet. Calcium has a direct link with phosphorus so extra calcium needs to be fed to make sure the calcium:phosphorus ratio is greater than 2:1. This will lower phosphorus excretion in the urine.

Another part of the problem is the nature of the diet. High roughage diets require chewing, which stimulates saliva flow. Phosphorus is excreted in the saliva, which is then swallowed, allowing phosphorus to be lost in the faeces rather than excreted by the kidney and hence to the urine. If roughage is fed *ad lib.* the amount of phosphorus in the urine is halved. Even feeding pellets rather than a coarse mix of concentrates has an adverse effect as loose concentrates increase saliva and hence increase faecal loss of phosphorus. Apart from the effect on phosphorus excretion, a high concentrate/low roughage diet has an effect on the excretion of urinary mucoproteins. These act as a nidus for phosphorus calculi formation in the kidney medulla.

Urinary volume has a direct effect on calculi formation. The higher the flow of urine the less likely calculi are to form. Urinary volume is obviously linked directly to water intake. Lambs must have a constant supply of clean water. This may well be compromised in sub-zero temperatures. The moisture content of the food has an effect, but the frequency of feeding has more effect. Intermittent feeding triggers a renal response, so that urine production is decreased and hence urine concentration is increased. Feeding roughage *ad lib.* stimulates urine production, which in turn stimulates thirst.

Abrupt weaning, which is to be encouraged to lessen the danger of ewe mastitis (see Chapter 13), will reduce both fluid intake and urine excretion. Studies in artificially reared lambs have shown that both are halved at weaning. Urinary concentrations have been shown in ewe-reared lambs to be up to three times their strength in the first month after weaning. Ewes with twins and triplets may not have sufficient milk and so fluid intake will be reduced in these lambs even though they are suckling their mothers.

High water intake and hence high urine output has a high heritability and is linked to the potassium composition of the RBC, so certain individuals will have a higher urine output and therefore will be less at risk. Certain breeds (e.g. Scottish Blackface) have been found to have a higher urine output.

The normal ruminant urine from animals fed on an *ad lib.* roughage diet is alkaline. On the other hand a high cereal diet lowers the pH, making the urine acid. This effect is beneficial to the lamb as an acid diet lessens the formation of calculi. The farmer therefore has a balancing act to perform, as high cereal diets are not necessarily going to have an adverse effect: they will cause the urine to be acid, but will increase its phosphate level.

Key factors to prevent urolithiasis

- Ensure a supply of fresh clean water from accessible drinkers *ad lib.*
- Make sure that artificially reared lambs are used to the supply of fresh water so that they can be weaned gradually. Making older lambs drink milk from a container rather than sucking allows a better transition.
- Wean lambs that are suckling from ewes when they are still on grass or outside on roots, and so on, rather than straight on to a cereal diet.
- Leave lambs entire if possible, as obstructive urolithiasis will occur in rams but it is much rarer.
- Select a suitable breed to fatten on a cereal diet.
- Do not supply free access to minerals containing phosphorus to lambs, except at grass.

- Add calcium carbonate, calcium chloride or calcium sulfate to the cereal diet to maintain a calcium:phosphorus ratio that is greater than 2:1.
- Feed palatable forage *ad lib.*
- Do not feed pellets.
- Feed cabbages and other brassicas. These are particularly useful for ram lambs being prepared for sale.
- Acidify the urine by adding ammonium chloride to the feed at the rate of 1 g per animal.
- Add salt to the diet at the rate of 2 g per animal to encourage water uptake.
- Give access to urea blocks to encourage water uptake provided they do not contain phosphorus or high magnesium.
- If the water supply has been inadequate do not handle lambs or move them violently as this may make a formed calculus move into an obstructive position.

Treatment of obstructive urolithiasis

The welfare of the lamb must be at the forefront of the clinician's mind. Lambs should not be put through painful surgical procedures just for monetary gain. Equally, very careful consideration must be given before undertaking surgery that may cause painful urine scalding and the risk of fly strike. Sadly, the use of muscle relaxants is very rarely successful. It is impossible to catheterize without severe damage to the urethra, so retrograde flushing is also impossible. Obstruction can occur at three points, and influences the surgical procedure. This must be performed as soon as possible on welfare grounds, for bladder rupture will occur within 48 h. Urethral rupture with urine escaping into the tissues may occur sooner than that.

Three options for surgery at the sigmoid flexure

Urethrostomy

This can be performed under a GA (see Chapter 8) or sedation and local anaesthesia. The penis is located just below the anus. A linear incision is made over the penis and it is drawn to through the incision by blunt dissection. The penis is then incised and the urethra within is located. The urethra is then sutured to the skin with multiple small sutures, leaving an orifice at least the size of a pencil. Urine will flow out and the bladder should be flushed with warm sterile water to remove any further stones. The animal should receive antibiotics and NSAID daily and the wound should be cleaned. Historically clinicians used to perform an urethrotomy rather than an urethrostomy, as the animal was sent for slaughter as soon as the withhold period had been reached for any medicines given, and when the smell of urine could no longer be detected. The author is concerned about the ethical and welfare issues around such a procedure, and advises immediate on-farm slaughter in such cases. In the UK the farmer is permitted to dress the carcass and use it for home consumption, but is not permitted to sell any part of the carcass. If the animal has received medicines or if the flesh smells of urine, the whole carcass should be sent for incineration.

Marsupialization

In theory this surgery could be performed under sedation and local anaesthesia. However in reality this would be very difficult, compromising both welfare and sterility, and therefore a GA must be advised. The lamb is placed in dorsal recumbency. A linear incision is made through the skin and abdominal muscles just anterior to the preputial orifice towards the umbilicus. The full bladder is drained by puncture through a sterile needle attached to a sterile piece of tube to the outside of the abdomen. The rostral end of the bladder is then drawn to just in front of the prepuce and anchored to the peritoneum, musculature and skin. A very small hole is pierced in the bladder and this is stitched with many small sutures to the peritoneum, musculature and skin. It is very important that there is a seal between the bladder and the peritoneum so that urine cannot leak into the peritoneum. The rest of the abdomen and skin is then closed in the normal manner. On recovery the lamb should be draining urine through the small hole in the skin, which should be at the lamb's lowest point on the ventral body wall.

Surgical tube cystotomy

This has been described by workers in India (Fazili *et al.*, 2010). It is a minimally invasive technique through the left paralumbar fossa that can be performed in lambs or kids. A catheter is placed in the bladder lumen through a metallic cannula, and fixed to the skin with a stay suture. The surgery can be performed with the animal either standing or in right lateral recumbency. With acidification of the urine the urinary crystals are dissolved, leading to the restoration of full urethral patency in successfully treated animals within a few days. No hospitalization is required and the catheter is removed after normal urination occurs. No recurrence of the condition was noted by the workers in a 6-month follow-up.

Surgery at the glans penis

Penile amputation has been described by other authors (Hay, 1990). The perineal area from the anus to the scrotum is clipped and prepared for surgery. The tail is held upwards and out of the way by an assistant or by anchoring in position to the pelvic fleece. A 4–5 cm vertical incision is made in the midline from the level of the tuber ischii downwards. Using blunt dissection the incision is deepened until the penis is identified as a firm, smooth, yellowish organ 1–2 cm in diameter. By blunt dissection and manual traction, isolate the penis and pull it outwards through the skin incision. Sever the penis at the lower end of the incision, but above any area of urethral obstruction, making sure that the proximal stump will be long enough to be fixed outside the wound, particularly in fatter animals. Non-absorbable simple interrupted stitches are used to suture the periurethral tissues to the dorsal end of the skin wound. Care must be taken not to puncture the urethra with sutures, or to occlude it by excessive dorsal flexion of the stump.

Surgery at the vermiform appendage

It the obstruction is seen in the vermiform appendage, this can be snipped off at its base with a pair of scissors. It is vital that all preventative measures are taken so that obstruction does not occur further up.

Tumours of the Urinary System

The most common tumours found in sheep and goats are in the bladder, and are all related to eating bracken. These tumours can block the ureters and cause nephrosis. Adenocarcinomas are seen in the kidneys of sheep and goats. They are highly malignant and will metastasize not only locally but also to other organs throughout the body.

13

Reproductive System

Congenital and Hereditary Conditions in Sheep

Daft lamb disease

The lambs show advanced neurological signs. These are as a result of degenerative changes in the Purkinje cells in various parts of the brain. The condition is caused by a recessive gene.

Hereditary chondrodysplasia

This has been termed the 'spider syndrome'. The lambs have twisted spines that cause considerable parturition problems. The condition, which is thought to be inherited, is common in Scottish Blackface sheep and was first reported in that breed in Minnesota in the USA. However it is also found in Down breeds in the UK.

Myodystrophia fetalis deformans

The lambs affected by this condition are often called stiffed-limbed lambs. There are often difficulties at parturition. It is mainly found in Welsh Mountain breeds. It is a lethal Mendelian recessive gene.

Congenital and Hereditary Conditions in Goats

Hermaphroditism

True hermaphroditism, when the goat has both ovarian and testicular tissue, is extremely rare. However pseudo-hermaphroditism is relatively common. It is linked with the poll gene in the following breeds: Alpine, Saanen, Shami and Toggenburg. It is not reported in Angora or Nubian goats. Modern terminology prefers to call both conditions 'intersex' as often the exact nature of the gonads is not known. Freemartins, when a female that is twin to a male is infertile, have been recorded but they are very rare. This is in contrast to the situation in cattle, when a female that is twinned to a bull calf is always infertile.

Medical Conditions of the Reproductive System in Sheep

Group infertility

This can be affected by a variety of conditions. Sudden changes of feed should be avoided before ram use. It is very common for shepherds to yard rams before tupping in order to prepare them, and then to turn them back out on grass with the ewes. This practice should be avoided. Rams should be turned out at least 3 weeks before running on a pasture with ewes. Obviously group fertility will be affected by long periods of either over- or underfeeding. Confinement and overfeeding before sales or showing will lower fertility, as will prolonged periods of travelling.

Individual infertility in rams

Individual fertility can be influenced by age. Both young and old rams (i.e. those over 5 years of age) can be unreliable. General health conditions, particularly diseases causing a fever, are particularly detrimental to fertility. Lameness in any form will lower fertility as will any skin disease causing pruritis. Headfly strike appears to cause particular problems to breeding rams. Any condition affecting the scrotum such as dermatitis or indeed heavy wool cover will adversely affect fertility. It is recognized among flock owners that levels of fertility within a group of rams can vary significantly. Unfortunately, there are no tests available that will accurately predict a ram's ability to put ewes in lamb. The only guarantee of a ram's breeding ability is the number and the quality of the progeny produced under normal breeding conditions. It is possible, however, to examine the different aspects of a ram's reproductive functions to estimate how closely it conforms to the generally accepted 'normal' standard and to define any abnormality that may be present (Boundy, 1993).

Poor libido in rams

One cause of individual poor libido is the raddle harness. Certain rams will not serve a ewe with the raddle harness in place. As soon as the harness is removed the ram will serve normally. Either the ram is used without any harness or marker, or the ram is used with a coloured paint on its brisket.

Poor libido will be shown by rams outside of their normal breeding season. Rams as well as ewes are influenced by length of daylight, and this is known as the photoperiodic effect. Rams can be trained to produce fertile semen throughout the year. Certain breeds such as the Suffolks are renowned in the UK for being early breeders, and others such as the Texels for being late breeders. In the northern hemisphere Finnish landrace, British Friesland and milk-sheep rams will be active early in the season, followed by Down breeds. These will be followed by such breeds as the Romney Marsh (Kents) or Border Leicester. French breeds including the Rouge de l'Ouest and Bleu de Maine will be later followed by hill breeds like Scottish Blackface and Cheviots. Herdwicks and Scottish island breeds will only be active late in the autumn. Horned breeds such as Jacobs and Dorset Horns are active throughout the year.

Some rams will show only a mild interest when joined with ewes in oestrus and this lack of libido may be permanent or temporary in nature. Over-the-fence examination of working rams should be stressed to flock owners, as a low-libido ram working with a group of rams could easily slip through the net and remain an uneconomical passenger for a considerable period of time.

Ram examination

Over 10% of rams may be infertile. This is likely to be the tip of the iceberg, with up to 30% being sub-fertile. Therefore routine physical clinical examination is well worthwhile. It is simple to perform and certainly cost effective (Fig. 13.1).

First of all it is important to identify each ram. In many countries all sheep will have ear tags, and some may have ear notches. It is quite acceptable with good shepherds for rams to have names or to be sprayed with coloured numbers. In the latter instance the numbers must be readable until the end of tupping.

Each ram should receive a general examination and a note made of his condition score. The ram should be examined standing, starting at his head. The clinician should examine the lips and incisor teeth. If the ram has a low condition score, the cheek teeth should be examined with the use of a gag.

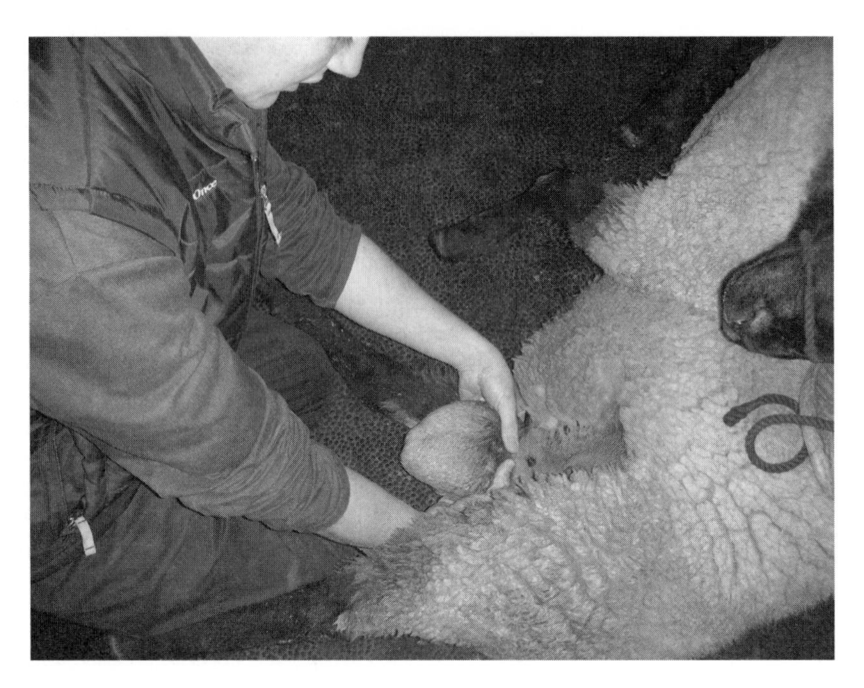

Fig. 13.1. Ram examination.

The whole head should be examined for swellings. The eyes should be checked visually and with an ophthalmoscope. Each leg should be checked for swellings and other abnormalities. Check the ram's gait before turning it over on to its rump.

Check all four feet before examining the genitalia. After examining the scrotum each testicle should be felt for resilience and abnormalities. The clinician should check for vasectomy scars and for inguinal herniation. The testicles should be symmetrical, ovoid and mobile within the scrotum. Tumours of the testicle have not been recorded in abattoir surveys in the UK (Head, 1990). Obviously old entire males are a rarity compared to cull ewes. It is thought by some shepherds that very woolly scrotums interfere with fertility as the testicles are too hot for spermatogenisis to occur normally, but there is no actual evidence for this and the amount of wool on the scrotum will vary enormously between breeds. Obviously the wool can be shorn off although it will regrow fairly rapidly. Spermatogenisis takes 6–8 weeks so shearing, if thought to be beneficial, should be carried out at least 2 months before tupping. The length and diameter of the testicles should be measured and recorded, then the epididymis tail should be examined and measured. The umbilicus should be examined for walled-off abscesses and herniation. After examining the prepuce the penis should be extruded and examined.

Semen collection

It should be remembered that rams should be removed from contact with ewes for 3 days before semen collection. Other stresses such as long travel or feed change should also be avoided.

There are three methods of collecting semen for evaluation:

- Semen can be collected immediately after natural service. A warm pipette can be inserted into the vagina through a warm speculum. Collection is not easy as a normal ejaculate is only 2 ml and this will be contaminated with female secretions, cells and even bacteria.
- Semen can be collected into an artificial vagina. This method has difficulties as

some rams will not serve such a device at all and others need a period of training.

- Semen can be collected by the use of an electro-ejaculator inserted into the rectum after the ram's prepuce has been cleaned (Fig. 13.2). This should be inserted 12–15 cm into the rectum with the probe tilted approximately 20° ventrally. Small electrical pulses are given rhythmically. This can be achieved by counting 'one, two, three, stop, one, two, three, start'. Normally a ram will ejaculate after four or five pulses. His abdominal muscles will contract but the stimulus does not appear to be painful as the rams readily submit to a second ejaculation. If semen has not been produced after 15 pulses the procedure should be abandoned. It can be repeated in 24 h. Most operators carry out this procedure with the ram standing, being held by the shepherd. One operator is required to work the electro-ejaculator and a second operator is required to collect the semen into a small polythene bag, which is kept warm in the hand. If a sterile sample of semen is required the ram has to be kept in lateral recumbency so that an operator can extrude the penis and hold it with a sterile swab. The semen can then be collected into a sterile container.

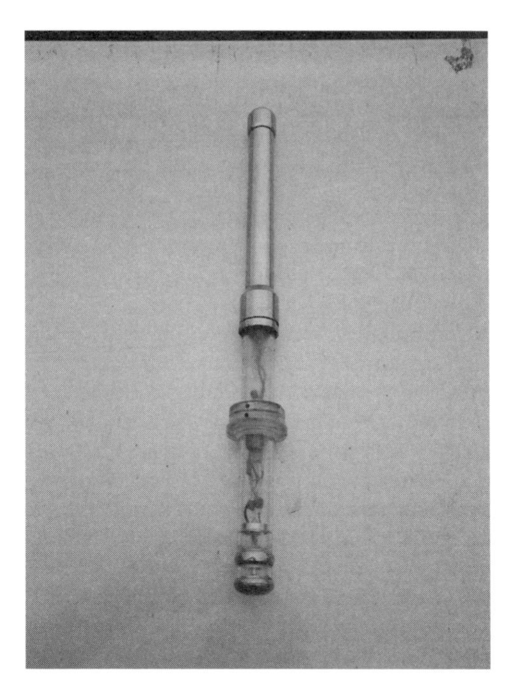

Fig. 13.2. Electro-ejaculator.

Semen examination and evaluation

Clinicians need to take care as semen is very sensitive to cold shock, bright light, detergents, blood, disinfectants, metals, cigarette smoke and temperatures above 40°C. Ideally it should be kept at 37°C. A hot-water bottle is ideal to achieve this goal. Before collection a microscope needs to be set up in a clean, warm, draught-free area. The focus needs to be adjusted to 100× initially. A heated microscope stage and a temperature-controlled water bath are very helpful, but not essential.

As stated earlier, except for bacteriological examination, the semen should be collected in a small warmed polythene bag, and with experience it is very easy to judge the approximate volume. Inexperienced clinicians can try out measured volumes of 1, 2 and 3 ml of liquid beforehand. The concentration of spermatozoa can be estimated by eye. A sample that is just watery will be very unlikely to contain any but a few spermatozoa. A cloudy sample will contain 1×10^9 spermatozoa/ml; a milky sample will contain 2.5×10^9 spermatozoa/ml; a thin creamy sample will contain 3.5×10^9 spermatozoa/ml; and a proper creamy sample will contain the desired concentration of $>4 \times 10^9$ spermatozoa/ml.

Wave motion can be assessed by directly examining the sample in the bag under 100× on the microscope. The requirement is for vigorous moving waves to be seen. If only slow small waves are seen, this is not ideal. Individual sperm motility requires dilution with warm 0.9% normal saline at 1:100 with the sample viewed under the 400× power. Ideally over half of the spermatozoa should be moving in a single direction.

To study spermatozoon morphology a slide of the diluted semen needs to be stained with a warmed 5% nigrosin and 1% eosin mixture. After 30 s the excess stain can be poured off and the slide examined under the oil immersion. Normal semen will often contain up to 30% abnormal cells. The normal abnormalities are: detached heads, detached tails, abnormal head shapes, abaxial tails, double heads, double tails and dag tails (tails curled tightly around the midpiece). The percentage of abnormal spermatozoa should be noted. This stain will also differentiate dead spermatozoa, which, unlike the live spermatozoa, will take up the nigrosin stain. Normally a sample will have up to 25% dead spermatozoa. The percentage should be noted and recorded.

A thin smear of semen can be air dried and stained with Leishman's stain. This is useful to evaluate any inflammatory response in rams that are suspected of being infertile. It is not required for routine fertility evaluation.

In conclusion it should be stressed that semen evaluation is a useful tool but has its limitations and is only a picture for that day, neither for the past nor the future. Clinicians must make sure every ram is identified carefully. Finally, it is of the utmost importance that welfare is always a consideration.

Artificial insemination and embryo transfer

The reproductive technologies of artificial insemination (AI) and multiple ovulation and embryo transfer (MOET) have made a significant impact on the UK sheep industry. Objective assessment of body composition has allowed a large genetic improvement. This improvement could have been obtained with normal breeding policy but it has been considerably speeded up by these reproductive technologies. The downside of these technologies is welfare. The improvements have become more efficient and acceptable, but researchers always need to have welfare at the forefront of their minds.

Causes of abortion in ewes

General

A low level of lamb loss from natural, uncontrollable causes is inevitable. Once the level of abortions reaches 2% (i.e. 1 in every 50 ewes), then the chances are an infection is present. This should be controlled, but a diagnosis needs to be made before control measures can be put in place. In the UK on average 6.3% of lowland flock ewes abort annually. If the top 10% of herds are studied, this figure drops to 3.3%. Labour costs are a significant factor for most sheep flocks. High abortion rates create a lot more work and stress at lambing time, which will increase the labour demands. *Chlamydophila* accounts for over half of infectious abortions and, together with toxoplasmosis, accounts for over 75% of the infectious causes of abortion in the UK. Both of these diseases can be controlled by vaccination (see Chapter 7). The other infectious causes are *Campylobacter* 9%, *Salmonella* 3%, *Listeria* 2% and other causes 10%.

Clinicians should advise their clients to isolate and mark ewes that abort (Fig. 13.3). They should submit freshly aborted lambs and placentae. Clinicians in their turn should submit placentae, abdominal fluid and abomasal fluid to a laboratory to obtain a diagnosis.

Farmers should adopt the following procedure when dealing with a ewe that aborts:

1. Immediately isolate an aborting ewe from the remaining ewes.
2. Ear tag and record which ewes have aborted on which date to help with possible blood sampling for serology later.
3. Remove all cleansings and fetuses.
4. Contact their practitioner to discuss which samples to collect for laboratory diagnosis.
5. Do not foster female lambs on to aborted ewes.
6. Do not allow any pregnant women anywhere near the aborting ewe, the products of abortion or their overalls.

Farmers should prepare for the worst long before lambing by preparing an area to isolate any ewes that abort.

Akabane

Akabane is an insect-transmitted virus that causes congenital abnormalities in the central nervous systems (CNS) of sheep and goats. It is spread by biting midges in Australia, Japan

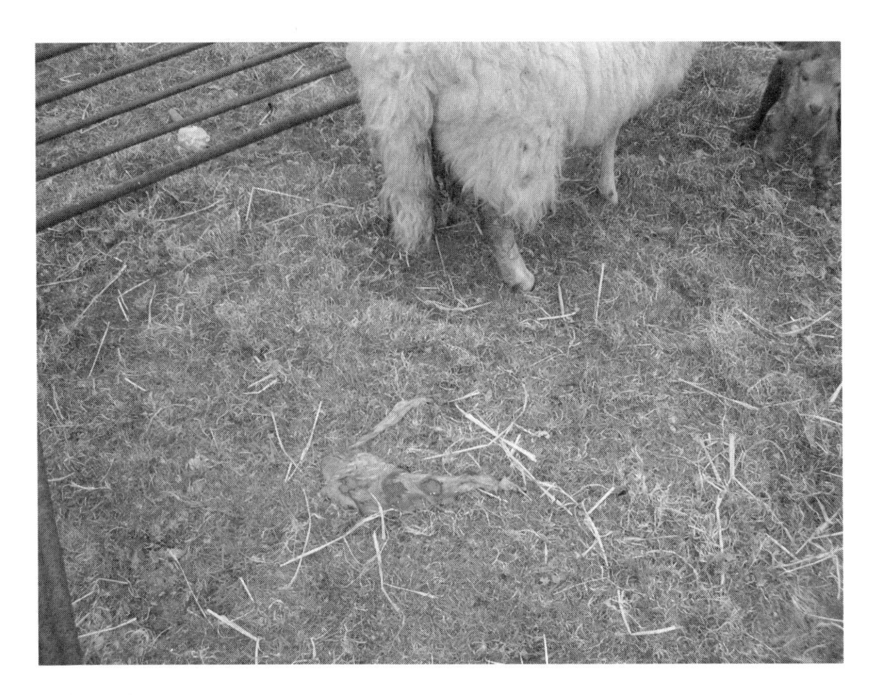

Fig. 13.3. Sheep abortion.

and Kenya. The author has had first-hand experience of the disease in Bahrain. It is a virus of the Bunyaviridae family and is mainly a disease of cattle, causing stillbirths and abortions in sheep and goats. The lambs and kids will show pulmonary hypoplasia and hypoplasia of the spinal cord. A presumptive diagnosis can be made on these gross pathological signs, and this can be confirmed by testing sera of unsuckled affected offspring and their dams for serum neutralizing antibodies. There is no specific treatment for affected animals, and measures should be directed at the prevention of infection of susceptible animals with Akabane virus during pregnancy. Introduction of stock from non-endemic areas should be done well before first breeding. A vaccine is available in Japan.

Border disease

This disease is caused by a *Pestivirus* very similar to BVD in cattle. It can occur at any stage of pregnancy. The disease should be suspected if live lambs are born showing the pathognomic signs of a hairy coat and trembling; shepherds call the lambs 'hairy shakers'. Other than abortion the ewes show no other signs. The only danger to the ewe is a metritis subsequent to a difficult lambing. Abortion storms can occur but they are rare, and are normally sporadic. The diagnostic sample of choice is a precolostral blood sample taken from an affected neonatal lamb. Affected lambs may be border disease virus (BDV) antigen positive, or BDV antibody positive and antigen negative. When a group of ewes from a flock experiencing a BDV outbreak is tested, a range of moderate to high antibody titres is likely to be seen in the ELISA test. However, the presence of antibody only indicates exposure to the virus and is not diagnostic of BDV-associated abortion. Testing a stratified 10% sample of ewes can be of some assistance in assessing the extent of infection within a lambed group. Ewes which produce lambs showing neurological signs may be BVD antibody negative but also be persistently infected with the virus (i.e. antigen positive). The condition is best controlled by management, mixing replacements with the ewe flock before tupping. BVD vaccines have been used but there is no evidence of their effectiveness in sheep.

Brucellosis

The main species causing abortion in sheep is *Brucella melitensis*; although this is mainly linked to goats, it has similar effects in both animals. The species *Brucella ovis* is more often found in sheep than in goats. It is an organism that causes infertility in rams and is not associated with abortion. It is occurs in east and southern Africa, as well as in the Middle East. *Brucella* spp. are zoonotic (see Chapter 19).

Cache Valley virus

This mosquito-transmitted viral disease causes infertility, abortions and stillbirths in sheep in Mexico, the USA and Canada. By the time the sheep has aborted it is no longer infective. The disease occurs as abortion storms and then appears to die down for several years. Diagnosis is by paired blood samples showing a rising titre. There is no vaccine or treatment available.

Campylobacteriosis

Campylobacter usually enters a flock through a carrier animal, normally a sheep; however it could be another mammal or a wild bird. The ewes pick up the infection from aborted fetuses, placenta or birth fluids. Abortion occurs 1–3 weeks after infection and there may be large numbers of abortions. Once a ewe is infected, she will develop a lifelong immunity to the disease and an abortion storm is very unlikely to recur in the same flock in the following year. A vaccine is available to protect against campylobacteriosis, but it is not very effective and so farmers have to rely on strict hygiene and biosecurity when dealing with an aborting ewe. Water sources should be protected from vermin. Some clinicians advise natural vaccination by mixing ewes that are known to have aborted from campylobacteriosis with ewes that have lambed normally to give immunity to the disease before next year's lambing.

Concurrent disease

Any disease that causes a high temperature (e.g. an early infected fly strike) is likely to cause an abortion. Multiple abortions will occur in any flock that is infected with a highly contagious disease (e.g. FMD) or by infectious diseases (e.g. blue tongue). Clinicians have a dilemma when asked to treat ewes with high temperatures. Obviously they must warn owners of the danger of an abortion, but equally the abortion may be blamed on their treatment. Antibiotics will not normally cause abortions nor will NSAID but many are not licensed for use in pregnant animals. However NSAID will reduce pyrexia rapidly and therefore the risk is worthwhile. Corticosteroids or prostaglandins should never be given to pregnant ewes.

Enzootic abortion of ewes

Enzootic abortion of ewes (EAE) is caused by ovine strains of the zoonotic microorganism *Chlamydophila psittaci* that exhibit a predilection for placental tissue. In a severe outbreak over 30% of ewes may abort, but the endemic situation is more common with 10% of naive ewes aborting. The infection is most commonly introduced into a clean flock by sheep carrying asymptomatic enteric infection. Some animals will then abort and spread the organism to in-contact ewe lambs and ewes. These in turn will then abort and spread the infection throughout the flock. Normally abortion occurs in the last 3 weeks of pregnancy, but there will also be stillborn full-term lambs. There will also be weak lambs that are reluctant to suck and soon die. Dead lambs will appear normal but there will be necrosis and thickening of the cotyledons and the rest of the placenta. Occasionally the ewes will have a transient metritis and be off colour. This is rare and usually they are normal and breed normally the next season.

It is vital to get a confirmation of the diagnosis, which is relatively straightforward using impression smears from affected areas of the placenta. The organisms will be revealed as red bodies among blue-staining cells. A retrospective diagnosis can be made by paired serum samples, the first of which should be taken at the time of abortion. The complement fixation test (CFT) is the standard screening test used. The Western blot test is more specific but is also more expensive. If adequate material (including placental tissues) from several ewes has been examined and found negative during an abortion outbreak there is little justification for further maternal serology. However, if abortion material submissions have been inadequate and suspicion of the disease remains, blood sampling of aborted females is advised. When there has been an abortion caused by EAE in late pregnancy there is a large multiplication of organisms in the placenta. This means aborting ewes commonly demonstrate high levels of circulating antibody to the organism in the period immediately following the abortion. Antibody titres will then tend to remain high for several months before declining steadily. Because of the relatively transient nature of this humoral response to infection, if a significant antibody titre is detected, it may be assumed that the ewe experienced an abortion due to EAE during her most recent pregnancy. Vaccination may confuse the serological picture to some extent, although generally vaccinated animals have lower antibody levels unless they have been exposed to field challenge of the disease.

Hygiene control is very important. As the dead lambs and the placentas have high numbers of organisms, they should be destroyed. The discharging ewes are also highly contagious and should be isolated until they have stopped discharging. They should not be used as foster mothers as the ewe lambs will become infected. There is good evidence that infection and abortion can occur within the same lambing period, so this isolation policy is particularly important in flocks with a long lambing period. The main period for the ewe to become infected is from the 11th to the 14th week of pregnancy. The ewes then abort 5–6 weeks later. The numbers of abortions can be greatly reduced if the ewes can be given long-acting tetracycline injections at 20mg/kg every 2 weeks during this period, although the best method of control is vaccination 1 month before tupping (see Chapter 7). This will almost totally eliminate abortions due to *Chlamydophila*. In following years all the replacements should be vaccinated prior to tupping. Vaccination can only cease if the sheep are kept as a closed flock.

The risk of human infection is real for pregnant women and so hygienic precautions should be taken (see Chapter 19). However mammalian *Chlamydophila* are much less virulent in humans when compared to avian organisms and so the risk should be analysed carefully.

Leptospirosis

The only really specific pathogen is *Leptospira interrogans* although many other *Leptospira* spp. have been found in aborted fetuses or placentas as opportunist pathogens.

Listeriosis

This is primarily a neurological disease (see Chapter 14), but the organism can cause abortion at any time in pregnancy. Abortion will usually occur approximately 7 days after infection. The organism can be found in the placenta or the fetus. Serology is unreliable as many normal sheep will show raised titres.

Neosporosis

The organism is *Neospora caninum*, and it is very similar to *Toxoplasma gondii*, being differentiated from *Toxoplasma* by electron microscopy. It can also be distinguished by serology by fluorescent antibody test (FAT). It is primarily a condition of cattle and dogs rather than sheep and cats, and it is thought that transmission from dogs is possible but rare. However, infected cows infect their fetuses, the majority of which will be born alive and healthy and in turn infect their fetuses. It is extremely rare in sheep, although one outbreak has been recorded in sheep in Brazil.

Nutrition

Theoretically starvation could be a cause of abortion. However in reality provided there is no problem of oxygen supply to the fetus, abortion does not appear to occur. Certain mineral deficiencies, e.g. iodine or selenium, will definitely cause abortion but general malnourishment does not.

Q fever

Q fever is a zoonosis caused by *Coxiella burnetii*. It is an obligate intracellular parasite with ruminants being the main reservoirs of infection, although other animals can be infected. Infected animals excrete *C. burnetii* in the placenta, vaginal mucus, faeces and milk. Human disease occurs from close animal contact or through contact with an infected environment. Many animals have a sub-clinical infection, and isolation of the organism is difficult and time consuming. The best diagnostic tool for abortion samples is a real-time PCR. There appear to be two circulation cycles. The first occurs in wild animals and ticks and the second in domestic animals. There is a small cell variant (SCV) that is very like a spore and is resistant to heat, pressure, desiccation and disinfectants. It will survive in a suitable environment for years. The large cell variant (LCV) multiplies and persists in host monocytes and macrophages. These localize in the mammary gland and placenta.

This condition is seen in sheep worldwide, particularly in milking sheep, and is a known cause of abortion and mastitis. Large numbers of seropositive sheep have been found in Germany and Cyprus, and significant numbers in Chad, Turkey and Italy. However it is primarily a disease found in goats. The disease is similar in both species and a vaccine is now available for both sheep and goats. Q fever is most likely to be spread from infected animals or samples to people by inhalation of infected aerosols and by splashing of infected fluids onto mucous membranes or non-intact skin.

Good hygienic practice should be adopted and the generation of aerosols should be kept to an absolute minimum, especially when examining and sampling aborted fetuses. Personal protective clothing should be commensurate with the risk, and one should consider the use of masks, eye shields and visors, as appropriate. Where the risk of Q fever is high then full respiratory protection by the use of a powered ventilator may be warranted. It is a serious zoonosis (see Chapter 19).

Rift Valley fever

RVF is a zoonosis (see Chapter 19). It is not found in the UK but it causes abortion in sheep in Africa, mainly south of the Sahara, and is also found in Egypt. Massive numbers of abortions, approaching 100%, is the typical picture when the virus hits a pregnant flock. It also causes deaths in lambs, which may die within hours. The main sign is haemorrhages and congestion in all the mucous membranes. Some orifices may even drip blood. The virus may even cause disease in adults with a mortality of up to 35%. Abortions may occur at any stage. The fetuses will be autolysed and the afterbirth will be retained. On post-mortem massive necrosis is seen in the livers of affected lambs. In adults there is also liver necrosis but this tends to more focal. Diagnosis in the live animal can be confirmed by virus isolation, AGID, CT and reverse transcriptase polymerase chain reaction (RT-PCR). The disease is mainly spread by mosquitoes (*Aedes* spp.) (see Chapter 10). Control is carried out by vaccination (see Chapter 7).

Salmonellosis

As a cause of ovine abortion in the UK this disease increased in importance in the 1960s and 1970s. It is not as important in the UK at the present time. It is normally caused by the specific serotype, *Salmonella abortus ovis*, a pathogen found in other places in northern Europe but not in the rest of the world. However abortions in sheep can be caused by other *Salmonella* spp., namely *S. dublin*, *S. montevideo*, *S. typhimurium* and *S. arizona*. These abortions occur worldwide. They may be the actual cause of the abortion (i.e. the organism will be found in the aborted placenta or fetus), or they may cause abortion by pyrexia. Abortions caused by these species of *Salmonella* may cause deaths and the morbidity may be high.

Abortions caused by *S. abortus ovis* rarely cause mortality. There is an initial abortion storm but after that the numbers of abortions are limited. Sadly there is no specific treatment or vaccination available. *Salmonella* spp. are zoonotic (see Chapter 19).

Sarcocystiosis

Various *Sarcocystis* spp. are found in sheep throughout the world. The most commonly reported is *S. tenella*, which is said to be a microcystic species. This is a cyst-forming coccidia in carnivores, mainly dogs, which are the definitive host. The sheep is an intermediate host. Macrocystic species are normally found in cats, where the cysts are visible to the naked eye. The role of the organism in sheep is far from clear. Massive infections will cause severe illness with a high fever and abortion, and death may follow. However most infections are low and cause no clinical signs. In fact the macrocystic species may not actually be pathogenic to sheep.

Schallemberg disease

This virus disease occurs in cattle, sheep and goats. It is caused by a virus very similar to the virus which causes Akabane. It is spread by midges and causes a transitory fever. The main problem with the condition is that if the disease infects animals during pregnancy it is liable to cause abortion and deformed fetuses. At the time of writing the disease has only been found in Germany, Belgium and Holland. However, since writing this we now have it in the UK (I have been dealing with an outbreak) and also in France.

Sporadic causes

The two most likely causes of sporadic abortions are *Bacillus licheniformis* and *Arcanobacterium pyogenes*. Rare isolates of *Staphylococcus* spp. and *Streptococcus* spp. are found in aborted fetuses. Extremely rarely *Yersinia* spp., *Fusibacterium necrophorum*, *Escherichia coli* (verotoxin producing) and *Pasteurella* spp. are found. Lastly, a variety of fungal organisms have been found but their significance is often in doubt.

Streptococcus pluranimalium

This organism has been isolated from the placenta of an aborted lamb (Foster *et al.*, 2010) and from a full-term lamb dead from a dystocia problem. The inference is that this organism may have been responsible for the abortion as no other pathogen was isolated. It has been associated with abortions in cattle and isolated from the tonsil of a goat but not associated with abortions in small ruminants before.

Stress

The part played by stress in causing abortions is very confusing, and clinicians should be very careful about blaming stress for an abortion storm in a flock of sheep. An infectious cause is very much more likely and strenuous efforts should be made to take adequate samples from the aborted lambs and their placentas so that a confirmed diagnosis is made. Stress from vaccinating heavily pregnant ewes for clostridial disease is likely to cause hypocalcaemia rather than abortion. Obviously if the hypocalcaemia is left untreated then an abortion is a likely sequel.

Heat stress may cause abortion. It is likely to occur in late pregnancy in housed ewes that are over-fat and have not been shorn. It does not seem to be a problem in the tropics in ewes that are native to the area.

Tick-borne fever

The disease itself is not the direct cause of the abortion that follows exposure of the susceptible pregnant ewe to the infection, but is the result of the biphasic pyrexia alone. This reaction to tick-borne fever (TBF) is seen in other species and also in other conditions in sheep such as pasteurellosis and sheep-pox.

TBF is seen throughout Europe where the sheep tick *Ixodes ricinus* is found. These areas are mainly in the colder parts of northern Europe or in the Alps. A similar condition has been described in India, where *I. ricinus* is not found. Another tick is thought to spread the disease but the agent causing the disease, *Ehrlichia phagocytophilia* (recently renamed *Cytoecetes phagocytophilia*), has not been isolated from any potential vectors. The disease has also been seen in goats.

Most stock will experience infection early in life, and life-long premunity will develop in acclimatized sheep on grazings that are heavily infected. Abortions are not seen in these stock, but are seen when naive pregnant ewes are exposed to the infection. Diagnosis is not easy: it is necessary to demonstrate the leucopoenia that follows primary infection, or the agent in the polymorphonuclear leucocytes. Often a presumptuous diagnosis is made from the history. Ticks can be newly spread on to a grazing, which may confuse the practitioner. The main method of control is to insure that all female stock are introduced to the infection before they become pregnant.

The organism is an extremely efficient parasite and infects most ticks, hence the infection can be transmitted by very few ticks. The duration of immunity following infection is variable and may last for as little as a few months or extend for more than 1 year, but resistance is generally maintained between periods of tick activity. There is no protection provided by colostral antibodies, so lambs can become infected as soon as they are exposed to ticks.

Achieving a satisfactory diagnosis in cases of abortion associated with TBF is a particular challenge. A positive TBF titre in the counter-immunoelectrophoresis test, or the demonstration of elementary bodies in peripheral blood smears, indicate recent exposure to the organism *C. phagocytophilia*. Single positive samples are of dubious value. If no other potential pathogen has been demonstrated, then the finding of a number of TBF antibody-positive animals within a group of aborted ewes is strong circumstantial evidence of the infection contributing to an abortion outbreak. A history of introduction of TBF-susceptible pregnant animals on to a known tick farm can also be helpful in confirming the diagnosis.

Toxoplasmosis

Toxoplasmosis causes perinatal mortality in sheep. It is of major economic importance and is a zoonosis (see Chapter 19). The disease is caused by an obligate intracellular protozoan parasite with a two-stage asexual life cycle that can take place in warm-blooded animals, and a coccidian-type sexual cycle that is confined to the intestine of members of the cat family. The domestic cat is the real zoonotic danger to man, but it is relevant to sheep that wild rodents and birds can harbour bradyzoites in tissue cysts within brain and muscle. In addition, infection in mice can also be passed vertically from generation to generation without causing significant illness, thus helping to maintain a long-lasting reservoir of infection for susceptible cats (Buxton, 1989).

The cat is also the main danger to sheep. Cats spread the disease in their faeces as very resistant oocysts. They contaminate concentrates, fodder and bedding. Young cats pose a significantly greater danger than older animals; a single young cat will produce 1 million oocysts/g of faeces. Only 200 oocysts are required to infect a single sheep.

After ingestion of feed or water contaminated with oocysts, naive animals become and remain infected for life. Infection of the placenta and conceptus occurs only when the initial infection establishes in susceptible pregnant animals following ingestion of oocysts. The oocysts encyst in the digestive tract and the released sporozoites penetrate the cells lining the gut so that tachyzoites eventually reach and infect the placenta and fetus. If this infection occurs before 2 months of the pregnancy the fetus will be resorbed and the ewe will appear barren. If the infection occurs between 2 and 4 months then the ewe will either abort, or have a stillborn or a very weak lamb. Ewes infected in the last month of pregnancy normally have normal, full-term lambs. Diagnosis of the condition can be carried out by histopathological examination of the cotyledons.

Once infected, ewes have life-long immunity. A good vaccine is available that should be injected into the ewes at least 2 weeks before tupping (see Chapter 7), but if natural exposure is likely to be sporadic a booster should be given every 3 years. Replacements should be vaccinated before they enter the breeding flock. If a clinician is faced with a confirmed outbreak, decoquinate can be given orally. However, to be fully effective it needs to be fed for the last 14 weeks of pregnancy. This is only practical on farms where there are two flocks, one of which is lambing much later than the other. The most practical manner to get decoquinate into the ewes is to have it in a palatable lick: 14-kg tubs are prepared with 4400 mg/kg of decoquinate and put out at the rate of 1 tub per 25 ewes. One tub per 7 ewes will cover a 14-week period.

If an unvaccinated flock develops the disease, the number of abortions can be lessened by feeding the ewes 15 mg of monensin daily from before the time susceptible pregnant sheep are exposed to infection. This preparation is not licensed in the UK.

Care must be taken when interpreting the results of serology on aborted ewes. The normal test is the Latex Agglutination Test (LAT). Antibodies persisting from an earlier infection and the use of the vaccine can both produce suspicious or weak positive titres. Conversely, since it may take 1 month for antibodies to appear in the serum, a negative LAT result does not necessarily rule out toxoplasmosis. However a strongly positive LAT titre from an aborted ewe, although not diagnostic, is still significant and generally indicates the need for further investigation. Examination of aborted and stillborn fetuses is still the gold standard. The duration of the antibody is prolonged and therefore a detectable titre is therefore not necessarily related to infection during the most recent pregnancy.

Thogotovirus

This virus was first reported to cause abortion in sheep in Kenya. The virus is spread by the brown ear tick *Rhipicephalus appendicularis*. It is only found in areas where this tick occurs in east Africa.

Tumours in ewes

Tumours of the female reproductive tract are extremely rare, and most are benign ovarian stromal tumours. Adenocarcinomas, which are highly malignant, are seen starting in the uterus. Adenomas will occur in the udder, but clinicians should not mistake granulomatous tissue in the udder (which is common) for neoplastic tissue (which is extremely rare).

Medical Conditions of the Reproductive System in Goats

Causes of abortion in goats

Akabane

This is primarily a virus that affects cattle, but it also causes abortions in sheep and goats.

Brucellosis

Brucella melitensis is a zoonosis (see Chapter 19). The disease is very common in southern Europe, Central Asia, India and Africa. It causes abortion in goats, normally in the fourth month of pregnancy. Affected animals retain their fetal membranes and often develop a serious metritis which may spread to the udder and cause mastitis. The organism is spread by fetal membranes and fluids. Outbreaks often occur as storms with nearly 100% abortion rates. Diagnosis can be made on the clinical appearance of the thickened leathery placenta, with necrosis of the cotyledons. The organism can be cultured from the placenta. Affected does will show a sharp serological response. There is a very effective vaccine available (see Chapter 7). Goats will abort if they are infected with *Brucella abortus*, which they can catch from cows, and with *Brucella ovis*, which they can catch from sheep.

Campylobacteriosis

Although *Campylobacter* spp. is a zoonosis, man normally becomes infected from the enteric form rather than the organism which causes abortion (see Chapter 19). This organism is rare in goats. Large doses of oxytetracycline will limit the number of abortions, unlike in sheep where it is not as effective. A vaccine is available but it is not very effective. Goats normally become infected when in mixed flocks with sheep, and occasionally abortion numbers may be high. Diagnosis can be made by seeing the bacteria in the abortion material on FAT.

Caprine herpes virus

This virus not only causes abortion but also vulvovaginitis and balanoposthetitis. It is spread venereally and is a virus of growing importance in southern Europe, as it links with *Mannheimia haemolytica* and causes fatal respiratory disease in young kids. In adults the main signs are related to the vulva, causing swelling and erosions of the mucosa. After 2 days a bloody discharge becomes purulent. The bucks show erosions on the prepuce and a discharge. Some authors claim that conception rates are not affected, but this has not been the author's experience. The lesions may appear during the next breeding season and cause further infertility. Abortions tend to occur in the first year that a herd has become infected. The virus can be isolated from dead kids and aborted fetuses and there is now a RT-PCR to help with diagnosis, although a diagnosis may be made on clinical grounds. Antibiotics certainly help the lesions to heal, and as the disease is spread by venereal contact, control can be carried out by starting a new herd and not using infected bucks on the clean does.

Concurrent disease

Any disease that causes pyrexia is liable to cause an abortion. This is very important in tropical countries where viral diseases and protozoal diseases are common.

Enzootic abortion of ewes

Although, as the name suggests, EAE is primarily a disease of ewes, it does occur in does. It is caused by *Chlamydophila abortus* (previously known as *Chlamydia psittaci*), and results in abortions in the last 2–3 weeks of pregnancy. In naive herds of goats it will cause abortion storms of up to 25% of affected does. The incubation period is a minimum of 6 weeks so does that are exposed to the infection close to term will not abort that year. However the bacterium remains latent in the body until the following pregnancy, when it will multiply in the placenta and cause abortion. Therefore when an abortion storm occurs, the infection may have actually come into the flock the year before. The rickettsia will be present in large numbers in the abortion products as well as in the placenta of live kids. These may be weak, and if they survive they will abort at the end of their first pregnancy. Goats are more likely to retain their placentas and get a resulting metritis than sheep. Treatment should be aggressive, with parenteral antibiotics and NSAID. Uterine washes with warm isotonic saline and soluble penicillin are useful, followed by 30 IU oxytocin injections intramuscularly. Clinicians should remember that this is a life-threatening condition, and should also check the tetanus status of the doe.

Diagnosis can be confirmed by examining the abortion products, particularly the placenta. A blood sample taken at the time will show antibodies, adding to confirmation of the diagnosis. Does that have contracted the disease late in pregnancy will not show a rise in antibody titre so that a blood test cannot be used to predict abortion. After an abortion the doe will have a solid immunity, but many shed the organism at oestrus and so are a direct threat to naive animals. An infected doe can also be an indirect threat as the buck will transfer the organism at mating. In the face of an outbreak some attempt can be made to control the numbers of abortions by injecting all the does with a long-acting tetracycline injection between 100 and 120 days of pregnancy. Sadly this will not eliminate the infection, but it will reduce not only the number of abortions but also increase the numbers of live viable kids. There are licensed vaccines for sheep in the UK. These can be used in goats and given as a single injection before mating (see Chapter 7).

It must be remembered that EAE is a zoonosis and so pregnant women should avoid does at kidding time. It is perhaps not quite the scourge that the media would have the UK population believe, but it is important that careful hygiene practices are carried out (see Chapter 19).

This is one of the diseases that goat keepers can certainly do without and so keeping a closed herd and only buying replacements from clean herds must be good advice.

Leptospirosis

Goats are affected by *Leptospira harjo*. This is a zoonosis (see Chapter 19) and is an organism that mainly infects cattle. However it will cause abortions in goats and also a 'milk drop' syndrome in dairy goats. Goats normally become infected from cattle but they may become infected from sheep or contaminated water courses.

Listeriosis

Abortion will occur after an infection of *Listeria monocytogenes* as a concurrent disease; however it would appear that the organism can be a specific cause of abortion in goats.

The normal route of infection is from badly made silage. Nevertheless there are a large number of organisms in the products of a *L. monocytogenes* abortion, and these may be a danger to pregnant does kept in close contact. It should be remembered that *L. monocytogenes* is a zoonosis (see Chapter 19).

Neospora caninum

This common protozoal parasite which causes abortion in cattle will infect goats. It may come from dogs initially, but then may well be passed from mother to daughter.

Q fever

Q fever is caused by the obligate intracellular rickettsial organism *Coxiella burnetii*. It is distributed worldwide and is a zoonosis but is not common in the UK (see Chapter 19). For example, in 2007 there were only four reported findings of Q fever in the UK from aborted farm animals and there were 62 human cases, which is about average for the previous few years. No deaths were reported. Q fever has been in the UK for a long time, usually at a low level. It has always been an occasional, though not regular, finding as a cause of abortion in cattle, sheep and goats, and can infect most other species, very often with no diagnosable signs.

The percentage of goats testing positive worldwide varies enormously. For example, 48.2% out of nearly 1000 were positive in Cyprus; 13% out of over 2000 were positive in Italy, and a similar percentage was found in Chad; but only 2.5% were positive in Germany.

When an animal becomes infected, Q fever can be shed via a variety of secretions, including faeces, urine, uterine fluids in particular and milk. It is also likely that the disease can be spread by ticks and even cats. It is killed by pasteurization. Once an animal is infected, the organism can be shed for several weeks or months, and in particular can be shed at two successive parturitions.

The organism can survive for several weeks in the environment, and survives best in dry and dusty conditions, where it can attach to dust particles. It is often via these dust particles blowing in the wind that infection is carried from animal to man, and as a result the disease is most common in the Mediterranean and Balkan areas where large numbers of farm animals are kept in relatively dry conditions, often being walked through a local village from pasture to be milked.

In 2008 there was an outbreak of Q fever in goats in the Netherlands. This continued through 2009, with over 2500 confirmed cases in humans and 11 deaths. Goats were the main problem but sheep were also implicated. Compulsory vaccination was carried out, which was then followed by a slaughter policy for all infected milking goats and sheep. Infection was monitored by bulk milk testing. In 2009, 63 herds were found to be infected, with a cull of 137,000 goats and sheep taking place. There are thought to be 400,000 goats and milking sheep in the country, a stocking rate of 30/km^2 (2½ square miles) compared to 1/km^2 (2½ square miles) in the UK. In the UK, goats are not kept in urban situations and so the spread to humans is limited, the disease only being notifiable in man and not in animals. Vaccination is not advised in the UK at the present time. Q fever is unlikely ever to be eradicated as it is found in too many species, but control should be carried out by targeting vaccination of humans and animals. It would appear that vaccination is the way forward in many countries.

Salmonellosis

Salmonella spp. will cause abortion in goats as a result of septicaemia and pyrexia, but *Salmonella abortus ovis* is a specific organism that will cause abortion in goats as well as in its primary host.

Schallemberg disease

This virus disease occurs in cattle, sheep and goats. It is caused by a virus very similar to the virus which causes Akabane. It is spread by midges and causes a transitory fever. The main problem with the condition is that if the disease infects animals during pregnancy it is liable to cause abortion and deformed fetuses. At the time of writing the disease has only been found in

Germany, Belgium and Holland. However, since writing this we now have it in the UK (I have been dealing with an outbreak) and also in France.

Tick-borne fever

This condition is seen in goats and the same advice given for sheep applies to goats.

Toxoplasmosis

This condition is common in goats. It has the same pathogenesis as in sheep.

Clostridium septicum metritis in goats

This bacterium causes a very serious metritis in goats that is likely to be fatal. High doses of penicillin should be given intravenously and the goat should be supported by NSAID, also given intravenously. The uterus should be washed with warm isotonic saline containing crystalline penicillin and then the goat should receive 30 IU of oxytocin intravenously. Goats should be protected by vaccination. Care should be taken, as some of the polyvalent vaccines do not contain cover for this disease.

False pregnancy in goats

False pregnancy or hydrometra (known as a 'cloudburst') is a unique condition to the goat and is not seen in sheep. It is relatively common and occurs in about 5–10% of females. It can be diagnosed from pregnancy by ultrasonography or a blood test for oestrone sulfate after 50 days. There is a persistent corpus luteum, so treatment relies on its regression, encouraged by prostaglandin injections. Dosages are empirical. A quarter of the cattle dose has been used successfully on many occasions. Dairy goat owners do not worry about this condition as the doe will have a rise in daily milk yield without any problems of parturition. On many dairy goat farms there is a surplus of kids, particularly males, and therefore kids are not desired.

Freemartins

These are infertile females that occur *in utero* when twinned with a male. However, unlike in cattle where they always occur in mixed sexed twins, they are rare in goats.

Intersex

This is a genetic condition often called pseudohermaphroditism. The dominant gene for polledness is linked with a recessive gene for intersex. Intersex is a recessive, sex-linked trait resulting from breeding to polled goats. Females are always heterozygotes. Males may be homozygotes or heterozygotes. A homozygote male bred on a heterozygote female will have 25% intersex offspring. On the other hand, a heterozygote male on a heterozygote female will only have 12.5% intersex offspring. Affected animals are genetically female, but show great variation phenotypically, from phenotypic female to phenotypic male.

Maiden milkers

Many young goats from heavy milking breeds may show udder development and milk production, particularly when they are on a high plane of nutrition. These animals should not be milked unless a maiden lactation is desired. This condition may be self-limiting, particularly if the plane of nutrition is reduced. Goat keepers should be very vigilant for signs of mastitis, which should be treated promptly. This is particularly common in the summer as bacteria will be spread by flies.

Problems with oestrus

Goats are seasonal breeders and come into oestrus when the day length starts reducing. Out-of-season breeding can be encouraged by the injection of PMSG. The expression of oestrus can be quite intense in goats and is often mistaken by owners as pain. Animals will visibly shake, and may take aggressive action against humans or other goats of both sexes. They may be very vocal.

Tumours

Cervical and vaginal neoplasia will occur in elderly females. The presenting sign will be a foul-smelling necrotic/haemorrhagic discharge. Effective radical surgery is impossible and euthanasia is indicated.

Surgical Conditions of the Reproductive System of the Male Sheep

Castration and tail docking

A recent small survey in Scotland has indicated that 100% of farms examined that have ceased both practices have had some substantial improvements. These farms have been breeding from their own ram lambs and have been getting better performance from them compared to bought-in animals. They report that none of the stock had dirty back ends and that fly strike was not a problem. By careful management, using dedicated grazing areas, crops and supplementation, all of the lambs are finished before 1 December. This finding puts the welfare of castration and tail docking in question.

Uncastrated lambs can reach an acceptable carcass size of better quality before they reach puberty and become sexually active. Uncastrated lambs generally grow faster and more efficiently, and produce leaner carcasses. Many types of husbandry do not, however, permit rapid growth, and castration may be the only way to avoid sexually based behaviour causing injuries together with damaged and tainted carcasses.

Some flocks manage well without tail docking. Good disease control, mainly helminth control and fly strike prevention, make the practice unnecessary.

There are three basic methods of castration and tail docking: surgical, ischaemic (by application of a rubber ring) and ischaemic (by application of a burdizzo clamp) (Fig. 13.4).

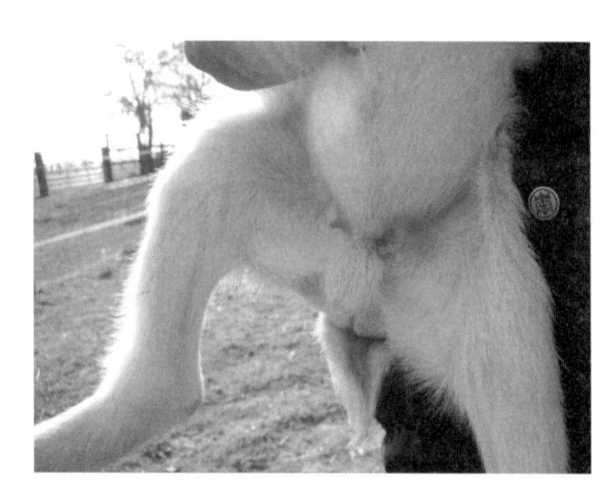

Fig. 13.4. Lamb rubber ring castration.

Surgical castration in rams can be carried out in many different ways. All of them may well be satisfactory from the aspect of preventing haemorrhage and infection but it should never be forgotten that they all will cause pain at the time and later. Pain can be lessened by local anaesthetic injected into the spermatic cord and into the scrotum. NSAID and antibiotics will aid pain management.

The normal surgical castration is an open method. The tip of the scrotum is removed or two lateral incisions are made to the tip, so that there is good drainage. The tunics are incised and the testicles drawn out with twisting traction for total removal. Oily antiseptic cream containing acriflavin and BHC is applied to the wounds. In pet sheep a closed method can be undertaken under a totally aseptic surgical technique. The scrotum is opened as in the open method but the testicles are left in the tunics. A transfixing ligature is applied to each testicle before removal, and the wounds are then closed with absorbable sutures.

Surgical tail docking can be carried out by cutting the tail with a scalpel after local anaesthesia has been given. The surgeon should try to cut between the coccygeal vertebrae and leave some skin in excess of the bone. The wound can be cauterized with a hot iron but this is not actually necessary as the haemorrhage will soon cease. Obviously in pet sheep the procedure can be carried out in a correct surgical manner and the skin sutured after the tail has been removed, making sure there is adequate covering of the bone. This is particularly important in older animals when the tail is removed because of damage.

The ischaemic method using a rubber ring is by far the most common. It is very important that both testicles are distal to the rubber elastrator ring. It is also important that rubber ring is not placed too high up the tail. The tail should be long enough to cover the vulva in a female lamb and a similar length should be left in males.

The ischaemic method of castration using a burdizzo clamp can be used in rams. The method described for goats should be used. If the clamp is used for tail docking the clamp should be applied first and then the tail is cut off.

It is extremely important, whatever method is used, that the lambs have received passive or active immunity against tetanus.

Shepherds are often not very well aware of the problems associated with castration and docking. They carry out the procedures just because they have always done them. They seldom consider the welfare of the animals or carry out a cost–benefit analysis. Clinicians have a duty to point out to shepherds the problems associated with castration and tail docking:

- The extra work and stress to the sheep of gathering them and handling them. Many shepherds try to minimize this by carrying out the tasks when the ewes are still penned up with their lambs straight after parturition. This is not without its dangers, because if the procedures are carried out too early the lambs may not get enough colostrum.
- Haemorrhage may not be life threatening, however there may be more than shepherds imagine, particularly as most of the haemorrhage will occur internally if the testicles are pulled.
- A rare but recorded outcome is strangulation of the small intestine by the spermatic cords, with fatal results.
- Herniation is also rare but it certainly does occur.

There definitely is acute pain that will cause a variety of problems. Lambs will lie down and get chilled. The ewe lamb of twins will not suffer the pain and can keep up with its mother and the male may get lost and be neglected. Certainly if lambs are older there will be a check in the growth rate. This will be more marked if the acute pain leads to chronic pain from an infected wound. Infection can occur even with ischaemic methods, and there will be a reduction in disease resistance.

For all these reasons shepherds should perhaps rethink their husbandry methods. It should be remembered that in the UK it is illegal to apply a rubber ring to a lamb older than 7 days of age without an anaesthetic. It is also illegal to castrate or dock a lamb surgically without anaesthetic if it is older than 3 months.

Castration of animals with a retained testicle

These are very rarely true 'rigs'. The common presentation is when the elastrator ring has been put on distal to one or both testicles. It is unlikely that such an animal will be fertile as the testicles, being close to the body, will be too hot to produce live sperm. Therefore the prudent and welfare-friendly approach is to fatten these animals as quickly as possible and send them to slaughter before they reach sexual maturity. The meat will then be wholesome and not have any ram taint. However in the case of pet sheep surgery may be demanded. In this case the ram should be restrained on its rump. After cleaning the area, local anaesthetic should be infiltrated where the scrotum should have been and in the spermatic cord near to the inguinal ring. The animal should be given antibiotics and NSAID, and its tetanus status should be checked. The whole area should be carefully checked to see whether there is a single testicle or if both testicles are present, as obviously in the latter case both will need to be removed. After surgical cleaning of the site the testicle should be pushed as caudally as possible before an incision is made over it. It is then twisted and pulled. The procedure is then repeated with the second testicle if it is present. The main problem with this surgical procedure is the lack of drainage from the incision. Antibiotics and NSAID should be continued for 7 days and the wound should be checked regularly. Fly control is essential. Castration of a true rig is very rare (see Chapter 8).

Surgical Conditions of the Reproductive System of the Male Goat

Normal castration

This can be performed surgically or by a bloodless method using a small pair of burdizzos (Fig. 13.5). The latter method is useful in areas where fly strike is a possibility. Both methods require the use of local anaesthetic placed in the neck of the scrotum (Fig. 13.6). The tetanus status of the animal must be checked. For surgical removal, after cleaning the scrotum, an incision is made in the scrotum laterally continuing down to the tip, just into the testicle. The testicle is then removed through the tunics using a twisting motion so that the cord is pulled out of the animal. This is repeated on the other side. With the bloodless method it is important that only one cord is crushed at a time. The cord should then be crushed a second time. The crushing lines of the second testicle should not be continuous with those of the first. Bucks should be examined 2 months after the bloodless method of castration to confirm that the testicles have regressed.

Castration of animals with a retained testicle

Unlike lambs, kids are not normally castrated using an elastrator and so problems with misplacement of the elastrator ring are very rare. Equally, true rigs are very rare. In these cases surgery is not easy and a general anaesthetic may be recommended. Often the testicle can be retrieved from the inguinal ring under heavy sedation with xylazine. The surgical procedure is the same as in rams (see Chapter 8).

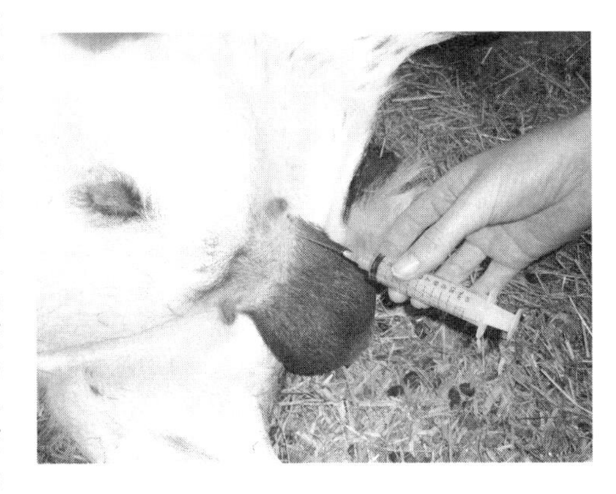

Fig. 13.6. Local anaesthetic injection for castration.

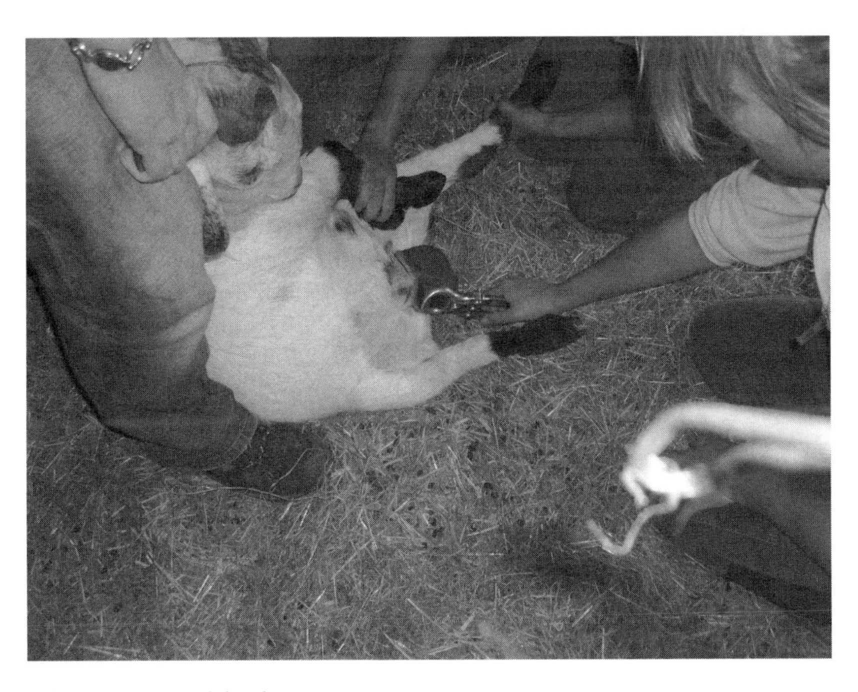

Fig. 13.5. Castrating goat with burdizzo.

Surgical Conditions of the Reproductive System of the Female Sheep

Reproductive ultrasonography

Ewes can be scanned for pregnancy and numbers of fetuses from 45 days onwards, and the age of the fetus can be judged fairly accurately using calipers. However, what is important is to use the information of pregnancy and numbers to the maximum advantage. Barren ewes should be removed from the lambing flock and ewes should be separated into three groups for feeding according to fetal numbers. Lambing assistance should be concentrated on those ewes with multiple fetuses. Hill ewes, which are often running with the tup, are normally scanned later, at approximately 90 days. This extended window picks up more late pregnancies. Twin-bearing hill ewes can be housed. Normally hill ewes that have twins one year, are so debilitated that the following year they have a single lamb or are barren. As the lambing will be stretched out in hill ewes, knowing the stage of pregnancy can be used to save feed. In lowland flocks which are totally housed for lambing, the ewes with triplets can be lambed next to those with singles to make fostering easier.

Accurate scanning and **recording** is the single most important management tool available to promote a successful enterprise.

Whenever high barren and/or low twinning rates are identified, the opportunity should be taken to investigate these problems, so that they can be avoided in the following year. High barren rates at scanning may be associated with:

- Ewes not showing behavioural oestrus at the time of tup introduction because the tup was put in too early or they were suffering from concurrent disease.
- Infertile rams.
- Early embryonic death from selenium or iodine deficiency, toxoplasmosis, border disease, severe under-nutrition or prolonged stressful husbandry.

Low twinning rates resulting from low ovulation rates may be due to:

- The tups going in too early.
- The tups going in too late.
- Ewes in poor condition at mating.
- The wrong breed of ewe for the type of farming.
- Mating ewe lambs.

Ram colour harnesses or keel marking will help to identify that the ram is working. If the colour is changed at 16 days it will also indicate that the ewes are returning to oestrus and therefore not in lamb that cycle. Ram harnesses must be a comfortable fit and checked regularly. Certain individuals may not work wearing a harness, and these rams will have to be keel marked. The crayons vary in hardness. The harder ones should be used in warmer weather and the softer ones during cold weather. Any soreness to the brisket must be treated promptly as if any sore is left it will be difficult to heal and become a welfare problem. Rams can easily be trained to a bucket of food so they can be gathered regularly to check harnesses without any stress.

Prolapse of the vagina cervix

Occurrence of this condition is very variable between flocks, and prevalence varies between 1 and 5%. There are significant differences between breeds. The worst breed combination to be affected is said to be Suffolk rams mating cross bred ewes (Fig. 13.7). However there are thought to be many other factors such as obesity, old age, bulky feeds, steep or hilly ground, and hormonal and mineral imbalances. These factors are thought to raise intra-abdominal pressure or increase the laxity of the vagina and its supporting structures.

Vaginal prolapse is a condition of the last 2 months of pregnancy, and most cases will occur in the last 3 weeks of pregnancy. Ewes that have experienced vaginal prolapse in a previous pregnancy appear to prolapse earlier in their subsequent pregnancies. Vaginal prolapse tends to develop over a few days. Peracute cases do occur when there is rupture of the vaginal wall. Prolapse of the vagina, cervix and uterus occurs post-partum and is sporadic, not a flock problem.

Initially the pink mucosa of the vagina may be noticed protruding slightly between the lips of the vulva in a ewe lying down, only to disappear from view when she stands up. Later the vagina fails to return to its normal position when the ewe stands and the prolapse progresses until the vagina is completely everted and the cervix is visible. Initially the vaginal mucosa is pink, moist and smooth but, if not treated, the vagina becomes swollen, oedematous and congested. It is very susceptible to injury. After prolonged exposure, the dried vaginal mucosa becomes rough and haemorrhagic. The ewe is now constantly straining as the urethra is kinked and the bladder is full and may even lie inside the prolapse. Trauma at this stage may lead to vaginal rupture, prolapse of the bowel and death.

All vaginal prolapses should be treated. This may be done by the shepherd by the use of a vaginal spoon. This is a plastic or stainless steel T-shaped device. The tongue is inserted into the vagina and the sides of the T are tied to a long piece of baler twine tied around the ewe just in front of the udder. If the case is treated early enough, this device is often successful, particularly if it is linked to a leather or webbing harness. In long-standing cases, however, veterinary intervention is required. With the ewe standing, a sacrococcygeal epidural anaesthetic should be administered (see Chapter 8). After replacing the vagina and cervix the lips of the vulva should be sutured with a single Buhner suture of uterine tape. A long Seton needle is inserted into the skin at the ventral end of the vulva. It is pushed carefully in a dorsal direction subcutaneously and slightly laterally to emerge ventral to the anus. The tape is threaded and withdrawn. This is repeated for the other side of the vulva. The two ends are tied with a bow so only two fingers can be inserted into the vulva (Fig. 13.8). The shepherd is advised to untie the bow but not remove the suture if the ewe is thought to be lambing. If this is the case the ewe may be lambed down by removing all the lambs and the suture removed, as the condition should not reoccur in the non-pregnant ewe. However if the cervix is closed and the ewe is not lambing then the suture should be re-tied, as the condition will reoccur until parturition has occurred.

Ewes should be marked and culled, as the condition will occur at any subsequent pregnancy. If flocks experience a high prevalence of vaginal prolapse, their nutrition

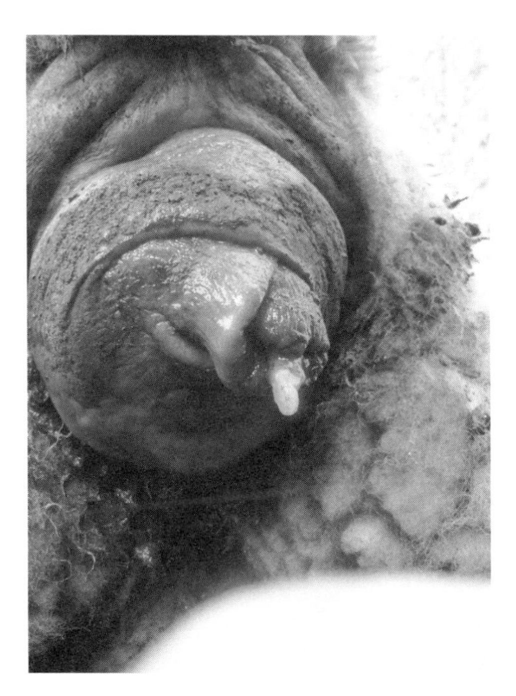

Fig. 13.7. Prolapsed cervix in a ewe.

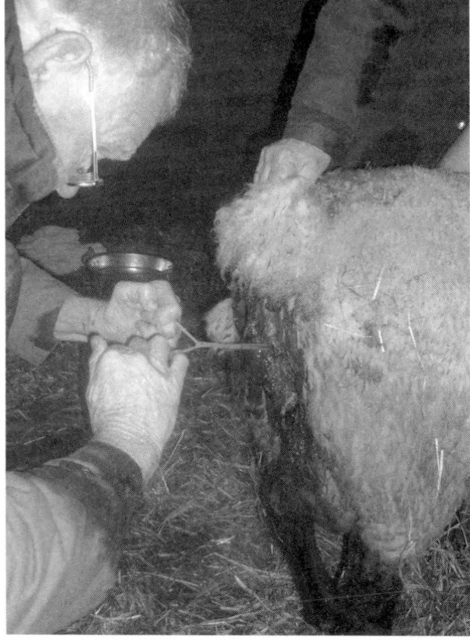

Fig. 13.8. Buhner suture.

should be investigated before tupping for the next lambing season and their body condition should be scored. Those overweight ewes should be dieted to bring them to a body condition score of 2.5 **before** tupping.

Prolapse of the uterus

Unlike a prolapsed vagina this is an emergency and occurs after lambing (Fig. 13.9). The normal cause is the birth of oversized lambs. Although the condition can reoccur at subsequent lambings, this is not the norm and therefore there is no reason to cull affected ewes. The clinicians must instruct inexperienced shepherds on the diagnosis of this condition, as retention of fetal membranes may in some instances resemble uterine prolapse. Normally the whole organ is prolapsed but occasionally the condition only affects one horn.

The ewe should be secured and given sacrococcygeal epidural anaesthesia. The fetal membranes should only be removed if they come away easily, otherwise they should be left *in situ*. The ewe should be given antibiotic cover and NSAID. If the ewe is still standing the uterus should be elevated and replaced. Old shepherds cover the organ with sugar to reduce the swelling, but the author has not found this to be advantageous. A second pair of hands is certainly useful: if the ewe is down an assistant can raise the pelvis of the ewe, and this helps replacement enormously. After replacement the lips of the vulva should be sutured with a single Buhner suture and the ewe should receive 20 IU of oxytocin intramuscularly. The suture should be left *in situ* for 48 h. Antibiotic cover and NSAID should be given for a minimum of 3 days.

Surgical Conditions of the Reproductive System of the Female Goat

Reproductive ultrasonography

Pregnancy diagnosis

Requests for pregnancy diagnosis in goats are, in the author's experience, rare. Transabdominal scanning is straightforward provided early pregnancy diagnosis (i.e. before 45

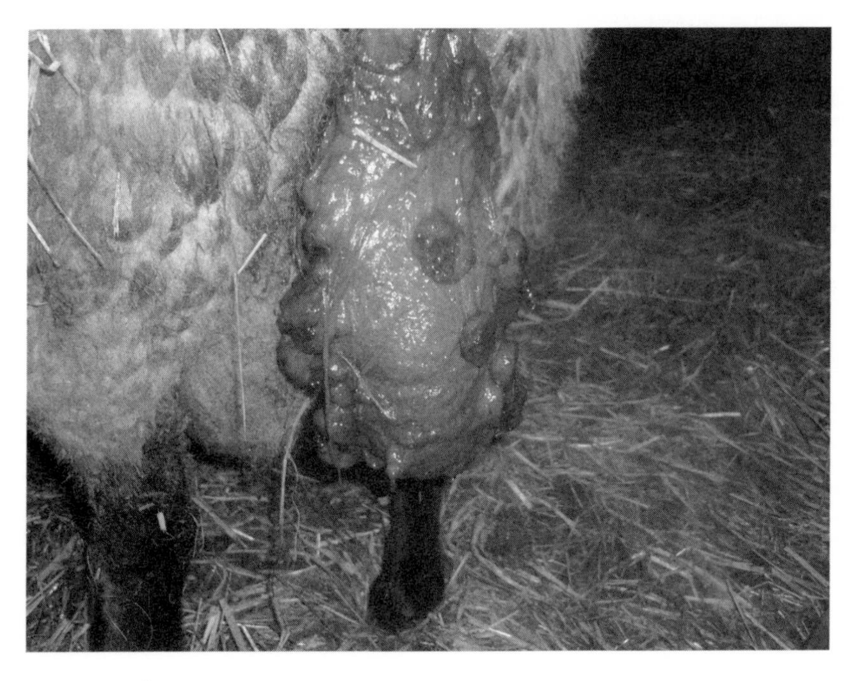

Fig. 13.9. Uterine prolapse in a ewe.

days) is not required. Prostaglandin injections should never be given before 45 days to a doe that is thought to be empty. A later check should always be performed, and the easiest method is with the doe standing. Some authorities recommend clipping the area on the right flank above the udder and using lubricant gel or vegetable oil. This is very messy and isopropyl alcohol is cleaner and will not damage the probe. There is no need for clipping if isopropyl alcohol is used.

Prolapse of the vagina cervix

Goats will suffer from this condition, but it is rare and does not occur as a herd problem as in sheep. However it will occur again in a subsequent kidding, and so affected goats should not be bred again. Surgical treatment is the same as for sheep, although vaginal spoons and leather harnesses are not used routinely in goats and suturing is the treatment of choice. Antibiotic cover and NSAID should be given and the tetanus status should be checked. It must be remembered that the condition normally occurs before parturition.

Prolapse of the uterus

There is some doubt about the cause of this condition. It can, as with sheep, be caused by relative fetal oversize. It is seen in pygmy goats with a single large kid. However it will also be seen in milking goats suffering from hypocalcaemia. In these cases it is important to treat the hypocalcaemia first as there is a danger that the stress of uterine replacement may cause death. Sacrococcygeal epidural anaesthetic should be administered and then the hindquarters of the goat should be raised. If that is difficult and is causing stress then the goat can be allowed to rest in sternal recumbency with its hind legs in extension directly behind it. This position greatly eases the replacement of the uterus. Antibiotics and NSAID should be given before replacement and 20 IU of oxytocin immediately after replacement. The tetanus status of the goat should be checked. In milking goats it is particularly important to check the udder for evidence of mastitis, which should be treated appropriately.

Normal Parturition in the Ewe

Birth injury and perinatal loss in lambs

The causes are interrelated but they can be attributed to the ewe, the lamb and the shepherd. The breed of the ewe is a factor particularly when linked to the breed of the ram and hence the breed of the lamb. Relative fetal oversize is important. The shape of the ewe's pelvis is also radically altered by the breed. The age of the ewe – or should we say ewe lamb or shearling – is important. Lambs must not be too immature. However with the correct sire there is no reason not to lamb down ewe lambs, but they should not be mated until they are 65% of their adult weight.

The ewe is considerably influenced by the level of nutrition. If they are on too good a plane of nutrition they will be too fat and the lambs at term will be too large. Fat deposits within the pelvis and fat around the posterior vagina will constrict the birth canal and cause dystocia. On the other hand, the undernourished ewe may be too weak to give birth and the fetus suffers birth injury caused by anoxia during prolonged parturition. In addition, clinical disorders (see Chapter 9) such as pregnancy toxaemia and, less commonly, hypocalcaemia, can lead to uterine inertia and consequent anoxia of the fetus, which frequently results in stillbirth (Wilsmore, 1989).

As well as fetal oversize, malpresentation of the lamb, if it is not corrected carefully and professionally, results in birth injury. Congenital abnormalities such as arthrogryposis may make it impossible for the lamb to be presented in a normal posture for delivery and therefore these cases also suffer injury.

The amount of input from the shepherd supervising lambing and their level of expertize are both major factors that influence the incidence of birthing injury.

Oedematous lesions, mainly of the head, are commonly seen following dystocia in cases of malpresentation (e.g. only the head is presented and not the legs). They are also seen in cases of relative fetal oversize. Oedema formed in this manner is colourless and should not be confused with accumulations of blood-stained extravasations of fluid under the skin and in the body cavities seen in autolytic lambs that die *in utero* before the birth process begins. In the latter cases fluid escapes from blood vessels and cells whose walls become permeable after death of the tissues. All the tissues and the transudates of these fetuses display red staining by haemoglobin from lysed erythrocytes (Wilsmore, 1989), unlike the birth-injured lambs. The reasons for the *in utero* deaths should be investigated by post-mortem and bacteriology. There is a simple method to see if a lamb was stillborn. A piece of lung is removed and dropped into water. If it sinks, this indicates that the lamb has never taken a breath. Conversely if it floats, the lamb has at least taken one breath. It is important to investigate perinatal deaths with an open mind. If there are other reasons other than shepherding these should be investigated and corrected. If there has been a lack of attention to detail by the shepherd, or if there has been undue force used, then careful education will be the way forward. Criticism will not be helpful and in the long term will cause even more welfare problems for the sheep. In large flocks extra help should be brought in to assist the shepherd. This can be in the form of unqualified assistants who will do the more straightforward tasks to allow the shepherd to carry out the actual lambing, or the help can be in the form of skilled people, such as experienced students who can work on a rota system. Either way the ewes need to have close supervision.

How much can we expect smallholders to do?

This is a very difficult question for clinicians to answer. It is important that all smallholders are urged to attend a lambing course (Fig. 13.10). However even then, those attending the course will have very varied abilities. The clinician must allow for the least confident and the least competent in the group. It is important to supply notes so they can refresh their memories when they get home. 'Hands on experience' is vital, using dead lambs. Hygiene must be stressed.

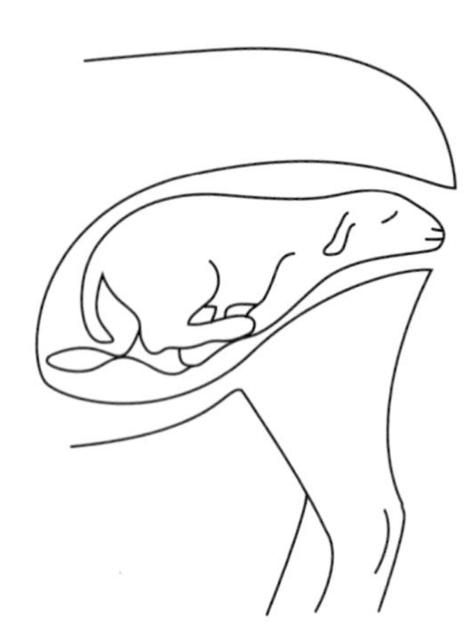

Fig. 13.10. Picture of a lambing.

The tasks they all should be able to perform are shown below:

- Put a halter on a ewe.
- Tag their sheep.
- Trim their ewes' feet.
- Dag their ewes.
- Differentiate between a fore and a hind limb of a lamb with their eyes shut.
- Put a lambing rope on a limb of a lamb above the fetlock with their eyes shut.
- Put a lambing rope on the head of a lamb with their eyes shut.
- Give a lamb a subcutaneous injection.
- Pass a lamb stomach tube.
- Take a lamb's rectal temperature.
- Give a lamb a peritoneal injection of glucose (it is vital they know when that is appropriate, compared to giving colostrum).
- Apply an elastrator ring to the tail and the scrotum.

It is important that they all have the equipment listed below:

- arm-length sleeves;
- lubricant;
- lambing ropes;
- a teat for feeding a lamb;
- a lamb stomach tube and 60 ml syringe with catheter tip;
- dried colostrum;
- thermometer;
- a marker spray;

- 21 G × 1 cm (½ inch) needles for injecting lambs with antibiotics;
- 19 G × 2.5 cm (1 inch) needles for injecting lambs intraperitoneally and ewes subcutaneously;
- an elastrator applicator and rubber rings;
- a pair of sheep hoof trimmers;
- a pair of dagging shears.

On the other hand in the UK the medicines shown below should only be supplied if the smallholding has been visited. However it is reasonable to supply these medicines on a regular basis, provided the smallholding receives an annual visit, ideally prior to lambing:

- Pen/Strep injectable suspension (see Chapter 6);
- long-acting Pen injectable suspension (see Chapter 6);
- antibiotic aerosol spray;
- 40% dextrose solution;
- an injectable NSAID (see Chapter 6).

There are certain tasks that clinicians should not encourage smallholders to perform:

1. Never supply eye ointment to smallholders, but insist that they bring any lambs with an eye 'infection' into the surgery. There are many causes of eye infections in sheep but in many flocks entropian is common. This is a welfare problem, and all the antibiotics in the world will not alleviate the condition. A useful treatment is to inject liquid paraffin into the affected eyelid, but this should be a task for a veterinarian.
2. Management of vaginal prolapse can be performed by a smallholder provided he or she has a harness and a suitable vaginal retainer or spoon. Giving an epidural injection of lignocaine and xylazine before replacement and a Buhner suture is definitely an act of veterinary surgery.

Normal Parturition in the Goat

Like the ewe, the doe likes to be separate from the rest of the herd. She should be left on her own without human interference to avoid interfering with a normal delivery. As in sheep, parturition occurs quicker in multiparous animals. Goats will vocalize as the cervix opens during the first stage and during the second stage as the fetus is delivered. The whole of the first and second stage lasts on average 2 h. The third stage of expulsion of the fetal membranes should be completed in less than 4 h. If the fetal membranes are not expelled there is no cause for alarm if the doe is well. The fetal membranes can be left to macerate, which may take several days. Antibiotics and NSAID should only be given if the doe is ill.

In normal sized goats 95% of kiddings do not require any assistance. The rate is not as high in pygmy goats, as parturition problems are more common. It is important that does are supervised by an experienced stock person. Clinicians should hold courses for both commercial goat keepers and pet goat owners.

Dystocia in the Ewe

General

A careful history should be taken before any examination takes place. The answers may be vague, but it is important that the clinician obtains as much information as possible. Is the fetus full term or is it an abortion? Is there a known infective agent in the flock causing abortions? If it is an abortion, extra precautions need to be taken on account of possible zoonotic problems, and sampling equipment will need to be prepared to collect placenta. Has the ewe been scanned for fetal numbers? Is she a maiden? If not, has she had problems before? What is the breed of the sire? This is important in cases of possible fetal oversize. Have fetal membranes been seen? If so, how long ago were they first seen? Has there been any interference by the shepherd? If so, how much traction was applied? Have any medications been given to the ewe?

The ewe should be given a general examination to see what state she is in. Is she bright, depressed, exhausted or suffering from any other condition (e.g. pregnancy toxaemia)? It is very important at this stage for the clinician to carry out a risk analysis, as if the animal is very ill or depressed then euthanasia must be carried out sooner rather than later on welfare grounds, quite apart from any economic considerations. The body condition score is important as over-fat ewes are likely to have large lambs and the pelvis may be obstructed with fat deposits. The udder should be checked for the presence of colostrum or mastitis. If there is an absence of colostrum this will give an indication of an abortion. The perineum and the vulva should be examined for signs of bruising. This will give an indication of the extent of any interference by the shepherd. Obviously any limbs or the head should be examined for signs of oedema. Whether the limbs are fore legs or back legs is important. Any ropes *in situ* should be noted. Any fetal membranes should be examined for evidence of autolysis. The presence of fresh blood giving evidence of trauma should be noted. The presence of meconium staining will give an indication of any distress in the lambs. An unpleasant sweetish odour will suggest either an abortion or that the lambs have been dead for a few hours. On the other hand, a putrid smell will indicate that they have been dead for longer than 24 h.

Before carrying out a vaginal examination the perineum of the ewe should be cleaned, and antibiotics and NSAID should be given at this stage. Initially the author uses a gloved hand and obstetric lubricant, but if manipulations are required the glove is often discarded. The hand and arm must be carefully cleaned and scrubbed. Examination of the cervix is crucial. Lack of dilation can indicate that the ewe is not yet ready to lamb or that there is a 'ring womb'. Clinicians will normally be able to distinguish the latter as it will feel harder and will show no elasticity. A caesarean section is the only option in cases of 'ring womb'. If the cervix feels normal the ewe should be left for further signs to develop. If a rifled effect is felt then this will indicate a uterine torsion. If the cervix is dilated the lamb or lambs will be felt. The joint flexion will inform the clinician whether a fore or a hind leg is being felt. If there is a combination of legs it is likely that they come from different lambs and twins should be anticipated. If the joints will not flex, this may indicate ankylosis and a possibly deformed lamb. If neither legs nor head can be felt then it is possible that a grossly deformed lamb is present. There may be two heads on one lamb, or extra legs; hydrocephalus, anasarca or ascites; schistoma reflexus lambs have been recorded – all things are possible. Clinicians should examine any small bowel presented to see if it is from a lamb or from the ewe. Obviously with the latter, immediate euthanasia is indicated. Experienced clinicians will be able to differentiate twins and be able to relate legs to torsos. They will also be aware that twins are much more common than monsters with multiple legs or two heads. Also, if there twins or triplets they will normally not be very large so there is much less likelihood of relative fetal oversize. This latter condition is usually in first-time ewes with a single fetus. Occasionally there may be damage to the pelvis of the ewe which reduces the size of the birth canal, and so the fetus will appear to be oversized. Various formulae have been put forward to suggest whether vaginal delivery is likely to be difficult, or indeed impossible. These formulae require knowledge of: the interischial diameter of the ewe and the digital diameter of the fetus at the fetlock, measured in centimetres; the parity and presentation (whether anterior or posterior); and the conformation of the ram (whether exaggerated muscle type). Such formulae are difficult to work out and therefore the clinician has to rely on experience. A useful yardstick is if traction cannot be accomplished by one person pulling with thin ropes wrapped around their hands, then it is likely that there will be severe damage to the ewe. Sadly this damage has often been already done by poor shepherding. Two other conditions should be mentioned. These are hydrops allantois, or a similar condition, hydrops amnion. They have a similar appearance. The ewe's abdomen will be very large but she will have a low condition score. When the fetal membranes rupture there will be a massive amount of fluid expelled, up to 10 l. The lamb or lambs will normally be rather small and very far back in the uterus. They will be difficult to retrieve and, like all lambs, must be delivered. Clinicians must always check the uterus after delivery is thought to have finished, to make certain that there is no damage to the birth canal and – more importantly – that there is no lamb left in the uterus.

The positioning of the ewe for parturition is very important. In most situations the ewe is most comfortable standing while an examination or a delivery is being carried out. In this position pressure is taken off the underside of her spine. The ewe is better on her back if she has a ventral hernia or if the lamb's head is flexed under the chest. If the ewe is exhausted and is lying in ventral recumbency it is best to roll her on to her side (Fig. 13.11). This is particularly helpful if the lamb has a leg back and the ewe is lying with the leg of the lamb that is back uppermost. Equally, if the head is back that needs to be on the upper side. Certain repositioning procedures require repulsion. This is best carried out with the hindquarters raised. However, this is uncomfortable for the ewe and puts pressure on her diaphragm, and so the length of time should be kept to a minimum.

With all manipulations great care and patience should be exercised. Obstetric lubricant is very important. With dead lambs which have become dry the insertion of some powdered J Lube™ (Dechra Veterinary Products Ltd, Shrewsbury, UK) can be very helpful. With twins it is often difficult to decide which lamb should be drawn first, and there are no hard and fast rules. However, normally if there is a lamb in posterior presentation, that should be drawn first, unless it is very large. Clinicians would be well advised to put ropes on to the two hind legs before drawing the lamb, for if it becomes stuck in the pelvis it will drown before ropes can be put on. If there is a lamb with its head back, a small lambing rope should be placed over the head and into the mouth so that the head can be drawn up before there is traction on the legs. Traction should never be applied to the lower jaw of a lamb unless it is definitely dead.

If the lambs are viable, clinicians should make an early decision about whether a vaginal delivery is possible. The lambs will quickly become weak and die and so the decision to carry out a caesarean must be made quickly. If the lambs are dead and putrid a caesarean is not an option. Welfare is extremely important and so if in any doubt the ewe should be destroyed. However, in certain instances an embryotomy is appropriate. It should be remembered that there is no bony attachment of the front legs and so with a rotten lamb

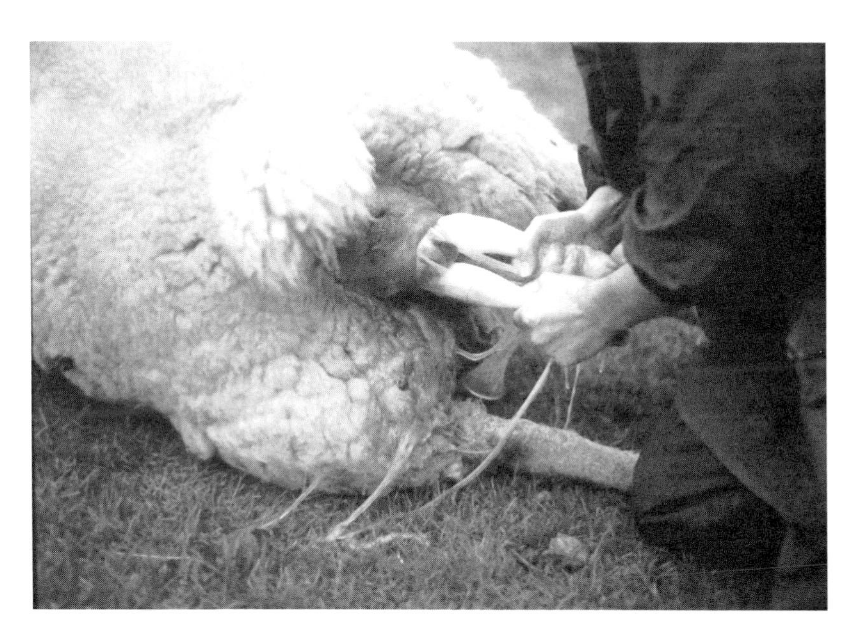

Fig. 13.11. Lambing (1).

these can be removed individually, then a noose can be put around the head and the rest of the lamb can be drawn.

With viable lambs it is important that they are revived as they are delivered (Fig. 13.12). Ideally this should be carried out by an assistant, allowing the clinician to deliver the next lamb. The nose and mouth of the lamb should be cleared of all fetal fluids, and this is easily performed with a paper towel. The use of suction may be appropriate, or the lamb can be held upside down to allow drainage. Breathing can be stimulated by rubbing the chest or tickling the nose. Chemicals such as doxapram may be useful. Hygiene and zoonoses should be considered before mouth-to-mouth resuscitation is performed. Small plastic pumps are available for this purpose.

After the clinician is fully satisfied that all the lambs have been removed, the ewe should be given 20 IU of oxytocin intramuscularly (Fig. 13.13).

Uterine torsion in the sheep

This is an extremely rare condition. It is not actually a torsion of the uterus but a torsion of the anterior vagina. Normally there is only a single lamb. Diagnosis is very simple as the rifling will be felt on vaginal examination. One authority (Scott, 2011) thinks that diagnosis may not be easy for shepherds and that the condition might be more common than previously thought. He advises that ultrasonography may aid diagnosis, as in some cases the torsion will be a true uterine torsion (i.e. it will occur cranial to the cervix). However, in the normal presentation of a torsion of the anterior vagina the history will be of a ewe looking as though she going to lamb but not getting on with parturition. If there is only 180° torsion the condition can normally be corrected *per vagina*. If this fails or there is a 360° torsion, the ewe will need to be rolled from a position of lateral recumbency in the direction of the twist. Two people are required to accomplish this manoeuvre. Further vaginal examination will reveal that the torsion has been corrected, but normally the cervix will then be only partially dilated. At that stage it is not a 'ring womb' but will become one in 30 min. To avoid this, the cervix should be carefully dilated manually and the lamb should be drawn. Obviously if the torsion cannot be corrected by rolling then a caesarean section is indicated.

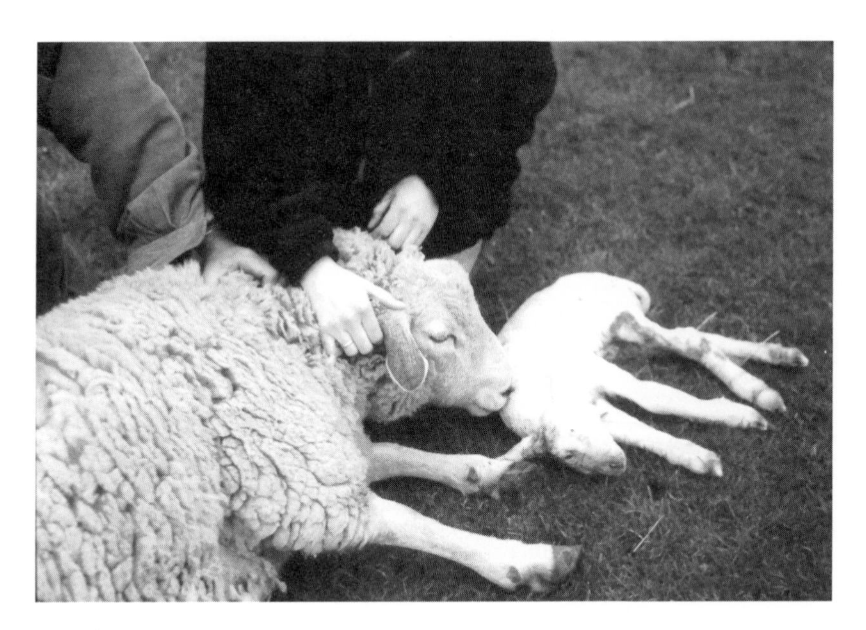

Fig.13.12. Lambing (2).

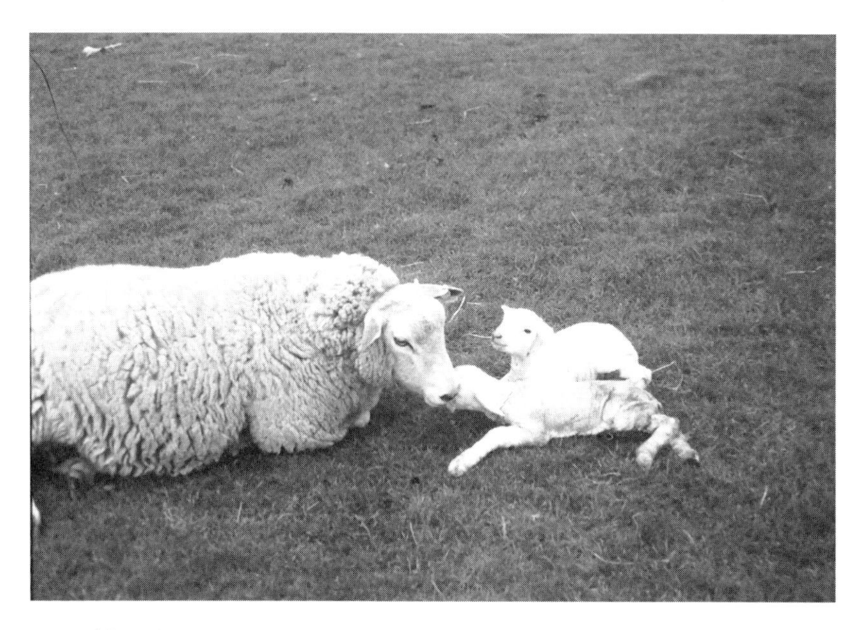

Fig. 13.13. Lambing (3).

Lamb survival

After delivery of the lambs and the initial revival it is vital that they are looked after properly. The ewe should be treated with all the appropriate medicines have her udder examined for mastitis and receive a general check. Then she should be allowed to lick the lambs while some colostrum is prepared. Each lamb should be given 100–180 ml of colostrum, depending on its weight, and then put with the ewe in a warm pen with straw bedding. If a caesarean or a lambing has been performed at a veterinary surgery it is vital that the lambs are kept in a warm box until the shepherd takes them home. They should not be left on a cold concrete floor.

Retained placenta

This is quite a common condition, which is more likely to occur after a difficult parturition, an abortion or an induced parturition. Historically shepherds used to try to manually remove retained placentae after inserting a pessary containing an antibiotic. This is not considered to be best practice nowadays. The ewe should be given antibiotics, penicillin being the antibiotic of choice on account of its good uptake by the uterus. NSAID should also be given. The placenta should be left *in situ* to rot away on its own. If the ewe is pyrexic the uterus can be flushed with 1 l of warm normal saline and the ewe given 20 IU of oxytocin intramuscularly. Antibiotics and NSAID should also be continued.

Dystocia in the Goat

General

Much of what is stated about dystocia in the sheep is applicable to the goat, although relative fetal oversize is more common in goats. This may be on account of the large size of male kids. Male kids in caesarean sections outnumber females by a ratio of 70:30. Pygmy goats also seem to have problems with relative fetal oversize.

Uterine torsion in the goat

In common with the sheep, this is an extremely rare condition. Correction by rolling is not easy in the goat and probably three or four people will be required to accomplish it. If rolling fails caesarean section is the sensible option.

Retained placenta

The condition in the goat is very similar to that in the sheep, although clinicians dealing with dairy goats will be put under more pressure to remove the placenta manually to maintain clean milk production. This pressure should be resisted, but uterine irrigation and oxytocin can be given early and more frequently if desired. Milk withdrawal with antibiotic treatment may be a problem. Clinicians may want to give ceftiofur type of antibiotics (see Chapter 6), which have a nil milk withdrawal period.

Caesarean Section in the Sheep

The main indication for performing a caesarean section is where there are live or freshly dead lambs. If considerable manipulation has been carried out, or if the lambs are dead and rotten the ewe should be destroyed on humane grounds. Clinicians should be aware that if the ewe is aborting and not full term then there is not the urgency to remove the lambs, and time, up to 48h, can be given for the cervix to dilate and for the macerated aborting lambs to be passed. Naturally the ewe should receive antibiotic and NSAID cover.

Main indications for caesarean section:

1. Failure of the cervix to dilate (the so-called 'ring womb').
2. Irreducible malpresentations.
3. Fetal oversize (particularly important if a large lamb is presented posteriorly).
4. Fetal abnormalities.
5. Maternal abnormalities.

Some clinicians administer an epidural before surgery to reduce straining. The author does not value this procedure, as straining normally ceases as soon as the lambs are removed from the uterus before stitching is started. Sedation is rarely necessary. However, the ewe should receive antibiotics and NSAID before surgery, and the tetanus status should be checked. The ewe is placed on an operating table on its right side with its head held and its legs tied individually to the table. The wool is shorn from a large area of the left flank and this area is cleaned. Local anaesthesia is instilled in an inverted L block in the lower left paralumbar fossa. The area then is prepared surgically. A 20–25-cm incision is made through the skin and the muscle layers, taking care not to incise the rumen. This is a definite danger in thin ewes. Having identified a limb of a lamb this should be exteriorized if possible before the uterus is incised, to lessen abdominal contamination. The uterus should be incised as far from the cervix as possible, but also without coming near to the ovary. As a rule of thumb the incision should be from the foot to the hock in a hind leg or the equivalent in a fore leg. All the lambs should be drawn out and passed to assistants to be revived. It is vital that a thorough check is made in the uterus to make absolutely certain that all the lambs have been removed. If the afterbirth can be removed easily this task should be carried out. If not it can easily be left in the uterus to be expelled later *per vagina*. The uterus should be closed with a single layer of uninterrupted inverting Lembert sutures, making sure no pieces of placenta are left protruding or included in the suture layer. A non-cutting needle should be used with no. 3 metric catgut or polyglactin 910. While an assistant gives the ewe 20 IU of oxytocin the uterus should be carefully replaced in the abdomen in its normal position. Instil 5 mega Crystapen™ (Intervet/Schering-Plough Animal Health, Milton Keynes, UK) dissolved in 20ml of sterile water into the abdomen and along both sides of the muscle incision. The muscle layers should then be sutured in two layers starting with the peritoneum and the deeper layer of muscle. Closure should be accomplished with a layer of continuous, inverted mattress sutures, making sure that the peritoneum is fully opposed from side to side. A cutting needle should be used with no. 3 metric catgut or polyglactin 910. The same suturing method should be used for the outer layer of muscle. The skin is then closed with interrupted mattress sutures using a cutting needle and monofilament nylon. After cleaning the area should be sprayed with antibiotic spray. The shepherd should be instructed to continue with the NSAID and antibiotic cover for a minimum of 4 more days.

Embryotomy

In cases where the lambs are putrid and rotten, the vagina will be dry and swollen. The lambs will be emphysematous and cannot be delivered *per vagina*. Caesarean section carries a very poor prognosis and therefore unless a decision is made to destroy the ewe on welfare grounds a simple embryotomy must be performed.

First give the ewe antibiotics and NSAID and check her tetanus status. If the lamb is in anterior presentation then, using a large amount of obstetrical lubricant or J lube put a rope around one carpus and draw it out as far as possible. Make an incision with a scalpel on the medial side of the leg to allow insertion of a disposable embryotomy knife. Put that up as far as possible to cut the skin up into the axilla and if possible over the shoulder joint up to the top of the scapula. With the open hand break down all the attachments of the shoulder blade to the chest wall, pulling the leg constantly. The whole front leg can then be removed after cutting the remaining skin. This process should be repeated on the opposite side. A rope is then placed on the head and the remainder of the lamb is removed.

In cases of a 'hung lamb' (i.e. when the head is out and the legs cannot be felt) it is vital to make absolutely certain that the lamb is dead. In these cases the head can be cut off as near to the body as possible to allow the fore legs to be located and extended. The lamb can then be drawn. If the lamb is alive it is usually possible to repel the head after putting a rope over the poll and into the mouth, and locate the legs. It is best if both legs are extended before drawing the lamb. However if one leg is in extension and the other is totally back against the body, it is normally possible to draw the lamb. Normally the lamb can be drawn if it is in posterior presentation. If it is dead and emphysematous an embryotomy may be required. The legs should be moved caudally and sectioned with embryotomy wire just distal to the hocks. The ropes can then be attached to the hock joint and the lamb can be drawn using a large amount of lubricant.

Caesarean Section in the Goat

Although classically 'ring womb' is a condition of sheep it also occurs in goats, and together with other birth canal obstructions such as vaginal prolapse and pelvic injuries, it is the most frequent reason for caesarean section. Relative fetal oversize is more common in goats than in sheep but is much less common than in cattle. Malpresentations can normally be corrected, as can uterine torsion. Fetal monsters are more common in goats than in sheep. Schistoma reflexus has been recorded in goats.

Although some surgeons have used a midline approach in goats under general anaesthesia, the author prefers a left flank approach with the doe in right lateral recumbency. If possible sedation should be avoided. Helpers should be warned of vocalization. Before surgery the doe should be given antibiotics, NSAID, and the tetanus status should be checked. Relaxation of the uterus is not as marked as in the ewe and so the use of a uterine relaxant such as clenbuterol is indicated.

Regional anaesthesia using an inverted L block should be carried out. There is a danger of using too large a volume of local anaesthetic solution, giving toxic effects. This is particularly true in pygmy goats, and in these animals it is highly recommended that the anaesthetic solution is diluted with sterile water for injection. Goats are very sensitive to hypothermia and so if the procedure is carried out in a cold place extra warmth in the form of hot water bottles should be placed around the doe.

The left flank should be clipped and surgically prepared. A 20-cm incision is made vertically between 5 and 10 cm below the transverse processes. Haemostasis is important as the doe is often shocked. Blood loss can be lessened by going through each muscle layer individually and keeping more in line with the muscle fibres rather than cutting in a straight line. If clembutoral has been given it is usually possible to exteriorize the uterus to some extent by grasping a leg through the uterine wall. Care should be taken, as the uterus is not as thick as in the cow and perforation is a danger. The uterus should be incised from the hoof of the kid to either the tarsus or carpus depending on the leg which is grasped. Ideally caruncles should be avoided, and the incision should be on the greater curvature of the uterus. Although it is easier to draw subsequent kids if the incision is in the body of the uterus, the closure of the uterine wound is harder and so the author favours a more cranial approach.

Assistants are required to revive the kids to allow the surgeon to close the uterus with a continuous layer of inverting Lembert sutures of either cat gut or a synthetic material such as polyglactin 910, as soon as a search of the uterus for further kids has been performed. The fetal membranes should be left *in situ* unless they can be removed very easily; however great care should be exercised to make sure that the membranes are not involved in the suture line. After checking the incision, the uterus should be returned to the abdomen and 5 mega Crystapen™ (Intervet/Schering-Plough Animal Health) dissolved in 20 ml sterile water should be instilled. An assistant should give 20 IU i/m oxytocin. The abdominal wound should be closed in two layers with continuous mattress sutures of dissolvable suture material. The skin should be closed with interrupted inverting vertical mattress sutures of monofilament nylon. After checking the skin wound it should be sprayed with antibiotic spray.

Aftercare of the doe is important, as infections are common. Antibiotics and NSAID should be given by injection for a minimum of 5 days and the udder should be constantly checked for mastitis. Even if the doe is a milking animal it is useful to allow the kids to stay with her to encourage her and to lessen stress in a potentially weakened animal.

Induction of Parturition in Sheep

This is not a common procedure. The major limitation to the technique in sheep is the poor survival of premature lambs and the frequent lack of precise information concerning the stage of gestation of ewes (Ingoldby and Jackson, 2001). There are only three indications: to synchronize lambing in flocks where tupping has been synchronized and lambing dates are known; to aid survival of a pregnant ewe; and to aid survival of unborn lambs. Ewes with pregnancy toxaemia are the most likely reasons for the latter two indications. Practitioners will have to use their clinical judgements. If the lambs are too premature their survival is unlikely. If the ewe is really sick the delay of 36–48 h will result in her death as well as the lambs, and so an elective caesarean is a better option provided the ewe is not more than 5 days from her due date. Dexamethazone given as far before surgery as possible will help dysmature lambs to survive.

Corticosteroids are the only reliable medicines to induce parturition in sheep. A dose of 16 mg of dexamethasone will bring about parturition in a mean of 42 h. Prostaglandins do not bring about parturition in sheep. Oxytocin will only speed up parturition and not initiate it. Antibiotics should be given with the corticosteroids to lessen the danger of infection likely to be caused by the increased susceptibility to disease.

Induction of Parturition in Goats

Relative fetal oversize is more common in goats than in sheep and therefore induction is often demanded by goat owners who are concerned when gestation lengths have become extended. If an elective caesarean is contemplated, induction should be carried out and surgery should be commenced at the start of cervical dilatation. The recommended induction method is a combination of corticosteroids such as dexamethazone at 3 mg/50 kg (as a lung surfactant) and prostaglandin at 250 μg/50 kg (to help luteolysis).

Diseases of the Mammary Gland

Removal of supernumerary teats

This seems only to be a problem in goats; the author has never found them in milking sheep. They should not be removed in goats unless they interfere with milking. A small amount of local anaesthetic should be injected into the base of the teat to be removed. Practitioners would be well advised to check with the owners to make absolutely certain that they are removing the required teat. A pair of small burdizzos is placed at the bottom of the spare teat and clamped shut. After 30 s they are removed and the spare teat is removed by cutting with a pair of curved scissors along the clamp line. The tetanus status of the animal should be checked and fly control should be implemented.

Mastitis in sheep

The incidence of clinical mastitis in sheep is usually below 5% in dairy sheep and lower still in sheep suckling lambs. Clinical cases are most often associated with *Mannheimia haemolytica*, *Staphylococcus aureus* and coagulase-negative staphylococci (C-NS), but *Streptococcus* spp. and enterobacteria have also been cultured (Koop *et al.*, 2010). Factors that have been associated with occurrence of clinical mastitis in sheep are parity, dystocia, breed, region and number of lambs born. Suckling two or three lambs is associated with a greater mastitis risk than suckling only one lamb per ewe. Several hypotheses have been proposed to explain why ewes suckling twins are at greater risk of developing mastitis than ewes suckling one lamb. Damage to the teats and udder by vigorous and more frequent sucking has been suggested as a possible cause of the higher incidence of clinical or subclinical mastitis. This is supported by the fact that experimental infection with *M. haemolytica* was facilitated by damage to the teats. A second possible explanation is an increased risk of teat contamination. The presence of *M. haemolytica* in the mouths of lambs, and transfer of these pathogens onto the teat skin, has been reported. On the other hand, in an outbreak of mastitis associated with *Staphylococcus aureus* it was shown that somehow there was a benefit to suckling twins. The conclusion must be that risk factors differ with pathogens. On reflection this is extremely likely when the cow is used as a model. One definite risk factor associated with twins is the method of weaning. This should be done abruptly, with ewes and lambs totally separated and the ewes moving on to a lower plane of nutrition. The worse scenario is for shepherds to draw off lambs from a flock as they become fat and ready for slaughter. Not only are the ewes which have been weaned kept on a higher plane of nutrition but also in many cases one of a set of twins will be selected, leaving the other twin suckling the ewe. This remaining twin will often avoid the second teat and the result is a considerable increase in the rate of mastitis. *M. haemolytica* and *S. aureus* account for the vast majority of mastitis infections, but some other bacteria, e.g. *Escherichia coli*, *Streptococcus* spp., *Pseudomonas aeruginosa* and *Listeria monocytogenes* have been isolated.

In southern Europe, the Middle East and Central Asia, *Mycoplasma agalactiae* will cause contagious agalactia. Other *Mycoplasma* spp. are also involved. These may normally be considered as goat pathogens, as is *Brucella melitensis*, but both will infect sheep.

Wet, dirty environments predispose sheep to mastitis. Animals should be provided with adequate shelter, dry lying areas and a good supply of dry bedding. Shepherds should be mindful of strict hygiene practices. Overcrowding, whether outside or inside, will increase the risk of mastitis. Mastitis in sheep requires aggressive antibiotic therapy as well as NSAID, as it is very painful and therefore there are welfare implications. Although mastitis in sheep is often described as acute or chronic, in the author's experience it is better described as peracute and acute. In peracute cases the animal may well die before there is real evidence of infection in the mammary gland. In acute cases there is marked pyrexia. The mammary gland or glands are very swollen and inflamed. Often the condition will turn gangrenous, even with aggressive therapy, and large amounts of mammary tissue and skin will slough (Fig. 13.14). Fly control is vital. The antibiotic of choice is a penicillin and streptomycin combination (see Chapter 6). This will be effective against *M. haemolytica* if given at the recommended dosage rate. It is also effective against *S. aureus*,

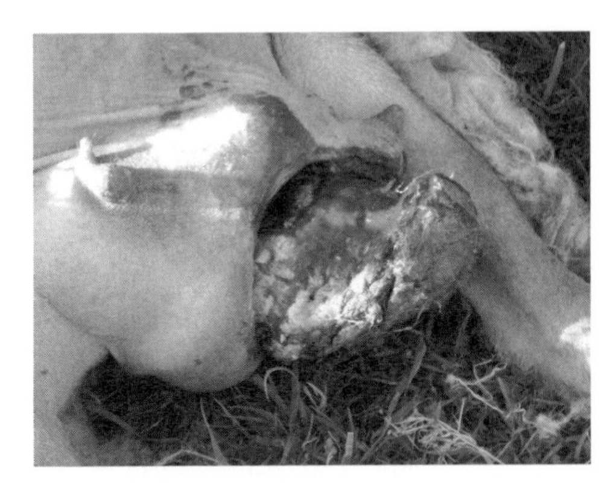

Fig. 13.14. Mastitis in a ewe.

as in the udder of the sheep these organisms are rarely resistant to penicillin. However, if there is any doubt about resistance, amoxicillin with clavulanic acid (see Chapter 6) should be used for a minimum of 5 days. Intramammary antibiotic treatment is not recommended as asepsis is difficult to maintain. It is also easy to injure the mucosa of the teat canal. Some clinicians recommend the use of cow intramammary drying-off tubes at weaning. However in the author's experience injections of penicillin and streptomycin or tylosin (see Chapter 6) are much more effective. Tilmicosin by injection is very effective but it must be remembered that in the UK it has to be injected by a veterinary surgeon (see Chapter 6). In other parts of the world where *Mycoplasma* spp. are involved in sheep mastitis, the drug of choice is oxytetracycline (see Chapter 6). This should also be used if *Brucella melitensis* or *Brucella ovis* is isolated.

Failure of lactation in sheep

The most obvious cause of lactation failure is mastitis, but there are many others that may be less obvious but still important. First of all are the physical factors. Ewe lambs may be too immature: it is important that ewe lambs reach two-thirds of their expected mature weight before they are served. Ewes must not be too poor at lambing. Not only is this a welfare issue, but it is also one of economics. There is no point in achieving a high lambing percentage measured as the number of lambs born per ewe if the real lambing percentage (i.e. the number of lambs weaned per ewe) is significantly lower.

All the factors which cause parturition difficulties will also lead on to lactation failure. One of the most important is post-parturition pain with oedema of the vulva and perineum. NSAID are an important therapy (see Chapter 6).

The environment will play a role in lactation failure if there is unexpected snowfall or heavy, unrelenting rain. However this relates to management, as these types of problems have to be allowed for and shepherds should be prepared. Shelter (remembering ventilation) and bedding are vital requirements. Underfeeding will cause milk loss and there must be adequate trough space. Arrangements for adequate, good quality forage must be arranged, together with concentrates stored ready for use and not relying on outside agencies for delivery. It goes without saying that there must be an adequate water supply. Frosts are the norm in many areas at lambing time and shepherds must have a fall-back plan.

Mastitis has already been considered. However any septic focus may lead to lactation failure; for example a cellulitis from a damaged perineal area will require prompt antibiotic therapy, as will any metritis that may or may not include retention of fetal membranes. Any lameness will also need to be addressed.

Finally, any undercurrent disease will cause lactation failure. This may not be the obvious type of disease causing abortion and stillbirths, but may be disease unrelated to parturition, such as pneumonia.

Mastitis in goats

In the UK mastitis in goats is less of a problem than in cows. This is particularly marked in milking goats where the incidence of mastitis is uncommon. The main pathogen is *S. aureus*. These are usually coagulase-positive. If the infection is recognized and treated quickly with injections of penicillin and streptomycin (see Chapter 6) there is a good cure rate. Resistance to penicillin and

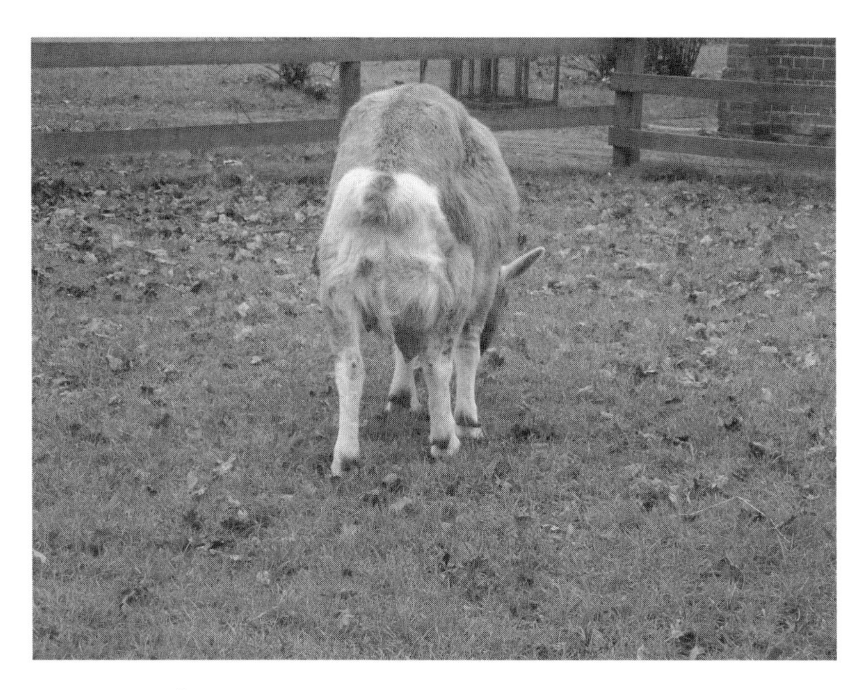

Fig. 13.15. Mastitis in a doe.

streptomycin is not common. However if there is a delay then induration and abscess formation occurs. These abscesses become thick walled and a source of infection to other goats. Initially the goats will be clinically ill with a pyrexia and hot swollen udder, but this quickly becomes a chronic condition. The goat will not be ill but the antibiotic cannot reach the bacteria in the abscesses and so the condition is rarely cured (Fig. 13.15). NSAID are helpful but in the author's experience using various different antibiotics does not seem to be worthwhile. *Streptococcus* spp. are rare but they respond well to antibiotic treatment and rarely cause systemic illness. The environmental mastitis as seen in cows and caused by *E. coli*, *Klebsiella* and *S. uberis* is not a real feature in goats although all three of these organisms have been isolated. There are rare periparturient cases which are very serious. These should be treated with intravenous fluids with intravenous flunixin (see Chapter 6) and intravenous enrofloxacin or marbofloxacin (see Chapter 6). Several other organisms will cause mastitis in goats in the UK, including *Arcanobacterium pyogenes*, *Listeria monocytogenes*, *Mannheimia haemolytica* and *Pseudomonas aeruginosa*, but they are all rare. They have all been found on culture. They also cause problems with treatment. Antibiotics need to be given for long periods and often have to be switched to effect a cure. Both *Corynebacterium pseudotuberculosis* and *Mycobacterium bovis* are very rare causes of mastitis in goats. Prompt euthanasia is required.

14

Neurological System

Neurological Diseases of Sheep in the UK

Introduction

It is prudent to consider neurological diseases in the different age groups of sheep, namely neonatal, unweaned lambs, older lambs and adults. The diseases can be infectious, developmental (obviously mainly seen in neonates), metabolic, nutritional and due to toxins and trauma. Trauma can be seen in all ages of sheep as a result of attacks from predators, and obviously neonates and younger lambs are the most vulnerable. Equally, all ages of sheep are likely to be involved in road traffic accidents and possibly involvement with trains. The most likely trauma to neonates occurs during parturition. This may be physical and so the lamb may be unable to stand as it has suffered a fracture, ligamental damage or peripheral nerve trauma (e.g. radial paralysis). The brain may be affected due to anoxia from prolonged parturition. Neonatal lambs can also sustain physical trauma from their mothers when they do not accept them. Neonatal lambs are very susceptible to trauma from other adult sheep from mis-mothering or a flight reaction. Over-aggressive sheep dogs will cause trauma. Shepherds themselves may cause trauma by poor injection technique either by injecting close to a major nerve or by bacterial contamination. Drenching gun damage to the pharynx can cause infection which may spread to the spinal cord.

Neurological diseases of neonatal lambs

Border disease

This disease is caused by a *Pestivirus* very similar to BVD in cattle. Some British strains of BVD are highly pathogenic for the sheep fetus (Terlecki *et al.*, 1980). It is a cause of abortion (see Chapter 13) and can occur at any stage of pregnancy. The disease should be suspected if live lambs (known by shepherds as 'hairy shakers') are born showing the pathognomic signs of a hairy coat and trembling. Other than abortion the ewes show no other signs. There is no treatment for the lambs and in most cases euthanasia is indicated. However, if they are not too badly affected they can survive and the neurological signs will gradually disappear. They will have significantly slower growth rates, so that at 20 weeks their body weights will be about 20% lower than normal lambs (Terlecki *et al.*, 1980). The carcass quality is also affected, so it must be suggested to farmers with infected flocks that they should slaughter their lambs as soon as they reach a commercially marketable weight, and before they start to lose weight. Although they may possibly develop a poorer breeding performance with age (Hughes *et al.*, 1959), ewes should be retained longer because they will acquire a degree of immunity.

Cerebellar hypoplasia

The shepherds' name for this is 'daft lamb disease'. The cause of the disease is unknown but it is thought to have a genetic origin. Affected lambs show opisthotonous, known as 'stargazing' by shepherds. The lambs have difficulty in maintaining their balance and their heads sway. Diagnosis should be made clinically. Histological examination at post-mortem may often be unrewarding. There is no treatment, although if the lambs can suckle they may survive. Otherwise euthanasia is indicated.

Dandy–Walker malformation

The hypertensive hydrocephalus and domed skull of this malformation is readily recognized at birth. Euthanasia is indicated.

Hypoglycaemia

Unfortunately this condition is very common (see Chapter 3) and occurs as a result of failure to suck. This may be due to dystocia, particularly with oversized lambs. It may occur as a result of extreme weather conditions, or in multiple births where a lamb is neglected by its mother. All of these instances can, in the main, be avoided by good shepherding. Treatment for the hypoglycaemic lamb is logical and straightforward. First the shepherd must decide if the lamb is older than 12h. If it is under 12h of age it should be given an adequate amount of good quality colostrum by stomach tube or by a teat if it is still able to suck. The amount of colostrum depends on the weight of the lamb. A lamb weighing 3kg or less requires 120ml of colostrum. Most lambs require 180ml of colostrum, although those over 5kg require 240ml. After the lamb has received this colostrum it should be warmed up to a core body temperature of 38°C (102°F). This can be accomplished in a variety of ways, either in a 'hot box' or with hot water bottles. Electric fan heaters should be avoided as initially they tend to reduce the core temperature further by causing latent heat loss. Colostrum can be warmed by conventional means or by the use of a microwave. The latter should be used on a very low setting (e.g. defrost), or it will denature the proteins. If the lamb is over 12h of age it is much more likely to be hypoglycaemic. If its body temperature is below 37°C (99°F), it must receive glucose by intraperitoneal injection **before** it is warmed up, or its last remaining reserves of glucose will be used up and the brain will be permanently damaged.

A 20% glucose or dextrose solution should be used. This is easily prepared at the correct temperature by drawing up half the quantity required of a 40% solution (this is the normal strength of glucose solution supplied) at room temperature, into a 60-ml syringe. The other half of the solution is sucked up from a pan of boiling water. This warm solution can then be injected into the flaccid lamb intraperitoneally using a 2.5-cm (1 inch) 19G needle. The site is one finger's width from the midline and two fingers' width below the navel. The lamb is held up by its fore legs with one hand (remember the lamb is nearly dead or it would not require this treatment) with its body hanging down. The correct spot is marked on the fleece with a dot of blue antibiotic spray. The injection is then made at 45° from above towards the tail of the lamb. In this manner the abdominal contents will not be damaged. It is sensible to give antibiotic cover by injection at this time. The volume of the fluid depends on the size of the lamb. This should be roughly 10ml/kg, that is, 30ml for a small lamb; 50ml for a standard size lamb; and 60ml for a big lamb. As soon as the injection has been completed the lamb should be warmed up to a core body temperature of 102°F.

Injury to the CNS at birth

This should not occur as a physical injury with correct lambing techniques. However lack of oxygen can readily occur during parturition, particularly to lambs presented in a posterior presentation.

Swayback

This condition is normally congenital although delayed swayback can occur. With congenital swayback the severity of the symptoms varies from mild hind limb ataxia to severe brain damage and death soon after birth. Post-mortem examination will show actual cavitation of the brain in severe cases. Milder cases will require histopathology of the spinal cord. The blood of either the lamb or its mother will show low copper levels, and the copper content of the lamb's liver will give a definitive diagnosis. There is no treatment as the demyelination is irreversible. However the mildly ataxic animals will live and fatten. The condition occurs in primary copper-deficient areas, or more commonly in areas with high molybdenum or sulfate, which binds up the copper so it is unavailable. The condition can be prevented by giving copper to the ewes between the 10th and 16th weeks of pregnancy (see Chapter 6). As excess of copper is toxic to sheep, it cannot be supplied by mineral blocks or licks. Before treating a flock it is advisable to take some blood samples from a selection of the ewes to confirm the need for treatment.

Neurological diseases of unweaned lambs

Introduction

The conditions affecting unweaned lambs may be the same as those affecting neonatal lambs, but might just have become more noticeable. Hypothermia may lead to hypoglycaemia and fits, and delayed swayback may become more apparent. However, lambs are exposed to a large number of bacteria which may affect the nervous system.

Listeriosis

This can occur in young lambs and is caused by *Listeria monocytogenes*. The lambs will be mentally abnormal and have a very high rectal temperature; their necks will be stiff, which may lead to opisthotonous. However *L. monocytogenes* in young lambs is more likely just to cause septicaemia. In theory the bacteria should be sensitive to penicillin, but in the author's experience oxytetracyclines are more likely to bring about a cure. Dexamethazone is useful if given at a high dosage rate of 1 mg/kg daily in the morning either intravenously or intramuscularly.

Meningitis/encephalitis

This does not occur in isolation but is normally associated with other conditions, such as navel infections, septicaemia, enteritis or polyarthritis. All these conditions result from poor hygiene at lambing. These conditions should be corrected. Shepherds should not rely on prophylactic broad-spectrum antibiotics.

Spinal abscess

Atlanto-occipital infection is very common in young lambs and should always be considered in the ataxic 2–4-week-old lamb. The lambs are mentally normal. Spinal abscesses may occur as a result of tail docking or infections originating in the navel or tonsil. Symptoms are progressive, beginning with slight ataxia which worsens over a few days to complete hind limb paralysis. There is quite a good response to antibiotic treatment if it is started early enough. NSAID should be given for pain relief.

Tetanus

This disease should always be suspected if a lamb is stiff, hyperaesthetic and showing spasms. The vaccination history should be checked as the organism is likely to have gained entry at castration or tail docking. High doses of penicillin may allow the lamb to survive, but welfare must always be considered.

Tick pyaemia

Tick pyaemia will obviously only be seen in tick areas. The lambs will be mentally normal but may show some degree of ataxia. There will be multiple abscesses caused by *Staphylococcus aureus*. Normally this bacterium is not resistant to penicillin so a penicillin and streptomycin mixture given by injection daily is the treatment of choice.

Neurological diseases of growing lambs

Introduction

Diagnosis of these diseases may be very difficult. The speed of onset may be helpful in reaching a cause for the neurological signs.

Cerebrocortical necrosis

Cerebrocortical necrosis (CCN) will have a sudden onset. Any lamb that is recumbent, blind, and showing strabismus and opisthotonous is likely to have CCN. There will be no pyrexia. Response to intravenous thiamine is the best pointer to a correct early diagnosis. A heparinized blood sample can be taken for transketolase estimation, a specific test for CCN. Thiaminase can best be estimated in a faecal sample or in rumen contents if the animal has died. The pathognomic sign at postmortem is seen in the brain. Macroscopically, the cerebral hemispheres will show a yellow discolouration and fluoresce under ultraviolet light.

Cervical injury

These injuries are likely to be seen in older entire rams which have been fighting. They will obviously have a sudden onset. They may be mentally normal showing paresis, and will be non-pyrexic. The head should be examined carefully to show any wounds or bruising. Valuable animals can be radiographed.

Delayed swayback

For swayback to be delayed as long as this would be exceptionally rare. It should only be suspected if there have been other cases of swayback earlier. It will have a gradual onset; the lamb will be mentally normal and slowly become ataxic. There will be no pyrexia.

Gid

The lambs will show visual deficits and postural deficits, with a slow onset. They may circle and show head aversion on account of a space-occupying lesion in the cerebral cortex. The lesion will be on the opposite side to the deficits. The cause is *Coenurus cerebralis*, the cyst of the tapeworm *Taenia multiceps*. In fact the same signs will be shown by any space-occupying lesion in the cerebral cortex (e.g. a haematoma or abscess), but these are extremely rare. Diagnosis will be difficult. A raised white cell count (WCC) would indicate an abscess. External injuries might indicate a haematoma. Softening of the skull in classical cases of gid only occurs in very advanced cases. In extremely rare cases the *C. cerebralis* cyst may form in the cerebellum. In these cases the lambs will show the cerebellar signs of tremor, dysmetria and nystagmus, and there will be a rapid deterioration. The cyst may be seen on radiographs. Surgical treatment is an option (see Chapter 8).

Lead poisoning

Chronic lead poisoning occurs in areas of high lead content (see Chapter 17). The animals will be ataxic and often have fractures on account of osteoporosis. Acute lead poisoning could occur in this age group of lambs if they have licked paint off old gates, but the author has never seen this acute poisoning in lambs, only in calves.

Louping ill

This disease is caused by a *Flavivirus* transmitted by ixodid ticks. The virus has been isolated in Norway, Spain, Turkey and Bulgaria. The clinical signs are considerably worse in the presence of *Anaplasma phagocytophilum*. It causes a diffuse, non-suppurative meningoencephalomyelitis. This is shown as a sudden onset incoordination progressing to paralysis in 24h followed by coma and death in a further 24h. Obviously the lamb needs to be in a tick area. Mortality will vary between 5 and 60%. Although the disease can occur in goats, only sheep and red grouse are infected by louping ill virus which is carried by ticks. Diagnosis would need virus isolation from heparinized blood or CSF from the live animal. The brain should be removed at postmortem. A small sample can be put in 50% glycerol saline for virus isolation, and – being extremely careful to avoid contamination – another sample can be preserved in formol saline for histology. There is a PCR test available for post-mortem material. Paired samples showing serum conversion may be helpful. The risk of louping ill is reduced by frequent acaricide treatments throughout the period of tick activity, but such gathering of hill sheep is rarely practical. Control is better with the effective killed louping ill virus vaccine. On farms where the disease is endemic, all ewe and ram lambs to be retained for breeding should be given a single subcutaneous injection of the vaccine in the autumn or during the following spring before the ticks become active. In addition, any introduced sheep should be vaccinated once, at least 28 days before exposure to the louping ill-infected ticks. When the disease occurs for the first time on a farm as a result of either new tick habitats or following the introduction of louping ill-infected ticks with introduced sheep, it may be necessary to vaccinate the entire flock. The high cost of this strategy is readily offset against potential losses. A second vaccine dose for breeding ewes should be given to stimulate the production of high antibody titres in colostrum, which is likely to maximize protection of young lambs.

Plant poisoning

The following plants may cause neurological signs if ingested (see Chapter 17):

- *Aconitum napellus* (aconite, monkshood);
- *Aethusa cynapium* (fool's parsley);
- *Cannabis sativa* (marijuana);
- *Cicuta virosa* (water hemlock);
- *Conium maculatum* (hemlock);
- *Dryopteris filix-mas* (male fern);
- *Equisetum* spp. (mare's tails);
- *Haplopappus heterophyllius* (golden rod);
- *Ipomoea muelleri* (poison morning glory);
- *Juncus* spp. (rushes);
- *Laburnum anagyroides* (laburnum);
- *Lolium* spp. (rye grass);
- *Lupinus* spp. (lupins);
- *Malva parviflora* (marsh mallow);
- *Nicotiana tabacum* (tobacco);
- *Oenathe crocata* (water dropwort);
- *Pteridium aquilinum* (bracken);
- *Stypandra glauca* (blind grass);
- *Trachyandra divaricata* (branched onion weed).

Pulpy kidney

This disease normally causes sudden death (see Chapter 18), but in rare cases the lamb will develop nephrosis and have fits before death occurs. The urine will be positive for sugar content. Serum will show a raised creatinine and urea level. This disease is a distinct possibility in unvaccinated pet sheep.

Rye grass staggers

This poisoning is reversible. Animals will show tremors and knuckling of the joints. They may even collapse but will recover after rest. The signs are caused by a toxin produced by a fungus living in the rye grass seeds (see Chapter 17).

Sarcocystosis

All ages of the flock may be affected but this is primarily a neurological disease of fattening lambs. The disease is caused in the UK by two microcystic species *Sarcocystis arieticanis* and *S. tenella*. These are obligate two-host parasites. The sheep is the intermediate host and the dog is the main final host although the fox may take on this role. There are macrocystic species but they appear not to be pathogenic.

Microcystic cysts are very common, with at least 85% of sheep showing them in either their myocardium or in striated muscle, but clinical signs are very rare. Affected sheep show muscle weakness and ataxia of variable severity, and hind limb paresis may sometimes progress to recumbency (Jeffrey, 1993). Some sheep may die without premonitory signs. Sheep with these nervous signs are usually still bright, alert and appetent. Less severely affected sheep may recover with supportive therapy.

Diagnosis is extremely difficult as most sheep show antibodies and the cysts are common at post-mortem. If several sheep are affected by a strange neurological condition this disease should be suspected.

Spinal abscess

The lambs will slowly become ataxic. They will be mentally alert and have a raised WCC.

They may be pyrexic. Antibiotics may be helpful, but animals showing an increased level of protein in a CSF sample are not likely to recover and euthanasia is indicated.

Tetanus

This condition should be extremely rare as there are very good vaccines available.

Neurological conditions of adult sheep

Introduction

Once again the speed of onset will be helpful in making a diagnosis. Naturally a really observant shepherd will notice the first animal to be affected, but if there is just an individual animal affected rather than several animals this fact will aid the clinician with a diagnosis. The level of protein in the CSF is a useful prognostic indicator in animals with a hind limb paralysis. If it is high the animal is very unlikely to recover and euthanasia is indicated. A post-mortem will then aid diagnosis.

Botulism

This condition has a worldwide distribution and is caused by *Clostridium botulinum* types C or D. There are likely to be several cases seen with a flock eating big-bale silage which has been badly made. It can be associated with carrion, as the organisms proliferate in decomposing carcasses. Access to broiler litter and the presence of a carcass in the water supply are risk factors. The signs will be muscular weakness leading to flaccid paralysis. This is progressive and symmetrical, involving cranial and peripheral nerves. Normally it begins with the hind legs and progresses cranially. No rectal tone will be seen when taking the animal's temperature. The speed of the progression of the disease is dose related. It may cause sudden death, be peracute, acute or even chronic, and mortality can be as high as 90%. In the early stages the animals will have an unusual stilted gait. Clinicians should note that pyrexia and a loss of sensibility are not features of the disease. The animals are not nervous or apprehensive, and there are no unilateral signs of neurological disease. Confirmation of the disease is challenging as demonstration of the toxin is difficult. There are no pathognomic gross pathological or histopathological features in cases of botulism, nor any useful specific treatment, but with careful nursing some animals may recover.

Cervical injury

This will occur from fighting in groups of adult rams. When mixing rams they should always be penned up in a tight bunch for 48 h so that they cannot reach a fast enough speed when head butting to cause severe trauma.

Cerebrocortical necrosis

This can occur in adults but is rare.

Concussion

The findings in concussion will mimic those of cervical injury. Treatment for concussion is large doses of corticosteroids with antibiotic cover.

Fibronecrotizing pachymeningitis

This condition is rare and is normally caused by *Arcanobacterium pyogenes*. There will be a raised WCC and pyrexia. Antibiotic treatment might be effective.

Gid

This condition is very rare in animals over 2 years of age. A cervical abscess is a more likely cause of cerebral or cerebellar deficits in an adult sheep.

Heartwater

This condition is caused by *Rickettsia ruminantium* (previously known as *Cowdria ruminantium*). It is transmitted by the larval or nymph stages of two species of tick, *Amblyomma hebraceum* in South Africa and *A. variegatum* in the rest of Africa south of the Sahara and in the Caribbean. The incubation period is approximately 2 weeks. The sheep are initially lethargic with a fever before showing neurological signs. They bleat continuously and will be seen to be constantly moving their tongues, and will circle before collapsing into convulsions and death. As the name suggests, on post-mortem there is an excess of pericardial fluid. Isolating the organism is not easy and so a definite diagnosis will not always be possible. Treatment with oxytetracyclines in large doses is often successful, provided the animal has not deteriorated into convulsions.

Hypocalcaemia

In sheep this is a condition occurring in the last third of pregnancy. There is a sudden onset after some type of stress such as gathering, housing, clostridial vaccination, copper supplementation or severe weather. Several ewes will be affected. There will be incoordination followed by recumbency. The rectal temperature will be sub-normal and there will be no rumen movement. If neglected they will die, so treatment with calcium borogluconate should be carried out as soon as possible. This will aid diagnosis as the response is within 30 min if given intravenously or within 4 h if given subcutaneously. The dose is 60 ml of a 20% solution for a 60-kg ewe. Shepherds should be supplied with bottles of 'calcium' and instructed on their use. They must take care as abscesses are common from needle contamination. If as a veterinary surgeon you are injecting 'calcium' you can have the head held and give the injection into the jugular. If you are on your own a convenient method of injection is to turn the ewe onto her rump and lean over her front legs. The mammary vein is easily located. Diagnosis can be confirmed by a serum sample. If there is doubt about the diagnosis, and pregnancy toxaemia is a possibility (indeed they may co-exist) then treatment with a glucose and calcium mixture is indicated (see Chapter 14). Normally the ewes affected with this condition are in adequate body condition. If they are in poor condition pregnancy toxaemia should be suspected.

Hypomagnesaemia

In sheep this is a condition of lactating ewes on good pasture. However, the author has wide experience with rams and non-lactating 'shearlings' being affected on very lush pastures due to heavy nitrogen use under fruit trees not only in Kent, but also in mountainous sub-tropical areas. The onset is extremely rapid. The animal will start to tremble and be hyperaesthetic. If initiated at this stage, treatment may be successful, but within minutes the animal will collapse and die. Treatment of collapsed animals is very rarely successful as, although the blood magnesium levels may be corrected, there is underlying brain damage, so the animals fail to stand again. Often the very act of treatment is enough to send the animal into a convulsion and initiate death. Clinicians should warn owners of this possibility. The best treatment is injecting a 25% solution of magnesium sulfate subcutaneously. Up to 75 ml can be injected into a large animal, and 50 ml is sufficient for a 60-kg ewe. It must never be injected intravenously. With care a mixture of 20% calcium and 5% magnesium may be given intravenously; 50 ml is sufficient for a 60-kg ewe. In the author's view, however, the stress to the animal is not warranted and so a subcutaneous injection is recommended. Diagnosis can be confirmed with a serum sample; however in the majority of cases these animals will be found dead. A sample from the aqueous humour from such animals will be diagnostic. Post-mortem examination is rarely helpful, as blood splashing under the endocardium or the pericardium is seen in any animal dying in a convulsion.

Listeriosis

This is mainly a disease of silage-fed sheep, but clinicians should be aware that sheep will contract listeriosis if they graze grass contaminated by sheep which have been fed silage. Affected animals will show marked depression and may circle. They will often show a raised rectal temperature, a useful diagnostic sign as a raised rectal temperature is not seen in many neurological conditions except in sheep suffering convulsions in hypomagnesaemia cases. As well as antibiosis, steroids are extremely useful. The latter should be given as dexamethasone at 1mg/kg intramuscularly every other day in the morning.

Louping ill

In a tick area this should always be a differential.

Maedi-Visna

In sheep flocks, clinical signs of Maedi-Visna (MV) usually only become evident when over 50% of the flock has become infected. The most efficient route for viral spread is through colostrum and milk from an infected ewe to its lambs or to fostered lambs, particularly soon after birth. It can also spread from the respiratory tract in the form of aerosol droplets but it only travels very short distances in the air so very close contact, probably nose to nose, is required. This is the likely route of spread between ram and ewe, although the virus has been found in the male reproductive tract so venereal spread is therefore a possibility. In milking sheep the virus can be spread at milking with a machine by backflow. It is unlikely to be spread by hand milking, but this is possible. It definitely can be spread by contaminated needles. Transplacental infection has been recorded, but this is extremely rare, and advantage can be taken of this to salvage unborn lambs from infected ewes. Infected ewes can be detected through blood testing before clinical signs are seen and hopefully before the disease has spread. There is no treatment. Culling all animals with a positive result on blood test is the way forward.

Plant poisoning

See Chapter 17 for a list of toxic plants causing neurological signs.

Pregnancy toxaemia

This is the most common condition seen in late pregnancy. It is also called 'twin lamb disease' as it is often associated with multiple fetuses. Ewes will be in poor condition or very fat and have suddenly gone on to a very low plain of nutrition. The cause is always related to inappropriate feeding in the preceding months. The ewes will be depressed, lag behind, be off their food and may become blind. If they are treated at this stage with an intravenous 40% glucose injection at 1 ml/kg they may respond, but if they become recumbent the chances of recovery are reduced. There is a wide range of treatment options which will be discussed below. Diagnosis can be confirmed by showing the presence of ketones in the urine, and a whole blood sample taken into oxalate fluoride (OxF) will show low glucose. However this needs to be tested quickly or stored in a fridge as the glucose levels will drop with time. A serum sample tested for beta-hydroxybutyrate (BHB) levels will give a more reliable diagnosis if levels are raised. Liver enzymes will also be raised in serum samples in cases of pregnancy toxaemia. The main post-mortem finding will be a pale fatty liver. This condition should be prevented by correct nutrition, and treatment – except in early cases – is problematic (see Chapter 9).

Scrapie

Scrapie is a primary spongiform encephalopathy of sheep and goats, which has been recognized in the UK since the mid-18th century. In other species, scrapie-contaminated material has been suggested as a cause of neurological disease such as transmissible mink encephalopathy and possibly bovine spongiform encephalopathy (BSE) (Sargison, 1995). Human Creutzfeldt-Jakob disease (CJD), kuru and chronic wasting disease of Rocky Mountain elk are similar but unrelated diseases. Scrapie in sheep and goats has been notifiable in the UK since 1 January 1993, and was known then to be widespread. In endemically infected and genetically susceptible flocks it was known to be an important cause of economic loss. The disease originated in Spanish Merino flocks and spread widely in Europe and North America. Although it was on occasions introduced to Australia and New Zealand, prompt identification and slaughter of imported sheep has kept these countries free from scrapie. The disease will be manifest in individual animals over 2 years old. Clinical signs are non-specific and variable. Any adult animal showing neurological signs, particularly excessive scratching, should be a suspect case. The pathognomic sign is lip nibbling when the back is scratched. Cases will show incoordination and abnormal behaviour, which will get steadily worse over a period of weeks. In younger sheep the clinical signs develop more quickly. If euthanasia is carried out it should be done chemically, not by shooting, as the head and ultimately the brain is required for histology to confirm the disease. Blood samples in EDTA (normally in a purple-topped vaccutainer) for genetic examination may point to the disease, particularly in pedigree flocks with familial relationships with other cases. UK samples should be sent to the Virology Department of the Central Veterinary Laboratory in Surrey, UK. It is known that the incubation period of scrapie is controlled by one major gene with two alleles. Homozygotes have the shortest incubation period. Heterozygotes have a longer incubation period and homozygotes are relatively resistant to the disease. However these animals may be carriers of the disease. The scrapie monitoring scheme in the UK is rapidly approaching eradication of the disease. However, recent research has demonstrated that scrapie prions can be demonstrated in the saliva of sheep up to at least 20 months before clinical disease. This is likely to be the same in goats. Prions can be detected in the milk of sheep long before clinical signs are seen. This too is likely to be the same in goats. So although the monitoring scheme is working well in the UK, it may have to be adjusted to reflect this recent research. There is an increased incidence of scrapie in the offspring of affected ewes, which may in part be due to transmission of infection from mother to offspring. A breeding policy that aims to decrease the genetic susceptibility of the population should decrease the incidence of scrapie, and removing the offspring of scrapie-affected animals from affected flocks could contribute to the control of the disease (Hoinville *et al.*, 2010).

Scrapie control policies, based on selecting animals with a scrapie-resistant genotype (*ARR/ARR*) for breeding can be used without the loss of genetic polymorphisms from sheep breeds (Nodelijk *et al.*, 2011).

Within the past decade, other scrapie-like conditions in sheep – described as Nor98, or atypical scrapie – have been reported in many parts of the world (Dawson and Del Rio Vilas, 2008). In the UK, the vast majority of such cases have been identified by active surveillance via the abattoir and fallen stock surveys following the introduction of sensitive immunoassays for prion protein (PrP) detection. Compared to classical scrapie, atypical cases have a different pattern of brain PrP deposition, do not show disease linkage to the same polymorphisms in the *PrP* gene and, in the UK at least, reports of clinical disease have been rare. Of the 190 cases of atypical scrapie confirmed in the UK from 2002 to the end of September 2007, only seven were reported as clinical suspects. At 5–6 years of age, these sheep were older than many classical cases. This is the norm with atypical cases. Both types of scrapie show a change of temperament, but with classical scrapie the cases show a fine body tremor which is not seen in atypical cases. There is ataxia with both types of scrapie but atypical cases sometimes show circling. There is loss of condition shown by both types but classical cases commonly show pruritus, usually with a scratch reflex, where this is not a consistent sign with atypical scrapie.

Spinal abscess

The sheep will slowly become ataxic. They will be mentally alert, have a raised WCC and may be pyrexic. Antibiotics may be helpful. Animals showing an increased level of protein in a CSF sample are not likely to recover and euthanasia is indicated.

Tetanus

This condition should be extremely rare as there are very good vaccines available (see Chapter 7).

Neurological Diseases of Goats

Introduction

Making a definitive diagnosis for neurological manifestations in goats is not easy. It is particularly important that a diagnosis is made where several animals are affected, as the disease may be associated with management practices which will have to be changed to prevent further cases. Equally, pet goats are much loved and clinicians will be put under pressure for a diagnosis when in reality one is only likely to be made on post-mortem.

As with any disease problem, a comprehensive history is vital. An individual's signs and their progression should be noted, and any response to treatment should be recorded. The social behaviour of the whole group should be observed before the individual is examined. Age is an important factor and it is often best to divide conditions into three age groups, e.g. neonates, kids and adults.

The initial observations of the individual should include:

- Head carriage, posture, and stance.
- Movement at walk and (if possible) at a faster speed.
- Does the animal circle? Is it always in the same direction?
- Is there any shaking or sign of weakness?
- Is the animal eating and is it eating in a normal manner?
- Does it appear to be blind or deaf?
- Is it vocalizing abnormally?

A more detailed examination should then be carried out. An examination should be performed to observe either trigeminal or facial paralysis and see whether it this unilateral or bilateral. The eyes should be examined for nystagmus, pupil dilation and constriction, and for menace and nictitating reflexes. The use of a swinging light is useful.

Both cutaneous and pedal reflexes should be examined.

Border disease

Congenital border disease is seen in kids born alive following *in utero* infection. The kids will show the typical nervous tremor but the hairy coat seen in affected lambs is not a feature.

Caprine arthritis encephalitis

CAE is caused by a retrovirus which is part of the lentivirus family. In common with other lentiviruses, CAE is a slow virus infection with a long incubation period and is very similar to the virus which causes MV in sheep. There is, in fact, compelling evidence that there is cross-species transmission; however CAE is primarily a disease of dairy goats. It is not a large problem in fibre goats and certainly not in meat-producing goats. When sheep and goats run together, as in so many tropical and subtropical areas of Asia and Africa, the sheep do not normally seroconvert to CAE but the lambs do seroconvert if they suckle goat's milk. So in 'natural' conditions the virus is host specific. Worldwide there are several genetically distinct isolates of the virus which differ in virulence. Care should be taken when mass inoculations are carried, because the virus can be carried on needles and so sheep could be infected from goats, and goats could be infected from other goats. There are even proposals that MV – which was described in South Africa about 100 years ago – may be the primary virus and that CAE is an adaption of the virus in goats. They certainly do have similar manifestations. Although the virus is related to the HIV virus in man, there are no zoonotic aspects.

Clinically the arthritis manifestation of the disease is seen in adults and is the most common and important aspect of the disease, so perhaps this disease should be discussed in the locomotory section of this book. However, the virus causes severe neurological signs in kids between 2 and 4 months of age and so I have decided to describe it in this section. In fact older kids and adults can show neurological signs, and these are invariably fatal. The neurological signs are progressive. The signs seen in kids are what the clinician would expect from a virus causing encephalomyelitis. They are ataxic with hind limb-placing deficits. These progress to paralysis, with the forelimbs involved. There is marked depression with a head tilt progressing to opisthotonous, torticollis and paddling. Euthanasia is the only cause of action. In older goats the normal presenting sign is arthritis. If they do show neurological signs these have a slower onset. The prognosis is extremely poor and euthanasia is indicated. It is usually a minimum of 2–3 years after infection is introduced to a herd before clinical signs are seen.

The most efficient route for viral spread is through colostrum and milk from an infected doe to its kid or to fostered kids, particularly soon after birth. Infected does will also spread the virus to lambs. It can also spread from the respiratory tract in the form of aerosol droplets, but it only travels very short distances in the air so very close contact, probably nose to nose, is required. This is the likely route of spread between billy and doe, although the virus has been found in the male reproductive tract and venereal spread is therefore a possibility. In milking goats the virus can be spread at milking with a machine by backflow. It is unlikely to be spread by hand milking but this is possible. It definitely can be spread on contaminated needles. Transplacental infection has been recorded but this is extremely rare, and advantage can be taken of this to salvage unborn kids from infected does.

Adult goats can develop a progressive interstitial pneumonitis, which will be manifest as a chronic respiratory disease with weight loss, although the animals appear alert and are not anorexic. Mastitis may be the most important clinical manifestation of the disease. A remarkable feature is that the disease can occur in the udder before puberty. Diffuse or nodular, indurative changes develop deep in the udder and gradually extend.

Infected goats can be detected through blood testing before clinical signs are seen and hopefully before the disease has spread. The virus can be killed in the colostrum by heat treatment of 56°C for 60 min without denaturing the immunoglobulins.

Cerebrocortical necrosis

This condition of obscure aetiology causes progressive neurological signs. CCN can occur in all ages of goat but is more common in growing kids. Thiamine deficiency is considered the cause of the disease. The aetiology is considered to be usually associated with the proliferation of excess populations of rumen bacteria that produce thiaminase, an enzyme which destroys thiamine (vitamin B1), and thereby reduces its availability to the goat. The conditions which favour thiaminase-producing bacteria are unclear and it is likely that the various feeds affect rumen flora differently. Outbreaks more commonly occur in housed animals fed concentrates but can also arise at pasture. Recently weaned kids are particularly at risk. Affected goats eventually become recumbent with opisthotonous. Even at this stage treatment is possible with intravenous injections of vitamin B1. These may have to be continued for several days. Sometimes goats will lose their sight, although this may even be restored with treatment. Definitive diagnosis can only be made on post-mortem when the brain will show characteristic autofluorescence under ultraviolet light.

Heartwater

This condition is exactly the same in goats as in sheep.

Listeriosis

This disease in goats is rare except in large, commercial, housed herds. Goats may exhibit these five signs:

1. The most common sign is encephalitis, seen early in the course of the disease. The head is turned and tilted to one side, with the neck held stiffly. The goat will become more incoordinate and will often start circling and end up leaning against a flat surface. All the muscles of the head and neck will be flaccid so the eyelids and ears will droop. The tongue will protrude and saliva and rumen contents will drool out as swallowing is impaired. This will be followed by recumbency, opisthotonous, convulsions and death.
2. Abortions will occur in what appear to be healthy goats. They will also occur in cases of encephalitis and septicaemia.
3. Vaginal discharge from metritis after abortion is common.
4. Septicaemia will occur as a result of encephalitis, abortion or metritis.
5. Keratoconjunctivitis as seen in cows is rare in goats but it will occur in animals showing septicaemia. It may also occur in animals which appear healthy in all other respects.

Treatment of the encephalitic or septicaemic forms needs to be carried out early in the course of the disease. Chloramphenicol used to be the antibiotic of choice, but in many countries (including the UK) it has been banned in goats as they are food-producing animals. The drug of choice would be trimethropin and sulfonamide given in high doses intravenously. High doses of tetracyclines given intravenously may be equally as effective. Supportive therapy should include NSAID and, if severe, intravenous fluids. If this is not possible then giving rehydration fluids by stomach tube will be helpful. The keratoconjunctivitis should be treated with sub-conjunctival injections of 20 mg dexamethasone and atropine sulfate in each eye.

The disease in goats is nearly always associated with feeding spoilt grass or maize silage. Any uneaten silage should be removed after 24 h. It was more common in the UK in 2005 and 2009 when poor quality silage was made in the previous summers.

Louping ill

This virus does occur in goats and has a similar manifestation to that found in sheep. The diagnosis can be confirmed by virus isolation, and a PCR is available.

Scrapie

Scrapie is a transmissible spongiform encephalopathy (TSE). In goats there are three recognized TSEs: classical scrapie, atypical scrapie and BSE. BSE was linked to variant CJD in humans in 1996. There is no evidence that classical scrapie or atypical scrapie pose a risk to human health. The EU has a surveillance scheme to monitor the numbers of scrapie cases, and in 2008 it detected 1202 cases of scrapie from 152,028 tests. There are large variations in the numbers of tests carried out in individual states and extremely wide differences in the number of positives. France carried out over half of all the tests in the EU that year (52%) and only recorded 22 positives (i.e. 3 scrapie cases in 10,000 tests). On the other hand Cyprus carried out 4% of the tests and recorded 1094 positive cases. In other words, if the figures are extrapolated there would have been 1991 scrapie cases in 10,000 tests. This is 44% of the total number of tests that were carried out in the rest of the EU. They yielded 86 positive cases (i.e. 13 scrapie cases in 10,000 tests). There are 318,000 goats in Cyprus showing this to be a very high rate of positives. The first recorded case of scrapie in a goat was in 1985. There are only 96,000 goats in the UK, and six herds have recorded cases since 2004. Two of these herds showing a rising incidence were culled in 2008. One new herd with some affected animals was detected in 2009. No cases of atypical scrapie have been recorded in the UK.

Swayback

This is often called enzootic ataxia and may not be directly comparable to swayback in lambs, although both congenital and delayed forms may occur. Kids may be born normally and show no clinical signs for 6 months, when forelimb weakness and anaemia may suddenly be seen. Very low copper levels will be seen in the blood and in liver samples at post-mortem. The typical histological signs of lack of myelination of the CNS will also be found at post-mortem. Goats seem to be more resistant to copper toxicity compared to sheep, however this condition can occur (Angora goats seem to be particularly susceptible) and great care should be exercised when composing goat rations. There is no treatment for copper toxicity or swayback, but kids may survive if they are not severely affected. It should be remembered that swayback is not the only manifestation of copper deficiency. Copper deficiency may be actual deficiency, or may be brought on by an excess of molybdenum or sulfur. Black goats will show bleached hair, as will cattle, when copper deficient. They will also show harsh coats, and Angora goats will show the classic 'steely' coat, as seen in sheep. Diarrhoea will also be shown by deficient goats. Blood tests on these animals will show a marked anaemia as well as low plasma copper levels.

Eyes

Introduction

Sheep and goats have horizontal slit-shaped pupils. The narrower the pupil, the more accurate the depth perception of peripheral vision is, so narrowing it in one direction would increase depth perception in that plane. Animals like sheep and goats may have evolved horizontal pupils because better vision in the vertical plane may be beneficial in mountainous environments.

Eye disorders and visual defects in general

As in all conditions a good history is vital. Eye disorders and visual defects may appear to have an obvious cause but the clinician must endeavour not only to make an actual diagnosis but also to find out the underlying cause of the condition. A corneal ulcer may appear obvious, but treating the ulcer without curing the entropian that is causing the ulcer will be at best a waste of time, and at worst a welfare issue resulting in the loss of an eye. Practitioners must be mindful that if an eye condition cannot be treated satisfactorily and is causing long-term pain, the eye should be removed.

The history should obviously include the age and the number of animals affected, and a record should be kept as to which eye is affected. Indeed if both eyes are affected that needs to be noted. If the eyes appear normal both from a normal visual examination and from an examination with an ophthalmoscope, then there is likely to be an underlying central lesion. Obviously the examination should include the eyelids and the other structures around the eye. The lens and the retina may well help with diagnosis, but oedema of the optic disc does not appear to be a useful sign in small ruminants, so a study of the optic disc will not reveal intracranial pressure. The visual pathways can be tested for integrity by the menace response or lack of it. This blink test needs to be carried out with care, and it must be remembered that if there is air movement the animal may well blink even if it cannot see in that eye. The swinging light test can be used to test brain-to-eye pathways. A light shining in one eye will make the pupil in that eye contract; the pupil in the other eye will also contract, but to a lesser degree. In a normal animal this will be reversed if the light is moved to the other eye. If there is a defect the pupil will not contract. It should be remembered that there is a crossover of the optic nerves. Depending on where the lesion is situated, effects will be seen in the opposite eye or in the same eye.

Eye disorders and visual defects in neonatal lambs

Congenital cataracts

These can occur from a genetic defect but more commonly from a border disease infection. There is no treatment. Often just one of a twin may be affected with genetic cataract and the condition will not be recognized until weaning as the semi- to totally blind lamb manages to use its twin as its eyes.

Entropian

This is the most common eye problem in neonatal lambs, but may go unnoticed by inexperienced shepherds, who will imagine that it has developed slowly. They may think it is contagious ophthalmia (New Forest eye). In fact it will have been present at birth and set up a secondary keratitis, which then in fact does develop quite quickly. This is an inherited condition and causes severe welfare problems if it is not treated promptly. Every effort should be made to stop using sires which have the gene. Often if the condition is observed at birth the curled-in eyelid can be immediately uncurled and an entropian will not develop, but if the condition is missed then treatment has to be initiated. Antibiotic eye ointment (provided no steroid is included) will help, but obviously will not influence the long-term disease; the turned-in eyelid needs to be turned out permanently. This can be accomplished in three ways. The simplest is to inject 0.5 ml of liquid paraffin, an inert oil, into the affected lids (normally only one lid but often the lids of both eyes). The oil will remain *in situ* for 24–48 h and keep the outside woolly eyelid away from the cornea. If there is keratitis, it will allow healing. The eye will heal and come back to its original size, which will keep the eyelid turned out in its correct position. The second simple treatment is to put a bleb of local anaesthetic under the skin of the eyelid, then a stitch can be put in to draw the eyelid back. This needs to be placed carefully or a cure will not be initiated. The suture needs to be removed in 48–72h. The final method is the best treatment, but a little time-consuming, and involves treating the lamb like a dog and carrying out a 'cake slice op'. After putting in the local anaesthetic, the area around the eye is clipped and prepared for surgery. A small slice of skin is then removed. The wound is then sutured with fine, interrupted simple sutures. The eyelid is then permanently in the correct position. The sutures need to be removed in 10 days.

Microphthalmia

This is usually a genetic defect and has been recorded in Kerry Hill, South Down and Texel sheep. It can occur in older sheep as a result of a vitamin A deficiency, but will not be seen in neonatal lambs with this cause.

Split eyelid syndrome

This defect is seen in the upper eyelid, and is a genetic defect linked to the four-horned gene. It is seen in Jacob, Jacob × Suffolk, Hebridean and Manx Loaghtan sheep. It is rarely seen in Norfolk Horn and Soay sheep.

Trauma at parturition

This is seen when a lamb with its head back has been roughly handled at delivery, or when there is a 'hung lamb' – a lamb which has only its head out of the vulva and the ewe has been in labour for some time, perhaps in brambles or some other thicket. The eyes should be bathed and antibiotic eye ointment applied.

Eye disorders and visual defects in older lambs and adult sheep

Blindness without obvious ocular involvement

There are many conditions which would be included in this classification, including pregnancy toxaemia, CCN and a space-occupying lesion in the brain. It is also reasonable to include progressive retinal atrophy (PRA), often termed 'bright blindness'. In reality this condition does affect the eye as the retinal damage can be seen with an ophthalmoscope. It is a symptom of bracken poisoning (see Chapter 17). Affected sheep have a high head carriage and high-stepping gait. The condition is irreversible; there is no treatment. It is not seen in sheep under 2 years of age.

Excess lacrimation without ocular disease

Large numbers of flies will cause excess lacrimation. This will occur more commonly in sheep that are ill and those that are pathologically thin. This may just be starvation or a specific condition e.g. cobalt deficiency (commonly called 'pine'). Naturally the underlying cause needs to be addressed. Practitioners must be aware of the welfare implications.

Foreign bodies

These should always be suspected in the individual case with a single eye affected (Fig. 14.1). Clinicians should bear in mind that if there is poor husbandry (e.g. poor placement of hay racks), more than one animal may be affected. If the eye has only recently been affected it should be irrigated with a human eye wash preparation; this is supplied in polythene bottles so some pressure can be applied. However if the lesion is of long standing the foreign body will have become incorporated into the inflammatory reaction. In this case the eye should be anaesthetised with local anaesthetic solution and the foreign body should be removed very

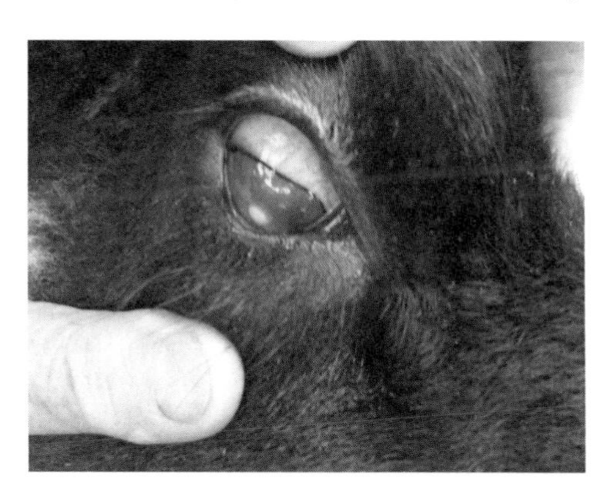

Fig. 14.1. Ewe with corneal damage.

carefully with fine forceps. Antibiotics should be instilled into the eye.

Infectious keratoconjunctivitis

This is the most common infectious ocular disease of sheep, known as 'pink eye' in the UK and 'contagious ophthalmia' in other parts of the world. The cause can be either *Mycoplasma conjunctivae* or *Chlamydophila psittaci*, or a combination of both. Reproducing Knock's postulates is not easy and there may well be another pathogen as yet not isolated. Many other organisms have been isolated from the eyes of sheep, but these have been found in healthy as well as diseased eyes. The list includes many *Mycoplasma* spp., which cause much more serious conditions in sheep, such as contagious agalactia (see Chapter 13). This condition has not been in the UK but it occurs in most other parts of the world. To isolate any *Mycoplasma* spp. special transport medium is required, and clinicians are advised to consult their laboratory for advice. *M. ovipneumoniae* and *M. arginini* definitely appear to be non-pathogenic. The role of *C. psittaci* is unclear, and deep conjunctival scraping is required to isolate the organism. Sheep can get ocular disease in outbreaks of abortion caused by *C. psittaci*. Equally, *C. psittaci* can be isolated as a cause of the abortion when there is no ocular disease. Other bacteria may be opportunist pathogens. These include *Escherichia coli, Branhamella ovis* and *Staphylococcus aureus*. *Listeria monocytogenes* will also cause ocular disease but is normally associated with parenteral disease, and normally causes uveitis rather than keratoconjunctivitis. Pathogens from other species such *Morexella bovis* have also been isolated. There is no doubt that there is a crossover infection between sheep and goats. However, the most likely cause is *M. conjunctivae*. This organism occurs in wild sheep and goats which act as a reservoir for the infection throughout the world. It is possible that deer may be the reservoir in the UK. In Kenya the nematode *Thelazia californiensis*, which is normally associated with cattle, has been found in the eyes of sheep. This is spread by flies, and it is likely that *M. conjunctivae* is also spread by flies in most parts of the world. In the UK it is also spread by close contact, particularly with the use of ring feeders.

Regardless of the cause of the disease, it always shows a sequential pathogenesis. As many animals are likely to be affected the clinician will see all the phases at one time. It is very rare, except with pet sheep, that the shepherd will be observant enough to consult the clinician when only the first phase is evident in a few animals. Initially there will be sclera inflammation, blepharospasm and an increase in lacrimation. This will lead to corneal inflammation and opacity, and there may or may not be corneal vascularization. Lastly there will be corneal ulceration. Antibiotic eye ointment should be applied to the eye, taking care to avoid actually spreading the disease with the tip of the eye ointment tube. Clinicians should read the data sheet of the eye ointment carefully as it is important that corticosteroids are not instilled at the same time. Antibiotics may also be given parenterally. Oxytetracyclines are ideal as they appear in the tears and have long-acting formulations. To help reduce the pain and inflammation NSAID can be given parenterally. NSAID in an eye ointment presentation are likely to be too expensive, except in a pet sheep scenario. If *Thelazia californiensis* is suspected, ivomectins should be given by parenteral injection.

Antibiotic eye ointment which will treat both *M. conjunctivae* and *C. psittaci* should be used, as making a clear diagnosis is difficult clinically without laboratory backup. Treatment should not be delayed waiting for results. As a rule of thumb, a diagnosis can be made between the two conditions by the following signs:

- Bilateral involvement will indicate *C. psittaci*.
- Severe corneal opacity will indicate *C. psittaci*.
- Good response to topical treatment will indicate *M. conjunctivae*.

Listeriosis

This condition can affect the eyes and cause conjunctivitis with excess lacrimation.

The animals will show systemic signs such as fever and neurological symptoms. Listeriosis will also cause the specific ocular disease of uveitis. This is commonly called 'silage eye' as it is linked with the feeding of silage in round-bale feeders. Several animals showing excess lacrimation will be affected, and careful examination with an ophthalmoscope will reveal a uveitis. The best treatment is a sub-conjunctival injection of 0.5 ml 2% dexamethasone and 0.5 of atropine. However, if treatment is going to be carried out by shepherds, both of these drugs can be given as eye drops. In this case treatment should be carried out daily for 3 days.

Trauma

This is likely to be self-mutilation from an irritant condition such as sheep scab, facial eczema or photosensitization. Obviously it is important to treat the underlying cause as well as the ocular condition.

Eye disorders and visual defects in neonatal goats

Entropian

This condition is seen in kids but it is extremely rare compared to its occurrence in lambs, so treatment by removal of an ellipse of skin below the eye is normally justified.

Eye disorders and visual defects in older kids and adult goats

Entropian

This condition may occur as a result of trauma, and corrective surgery will be required.

Tumours of the eyelids

The most common are squamous cell carcinomas of the third eyelid. These have a good prognosis if they can be removed before the tumour has invaded the conjunctiva. Surgery is straightforward as the eyelid can be removed with a pair of scissors under anaesthesia. Haemorrhage is minimal and suturing is not required.

A haemangioma of the third eyelid may occur but these are rare. Papilloma of viral origin will occur on the eyelids. These should not be treated as they will regress spontaneously.

Infectious keratoconjunctivitis

The most common infectious agent isolated from this condition is *Chlamydophila decorum*. This organism is thought to have come from sheep. A variety of other infectious agents has been isolated from the eyes of affected goats: *M. conjunctivae*, *Colesiota conjunctivae*, *Moraxella caprice* and *S. aureus*, but these organisms are also isolated from the eyes of healthy goats. Small nematodes are seen in affected eyes. They are normally *Thelazia* spp.

After careful examination of the eye for foreign bodies, cases should be treated with antibiotics locally and parenterally. The antibiotic of choice is oxytetracycline. If nematodes are seen, parenteral ivomectin should be injected twice separated by 7 days. If the condition continues further treatment should only be carried out after a further examination. Mycotic infections have not been reported in goats but there is always such a possibility.

Silage eye

The agent causing this condition is *Listeria monocytogenes*. Treatment is with atropine, dexamethasone and gentamicin eye drops. It only occurs in goats eating silage in round racks.

Yersiniosis

Yersinia pseudotuberculosis is a significant cause of ocular disease in goats (Wessels *et al.*, 2010). It also causes enterocolitis, mesenteric lymphadenitis, septicaemia, placentitis/abortion and mastitis. It is also a zoonotic infection (see Chapter 19).

Adult and post-weaned goats are affected and present with a sudden onset mucopurulent ocular discharge, blepharospasm, moderate to marked chemosis and conjunctival hyperaemia with corneal opacity and neovascularization (Fig. 14.2). The organism spreads to the parotid and submandibular lymph nodes, which may lead to abscessation. The goats remain bright, alert and non-pyrexic. In commercial dairy herds morbidity varies from

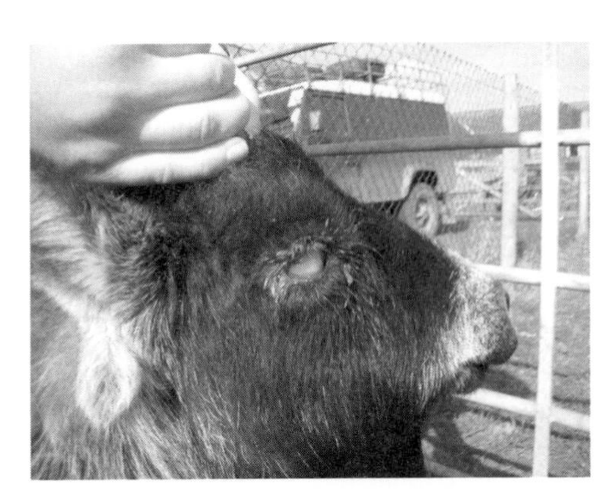

Fig. 14.2. Yersinia infection.

2–5% with no mortality. A dusty environment and diarrhoea caused by *Y. pseudotuberculosis* are predisposing risk factors. Diagnosis is by direct culture of swabs.

Enucleation of the Eye

In all cases where there is no chance of recovery from the eye condition in any disease or traumatic problem, enucleation should be considered on welfare grounds. It can be carried out under heavy sedation, normally with xylazine.

Local anaesthetic should be instilled all around the orbit, not only under the skin but into the deeper tissues with a single very deep injection of 5 ml behind the eye to block the optic nerve. The eyelids should then be sutured together and the whole area clipped and prepared aseptically. A careful incision is then made through the skin parallel to the upper eyelid margin but not entering the conjunctival sac. Using blunt dissection the eye muscles are sectioned around that half of the eye. The same procedure is then carried out to the lower half. Eventually a pair of curved scissors can be used to section the optic nerve and the eye can be removed. The remaining socket can then be obliterated with sub-cuticular suturing with absorbable material and the remaining eyelids can be sutured with non-absorbable material. The animal should receive antibiotics and NSAID for a minimum of 5 days.

15

Locomotory System

Conditions of the Limbs

Introduction

Lambs and kids need adequate amounts of calcium, phosphorus, protein and vitamin D for their skeletons to grow properly. While there will always be occasional animals that accidently break a leg, there are certain problems that increase the risk of fractures. If practitioners have the slightest doubt about the presence of a fracture, the limb should be splinted (Fig. 15.1). Welfare is paramount. Radiographs should be taken, and treatment or euthanasia carried out promptly. Animals should not be transported for slaughter but destroyed on site.

Increased risks of fractures may develop over long periods of time. The bones may become increasingly fragile. Severe copper deficiency has been reported to cause fractures, as copper is needed for development of a normal framework within the bone. Long-standing parasitic infections, particularly those involving intestinal nematodes, also predispose to fractures because damage to the gut wall prevents the young animal absorbing enough phosphorus. Where animals are kept in areas of old lead mining the continual daily intake of small amounts of lead as they graze makes the bones liable to fracture. With all three conditions the young animals will be ill thriven. Problems with rickets can occur in hill lambs that are wintered away on dairy farms. Following the move from the hill to lush grass the lambs and their bones grow quickly. Vitamin D is required for new bone to calcify properly and become strong. Unfortunately in the UK and particularly in Scotland sunlight only provides sufficient vitamin D between mid-March and mid-September. Affected lambs appear stiff or lame and will walk on their toes. There can be obvious bowing of the front legs and the worst affected lambs will not recover enough to be kept as replacements. Rickets can be prevented by injecting or drenching lambs with vitamin D before they go to wintering.

Flying scapula

This is a very rare condition which may occur in sheep and goats, normally after weaning, but before maturity. The muscles securing the scapula to the rib cage become weak and rupture to some extent so that the rib cage drops. The spine is then lower in the thoracic area compared to the lumbar–sacral area. The animal is still mobile. The condition is irreversible.

Fractures

Practitioners should always look out for fractures in small ruminants.

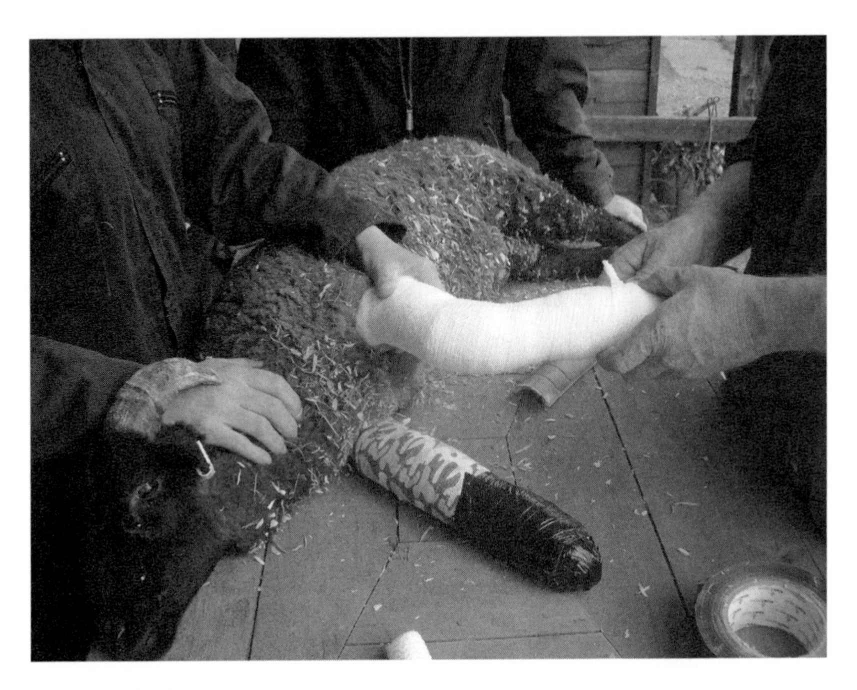

Fig. 15.1. Cast on a lamb.

Conditions of the Hooves

Foot-related lameness in individual sheep or goats

It might be said that there are only two certainties in life: death, and a lame sheep. However, although death is a certainty, I do not think lameness in sheep needs to happen. To prevent lameness we need to know its cause. Most, but not all, lameness in sheep and goats is associated with the feet, but it is often quite difficult to find the seat of lameness. Obviously the most common site is in the foot and we will be studying foot lameness in considerable detail, but causes of lameness higher up the leg should not be forgotten and are particularly important from a welfare point of view. Traditional sheep management is still carried out by many practitioners, but there is a massive increase in the new sheep practice. These new sheep keepers might be hobby farmers, rare breed savers, they might be trying to save the planet by no longer mowing the lawn, and they might even be running sanctuaries for rescued sheep! One thing that is certain is that they will expect the clinician to adopt a small animal practice approach, and our method must be as sophisticated. A proper diagnosis needs to be made. If there is a possibility of a fracture, radiographs will be required. Obviously the less dramatic causes of traumatic lameness need to be considered. Welfare needs to be always in the clinician's mind. No NSAID are licensed for sheep in the UK, so it is a matter of using cattle medicines following the cascade principle. There is no doubt that these NSAID will be helpful in controlling pain in old pet sheep with non-septic arthritis. It is important for clinicians to counsel these sheep keepers very carefully on welfare.

Foot lameness

The bacteria causing foot lameness in sheep are very confusing. Isolation, particularly in pure culture, is impossible. *Dichelobacter nodosus* (formerly known as *Bacteriodes nodosus*) may be found in traditional foot rot. There are said to be ten strains in the commercially available vaccine. Treatment with injectable preparations of penicillin and streptomycin combinations seems to be the best advice for the more old-fashioned foot rot. A more severe form, contagious ovine digital dermatitis (CODD) is now recognized. It is mistakenly called 'super virulent foot rot', but is actually not a form of foot rot at all because genuine cases are not infected with the foot rot-causing bacterium *Dichelobacter nodosus*; a *Spirochete* sp. has been implicated in this disease. CODD is the sheep equivalent of digital dermatitis in cattle. CODD infections differ from scald and foot rot in that the infection usually begins at the top of the hoof, in the area of the coronary band, rather than between the toes. The infection starts as small, ulcerated areas that quickly merge as the infection penetrates under the horn and spreads down towards the toe. Animals quickly become very lame on infected feet, although usually only one or two claws on each animal are affected at any one time. As the infection spreads, the underlying tissues anchoring the horn to the toe break down and it is not uncommon for the horn to separate completely leaving a raw stump. Euthanasia is indicated at this stage as the condition is extremely painful and the sheep is really suffering. As the coronary band has been damaged, any regrowth of horn is weak and deformed giving the foot a claw-like appearance. Treatment with oxytetracycline seems to be beneficial, particularly with zinc sulfate solution applied topically. However for flock treatment, antibiotic foot baths are required. Lincomycin on its own may be helpful but is better in combination with spectinomycin. Erythromycin has also been used successfully. Practitioners are allowed to inject tilmicosin, but this very effective antibiotic is not available to farmers. It has a 42-day meat withhold period, which causes major problems. No vaccine is available.

Strawberry foot rot, a crusty condition of the skin around the pastern is caused by a *Dermatophilus* spp. infection. This will certainly cause lameness. If it is linked with contagious viral pustular dermatitis (orf) it is extremely painful. The condition is made worse by grazing in long grass and is spread more rapidly if there are thistles or brambles in the pasture.

Scald is a painful condition of the skin between the digits caused by either *Fusobacterium necrophorum* or *Staphylococcus aureus*. It is more common in lambs and will appear as outbreaks. Treatment will vary with the organism involved. *F. necrophorum* is the most common, so the starting treatment should be a 3-day course of an injectable preparation of penicillin and streptomycin mixture and topical oxytetracycline spray. Should there be a poor response, then it is likely that there is a particular *S. aureus* infection which is resistant to penicillin. If that occurs clinicians should change to a 3-day course of amoxicillin with clavulanic acid.

Foot abscesses are normally caused by *Arcanobacterium pyogenes*. Poulticing with magnesium sulfate paste on cotton gauze kept in place with waterproof gutter tape is a useful treatment when combined with a subcutaneous injection of tilmicosin. In the UK it is only licensed for veterinary administration and must not be used by non-veterinarians. If the owner is going to treat the animal, injections of either tylosin sulfate or lincomycin hydrochloride can be used.

Chorioptic mange can cause lesions on the lower limbs of sheep. There is intense pruritus, as found with *Psoroptes ovis*. It is difficult to differentiate the conditions clinically but a diagnosis can be made from a skin scrape examined under the lower power on the microscope, for psoroptic mites are twice as large as chorioptic mites. Sarcoptic mites have been reported on a sheep but they are very rare. The mites are an intermediate size between the other two species. There are morphological differences, which a trained parasitologist can evaluate. As a rule of thumb, if the body of the sheep is infested then it is likely to be *P. ovis* (sheep scab); if it is just on the lower legs it is likely to be *Chorioptes* spp. (foot mange).

Other causes of foot lameness

Soil balling

This occurs when sheep are kept on a sea of mud during severe wet weather and then there is a drying wind. The soil will harden between the two claws. Treatment is straightforward and should be carried out immediately or there will be a welfare issue.

Interdigital hyperplasia

This condition is seen in older rams. It does not seem to cause lameness unless there is an accompanying infection. Normally if this can be controlled the lameness will disappear so that the need for radical surgery is avoided. In my experience surgery for this condition in bulls is very worthwhile and is usually straightforward. This is not so in the ram, which seems even more susceptible to infections after the surgery than before.

Excess granulation tissue forming from a solar abscess

Care must be taken when draining these abscesses not to remove too much horn tissue. If the granulation tissue bubbles out from the hole, the hard horn tissue cannot grow over the top. The granulation tissue then grows more, in a vicious cycle. The granulation tissue, which is very vascular but free of nerve endings, needs to be pared back and the whole foot bandaged. This should be changed twice weekly for at least 2 weeks.

White line abscesses

These are normally a sequel to foot rot. The underlying infection needs to be exposed but as much horn should be saved on the wall as possible. Lincomycin hydrochloride injections for 5 days help remove any bacterial problems. Topical spraying with the ubiquitous oxytetracycline spray is useful.

Viruses

Viruses which cause lameness in sheep and goats are notifiable in the UK. Blue tongue virus will cause sheep to be stiff or lame. They will be reluctant to move. They will have a high fever. The pathognomic foot lesion is a dark red or purple band in the skin just above the coronet. If clinicians are suspicious they should stay on the farm and contact DEFRA. Depending on the risk, DEFRA may allow the clinician to leave the premises. Foot and mouth disease will cause lameness in sheep and goats. The clinician in the UK must NEVER leave the farm, if FMD is suspected. Sheep will show a transitory fever and lameness. Unlike Blue tongue the coronet is ulcerated.

Treatment and control of foot-related lameness in sheep flocks

In recent years there have been radical changes in the veterinary advice given to shepherds on foot trimming. The new philosophy is 'little is good'. Excessive paring of feet should be avoided, and only the excess horn should be removed (Fig. 15.2). Any haemorrhage, in fact any paring to reveal any sensitive tissue is not only a welfare issue, but also will do more harm than good. It will lead to granulomatous lesions and malformed feet as well as pain and lameness.

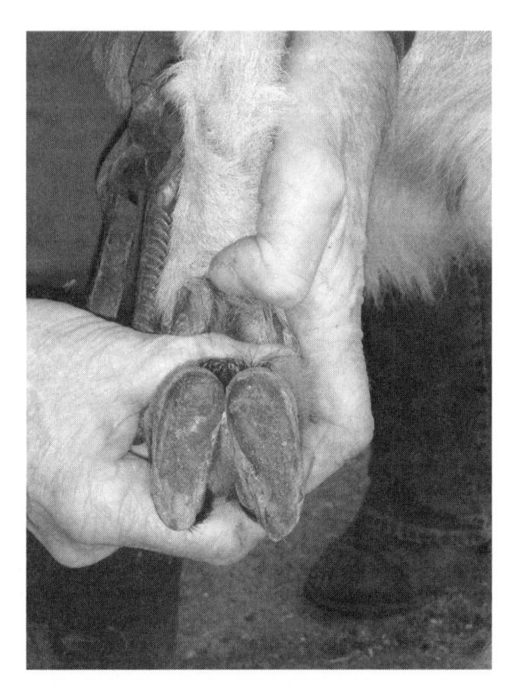

Fig. 15.2. Normal sheep's foot.

Trimming should only be carried out for the following reasons (Winter, 2004):

- To help make a diagnosis.
- To remove obviously loose horn before foot-bathing or applying other topical treatment.
- To improve foot shape when horn is grossly overgrown (Fig. 15.3).

Mild overgrowth of the wall is usually not a problem and, in any case, trimmed horn often regrows quickly.

Trimming should be carried out with foot shears. A very sharp searcher-type hoof knife will be useful for very precise paring. Equipment needs to be cleaned between animals unless they are going to be dressed or put through a foot bath immediately. All equipment must be thoroughly disinfected and oiled between flocks.

Attention to a sheep's feet is a labour-intensive, back-breaking job, and every effort should be made to make it easier. Equipment for individual sheep and handling facilities for the groups of sheep must be tailored to the individual holding to make the job easier; however the welfare of the sheep must be paramount. Foot baths must be kept clean; hoof dip must not splash into a sheep's eyes; and there must be no protrusions. Cradles are helpful for larger sheep, particularly rams. However if they are making the animal sit up they must not be used for too long or the cardiovascular system may be compromised.

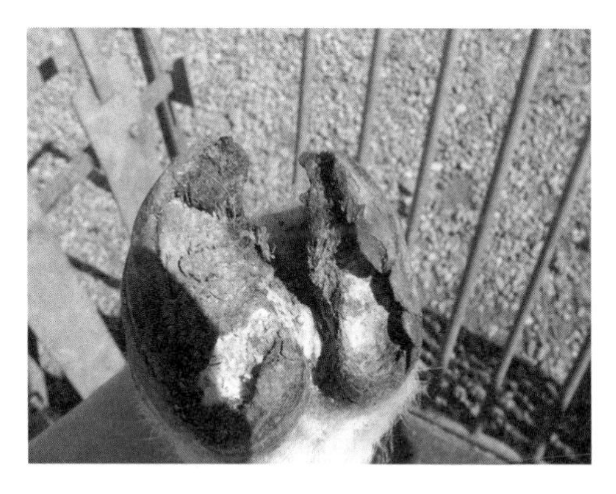

Fig. 15.3. Overgrown foot.

Footbaths are vital to treat scald or foot rot in all but the smallest flock. Careful design is very important. Footbaths may be moveable using big 'Heston straw bales' or sheeted gates, or they can be a permanent fixture. The size of the bath is only partly governed by the size of the flock, for the cost of filling the bath is also a factor. The material of the bath is important as certain footbath chemicals may be corrosive to galvanized iron or can damage concrete. In many ways what happens to the sheep before and after the footbath is as important as the bath itself. Ideally the sheep should run through a bath of plain water to clean their feet before going through the bath. When they come out there should be a dry 'landing area' where the animals wait while the chemical acts on the feet before being lost in the mud, muck or grass. If a moveable foot bath is being used a customized mat can be used or a large square plastic floor can be surrounded by gates. There are several different footbath chemicals; their advantages and disadvantages are shown in Table 15.1.

Great care should be taken with the disposal of footbath solutions. Formalin is quickly denatured but copper sulfate and zinc sulfate will persist for a very long time. Equally, antibiotics are hazardous in the environment. The main thing is not to dispose of them near a water course, but in a pit for the purpose.

There are a variety of control methods for scald. The grass should be kept short (i.e. 4–6 cm) by controlling stocking density. Muddy areas around watering points, feeding points and gateways should be avoided. However care should be taken that conditions are not made worse by the use of unsuitable 'hardcore'. Lime, which increases the pH, may help to reduce bacterial numbers in these areas, but once again care should be exercised as lime itself is an irritant.

Foot rot can be controlled only if it is recognized as an infectious disease. Careful attention to detail must be given if it is to be reduced and ultimately eliminated. Sheep should be bred for soundness; both individuals and breeds vary enormously in their susceptibility to foot rot, and this should be exploited. Control of the disease between flocks must be carried out. It should

Table 15.1. Footbath chemicals.

Name of chemical	Advantages	Disadvantages
Formalin (normally 2%, never more than 5%)	Cheap	Irritant and denatured by muck and mud
Copper sulfate (normally 10%)	Cheap	Toxic to sheep and wildlife **Do not use** except in the desert
Zinc sulfate (normally 10%)	Good to work with	Expensive, needs time
Zinc sulfate with a surfactant	Good to work with and works in a shorter time than without surfactant	Very expensive
Antibiotics e.g. lincomycin and spectinomycin soluble powder 100g/200l or tylosin soluble powder at same dilution	Excellent effects and ideal for treating CODD	Very expensive; long withdrawal time (28 days) in the UK
Proprietary mixtures e.g. benzalkonium or organic acids	Normally cheap	Unknown effectiveness

be recognized that the disease spreads most readily during warm, damp weather. Transmission does not occur below 10°C or in hot, dry weather.

All animals in a group or flock should be examined and infected animals should be treated and separated. Culling should be carried out in chronically infected sheep or those with misshapen or cracked feet. Vaccination, which is both preventative and curative, should be carried out. Timing should be linked with the times of greatest susceptibility. Both the infected and the non-infected groups should be regularly inspected and treated; regular foot bathing should be carried out. Fields grazed by infected sheep should be rested for a minimum of 2 weeks. It should be remembered that this 2-week rule should be applied to **all** walkways. All replacement animals (including rams) should be inspected on arrival, quarantined for 3 weeks and then re-inspected before being allowed into the flock.

Lameness in lambs and kids

Foot lameness

The causes of foot lameness in adult sheep and goats will also cause problems in lambs and kids, particularly if they are older, but they are very rare in very young animals.

Joint ill

This infection is common in young lambs and kids, particularly if they do not receive enough good quality colostrum. The most common organism is *Pasteurella haemolytica. P. multocida* has been reported in an outbreak in Greece (Petridou *et al.*, 2011). It should be remembered that the organism can enter the body through the tonsil as well as the navel, and is also much more prevalent if the lambing pens are dirty. Treating the navels with iodine or oxytetracycline rarely stops the disease if the ewe's udders are dirty. Treatment should be carried out with penicillin–streptomycin injections daily for a minimum of 5 days, and NSAID should also be given.

Laminitis

This has been reported in very fast-growing older lambs. It is extremely rare as very large numbers of lambs are given creep feed *ad lib.* with no ill effects. Ram lambs and shearlings are also given large quantities of food to get them ready for sale without ill effects.

Post-dipping septic arthritis

This is a condition of older lambs and is seen 2–5 days after dipping in a contaminated dip solution. The organism involved is *Erysipelothrix rhusiopathiae*. This is now a rare condition as dipping is confined to large flocks and shepherds are normally well aware of the danger of a contaminated dip.

Primary irritant contact dermatitis

This may catch out the unwary. It is relatively common in pet sheep in back gardens and on old waste ground. Treatment with bland oily cream is straightforward after the feet have been hosed down. Obviously the sheep need to be removed from the irritant.

Rickets

This is a rare condition in lambs and kids.

Swayback

This condition occurs if ewes are deficient in copper. Rarely, this may be a true deficiency, but more commonly the deficiency is brought on by an excess of molybdenum or sulfur in the diet. The condition is seen mainly when ewes are fed a diet of grass or preserved grass. It can be controlled by treating the ewes with copper between the 10th and 16th weeks of pregnancy. It is an easy disease to diagnose clinically, as the incoordination behind in an otherwise bright lamb is pathognomic. If the lambs that are born like this somehow manage to reach up and suck, they can survive. Delayed swayback has been reported but it is extremely rare. The aetiology is difficult to understand. If the myelin is damaged in the womb the lamb will be affected at birth. Suspect cases are perhaps missed at birth. Blood sampling the ewes is useful, although copper is stored in the liver and so ewes may be deficient but not show low blood levels until copper in the liver is depleted. Copper analysis of liver samples from culled ewes gives a more accurate picture of the copper status of the flock. It must be remembered that copper is also toxic to sheep, and there is only a narrow safety margin. The condition will occur in goats.

Tetanus

This disease is a thing of the past in most commercial flocks, even organic ones, as the sheep are fully vaccinated against clostridial diseases. This is certainly not the case with pet sheep or goats. The root of infection in young animals is the navel, and the sites of docking or castration. It is a welfare issue as it is so easily prevented; the vaccine is very inexpensive and effective. Treatment is possible if the disease is caught early enough. A large subcutaneous dose of TAT (e.g. 6000 IU) should be given immediately and penicillin should be given daily. Although acetyl promazine is recommended to relax the muscles, if there is that extent of tetanic spasm then euthanasia should be carried out on welfare grounds.

White muscle disease

This is not an uncommon condition. The lambs and kids are like rag dolls. They are weak and do not appear bright like swayback lambs. The actual aetiology is confusing: it is suspected that there are actually two forms, selenium deficient and vitamin E deficient. The treatment is the same however, with the commercial injection containing both selenium and vitamin E. If several cases are being seen, it is justifiable to inject each lamb as a preventative as soon after birth as possible. This injection should not be delayed until the rubber ring is put on the tail.

Surgical removal of the digit of small ruminants

Septic pedal arthritis does occur in both species, but it is rare. Antibiotic treatment, even if prolonged, is rarely successful and welfare must always be considered. Euthanasia is certainly an option to relieve further suffering. Full drainage of the distal phalangeal joint with subsequent arthrodesis may be considered. However this will result in a long period of severe pain, and surgical removal of the digit is a more humane option. However it is vital that this surgery is not attempted if there is sepsis in the proximal joints as pain will persist. If clinicians are in any doubt, radiography should be carried out.

Regional anaesthesia can be used (see Chapter 8). The distal limb can be cleaned but full asepsis is not required. A length of embryotomy wire is placed between the digits. The sawing direction should be at an angle of 45°

above the horizontal. The skin, soft tissue and half the second phalanx should be removed. The foot should then be bandaged before removal of the tourniquet. The animal should be given antibiotic and NSAID cover for a minimum of 1 week. The bandage should be removed every third day until clean granulation tissue is seen.

Hidden costs of lame sheep

The visible costs are extra labour, footbath chemicals, antibiotics, NSAID and foot rot vaccine. Store lambs will take longer to finish. A store lamb will start to lose weight within 48 h of the start of lameness. Obviously lame rams, particularly if they are lame behind, will have lower fertility rates or may actually fail to get any ewes in lamb. What is not so obvious is that lame ewes will lie down more and not seek the tup. The prolonged stress of lameness in early pregnancy will increase early fetal death. Lame ewes in the last 6 weeks of pregnancy will be thinner and more prone to metabolic disease. This may be hypocalcaemia, hypomagnesaemia or pregnancy toxaemia. After parturition ewes will show poor mothering qualities so there will be higher lamb mortality. Lame ewes will not compete at the trough and their milk yield will be reduced. They will lie down more and therefore reduce sucking times, and the lambs will put on less weight.

Tumours of the skeletal system

Bone tumours are exceptionally rare in sheep and goats and are only really seen as a metastasis of a melanoma in the mandible. However, tumours of the cartilage of the ribs are not so unusual. Diagnosis may be challenging as it is often difficult to find out how long the tumour has been present. It may resemble an old fracture occurring as early as at parturition, or trauma to the ribs later in life. If several sheep are affected, clinicians should question farm staff carefully as the animals may have been kicked. However a definitive diagnosis can be made with a biopsy or at post-mortem. Treatment is not effective but as they are normally benign the sheep may live for months or years after the initial diagnosis. Subcutaneous fibromas and fibrosarcomas may occur in rams around the horns, or even in polled animals.

16

Skin Conditions

Introduction

When dealing with skin conditions it is important not to only obtain a full history (e.g. species, age groups and genders affected; new animals brought on to the holding, etc.), but also to carry out a full clinical examination of the animal. Careful observation is required to check for pruritus, and if this is observed the clinician needs to eliminate ectoparasites before investigating other conditions. Direct visual examination should be carried out with the naked eye and with a magnifying glass, when many larger parasites may be seen. Skin scrapings can be taken from the moister marginal areas of lesions after clipping away the hair or wool. The scrapings can be softened and clarified with 1 or 2 drops of 10% potassium hydroxide solution before direct microscopic examination for ectoparasites or fungal hyphae/spores. Skin scrapings, plucked hair or moist material from lesions can be cultured. Direct impression smears can be stained with Gram, Giemsa or a modified Wright's stain such as a microscope slide already prepared with Giemsa stain. Scabs covering active, rather than healing lesions can be taken, kept dry and referred for further investigation. It should be remembered that it is dangerous to include scalpel blades with referred samples.

The ultimate diagnostic tool is the skin biopsy. When skin is processed for histopathology some potentially important surface features may be partially lost through the chemical processing. Consequently there should be no surface preparation of the skin prior to collecting a skin biopsy, although it is quite correct to clip the surrounding hair. If an entire nodule is to be removed then it should be sent in sufficient formal saline to preserve it. If it is large it should be cut in half to allow the formal saline to penetrate it. If just a biopsy is to be taken it is best to use a specially prepared 6-mm biopsy punch. Multiple biopsies may be taken and sent, recording the sites of each. A biopsy may be taken and labelled from normal skin, but it is best not to include too much normal skin with the biopsy as when the section is prepared it may not be apparent which is normal and which is diseased skin. It is very important to give a full report to the pathologist so this individual is aware of the extent of the diseased tissue and the timescale of the changes. It is also important to select the pathologist carefully; he not only needs to be familiar with skin disease, but also with sheep and goats.

Inherited Skin Diseases

Redfoot

This inherited condition is restricted to Blackface sheep and their crosses and occurs in the first few weeks of life. The progressive signs are ulceration of the oral mucous membranes and corneal opacity accompanying the loss of hoof horn. The exact nature of the hereditary link remains obscure. If particular sires are indicated as carriers of any genetic link, they should be culled. Death of the lambs is inevitable and euthanasia is recommended.

Sticky goat syndrome

This is restricted to Golden Guernsey goats, a dying rare breed. This fatal condition is common as close inbreeding is practised. It only occurs in purebreds and not in crossbreds.

Viral Skin Diseases

Blue tongue virus

BTV causes hyperaemia of the oral mucosa with excoriations of the tongue, lips and gums that become ulcerative and necrotic. There is also a coronitis with hyperaemia and swelling around the coronet leading to obvious lameness (see Chapter 10). It is only included as a skin disease for completeness.

Border disease

This disease is caused by a *Pestivirus* and is common in parts of the UK. It is primarily a neurological condition (see Chapter 14) and also causes pathological changes to the skin. The virus affects lambs *in utero* and they may be aborted (see Chapter 13). If the lambs reach term they may be alive or stillborn. They have a characteristic hairy coat, which may be pigmented and contain long, fine 'halo' hairs particularly in the neck region. The lambs have severe muscle tremors with erratic gait and incoordination. 'Hairy shakers' is a very apt descriptive name.

There is hypomyelinogenesis in the brain and spinal cord. The skin abnormalities are related to the action of the virus on fetal ectoderm resulting in hypertrophy of the primary hair follicles with medullation and a relative decrease in the number of secondary follicles.

The diagnosis can be made clinically and confirmed by histopathology; the virus can be isolated from infected lambs. Retrospective confirmation can be obtained by paired blood samples from ewes which have aborted. There is no treatment.

Caprine herpesvirus

As the name suggests this condition is a disease of goats. The disease might causes confusion, as there are lesions on the feet as well as on the lips, and these look like FMD. Both conditions produce vesicles and have a very low mortality. Unlike FMD, caprine herpesvirus has a very low morbidity, but the main problem with this virus is that it can cause venereal disease affecting the vulva and penis. The main signs in the individual animal disappear in 2 weeks unless there is a secondary infection. This should be controlled with antibiotics. The virus will also cause abortions but these are rare. Kids from infected mothers do not become infected until they are bred. Control can be achieved by separating young breeding stock from old breeding stock. The disease probably occurs worldwide. It has not been found in the UK but is definitely present on mainland Europe. There is no vaccine. The disease may be confused with venereal orf.

Caprine viral dermatitis

This is a separate viral condition caused by a pox virus. It is rare and restricted, as far as I am aware, to Central Asia. Lesions are seen all over the body; these are deep ulcers and are slow to heal. Antibiotics by injection and local creams are used in treatment. Mortality and morbidity are low. Fly control is vital.

Capripoxvirus

This is the true goat pox and is not related to orf. It can occur in sheep, when it is called sheep pox. It occurs in eastern Europe, the

Middle East, Central Asia and Africa, and it is possible that there is an insect vector. It is not just a skin disease and causes a high mortality in young animals. There is a high fever and pneumonia. The skin lesions are mainly seen in the mouth and around the nose; lymph nodes show painful swellings. There are pus-filled papules which only look like orf in the later stages, but unlike in orf, antibiotics do not appear to help healing. A vaccine is available that is very useful in preventing the spread of the disease. There are different strains of the virus, so, in some cases, the disease is of very limited severity. This does not appear to be a zoonotic disease; however clinicians should take care as there are some authorities who consider it is a zoonosis.

Contagious pustular dermatitis

This is primarily a disease of sheep, but will affect goats. Caused by a *Parapox* virus, it is perhaps the most important viral skin disease of sheep and is also called orf. It is highly contagious and is found worldwide. The lesions most commonly occur on the commissures of the lips, muzzle and occasionally on the feet and genitalia. It can be manifest as a flock outbreak or can be seen in the lambs in spring and summer. If the lambs are still sucking, the teats and udder of the ewes become infected, with disastrous results.

The initial lesion consists of a number of red papules within which vesicles develop and rupture, and a thick scab is formed. Proliferative changes may then occur resulting in papillomatous lesions. Secondary bacterial infection is common and in ewes mastitis may occur. Difficulty in sucking may cause weight restriction in lambs, and lesions on the coronary band may result in lameness.

Diagnosis should be straightforward clinically and can be confirmed by virus isolation. The disease will spread rapidly, and although it is a virus (Gallina and Scagliarini, 2010), antibiotics are useful. A blanket dose of a penicillin and streptomycin injection is very helpful. Really bad lesions should be treated with oily creams. Antibiotic aerosols should be avoided as they tend to cause the scabs to harden. When these scabs are knocked off there are large eroded areas underneath.

A live vaccine is available for sheep. This is licensed to be applied to a scarified area in the inner thigh. Vaccination should be carried out at least 6 weeks before lambing. It is vital not to allow infected lambs to suck ewes and cause mastitis. There is no colostral immunity. Normally lambs do not become infected until they are at weaning age. The vaccine should not be used in goats; it is a live vaccine and very bad reactions have been reported.

Foot and mouth disease

Vesicle lesions of FMD are found on the oral mucosa and the coronary band. The condition is included under skin disease for completeness (see Chapter 10).

Malignant catarrhal fever

In the UK, MCF is caused by ovine herpes type 2 virus (Ov-VH2). The sheep is thought to be the natural host. In Africa the natural host is the wildebeest. It is thought to cause cutaneous manifestations in goats. The lesions are a severe generalized alopecia with granulomatous mural folliculitis. A definitive diagnosis may be made with PCR. The condition is normally fatal. There is no treatment and so euthanasia is recommended if a definitive diagnosis has been made.

Peste des petits ruminants

This disease is caused by a *Morbillivirus* and is related to rinderpest. However, unlike rinderpest, it is not contagious to cattle. On the other hand rinderpest can affect goats but appears to be less virulent as the mortality rate may be as low as 50%, whereas in the author's experience the disease in cattle causes 100% mortality. It is hoped that rinderpest has been totally eradicated. The world was pronounced as free of the disease by the OIE on 25 May 2011, but the author has reservations as there are still 'no go' areas in the Sudan and Somalia where the disease might still be present. PPR is termed goat plaque. It is a disease with a high morbidity and mortality in goats. Clinicians should not be concerned that they will miss this disease, as the signs are very obvious. There is high fever with erosions on the mucous membranes of the mouth and eyes; acute bloody diarrhoea; and also signs of pneumonia. Whole herds will quickly become infected and the majority will die. There is no specific treatment, but oxytetracycline injections seem to reduce the number of deaths. NSAID may be helpful. No vaccine appears to be available but the literature claims that one has been developed.

Pseudorabies

Often called Aujeszky's disease, this is primarily a virus affecting swine. It is mainly a neurological disease (see Chapter 14).

Rabies

This virus disease affects sheep and goats and is primarily a neurological disease (see Chapter 14).

Rinderpest

It is hoped that this has been eradicated from the world thanks to the excellent vaccine prepared by Sir Walter Plowright. It is caused by a *Morbillivirus* and the primary host is cattle, although on rare occasions goats have been affected.

Scrapie

This virus is mainly associated with sheep but goats have a similar condition. It is primarily a neurological disease (see Chapter 14).

Venereal orf

This relatively rare condition is caused by two viruses, those causing contagious pustular dermatitis and ulcerative dermatosis. It is not entirely clear whether the presence of both viruses is required to give signs of the disease, however the presence of *Fusiformis necrophorus* certainly makes the lesions more severe. They are seen on the vulva and perineum of the ewe and the prepuce and penis of the ram. The disease is called 'pissile-rot' by shepherds in the UK. It appears at mating time and is spread by mating. It can result in a failure to mate with resultant late service or failure in conception, entailing many barren ewes and a drawn-out lambing period. It should not be confused with vulvitis. This condition has been recorded in the later summer months when 'fly worry' is at its worst. It is only seen in female animals which have been 'short docked', leaving the vulva unprotected. No virus has been isolated. Flies are the cause and should be controlled, even to the extent of housing ewes. **Sheep should not be short docked**.

Often the first sign of venereal orf is when a ram newly put out with the ewes is seen to be off colour. On examination it will be seen to have proliferative and crusted lesions on the penis and prepuce. When further rams are caught and examined they will be found to have similar lesions but to a lesser extent. All the rams should be withdrawn and examined. The affected rams should be immediately separated and treated with daily injections of a mixture of penicillin and streptomycin. An initial injection of a NSAID will be helpful. The penis and prepuce should also be treated topically each day with an oily cream (cream containing a mixture of benzene hexachloride (BHC) and acriflavin is ideal). This cream should be applied using rubber gloves as the contagious pustular dermatitis virus is contagious to man. Aerosols containing coloured sprays and antibiotics should not be used as they tend to desiccate the lesions, scabs then form, drop off and leave raw sore areas. The ewes should also be examined and those affected should be separated. Any badly affected animals should be treated daily with injections of penicillin and streptomycin and topically with oily creams.

This process should be repeated in 7 days and the dates should be recorded to help organize lambing later. The clean rams may then be admitted to the clean ewes. The affected ewes can be allowed to run with affected rams. As with all control measures based on identification and isolation, failures will occur. The labour involved, the chances of success as measured by the ability of the shepherd and the fact that lambing will be delayed by at least 2 weeks, must be measured against the disadvantages of a long-drawn-out lambing and a rather high prevalence of barren ewes. There are vaccines available against contagious pustular dermatitis that are licensed in the UK. They are live vaccines and should not be considered at tupping time, or indeed at lambing time, but only after weaning. Some authorities recommend preparation of an autogenous vaccine. In the author's experience this does not speed up the course of the disease, and the disease does not appear at subsequent seasons. Naturally care should be taken when bringing in new stock, whether rams or ewes; ideally this should not be encouraged. However, in most situations it is inevitable and farmers should make sure all the incoming animals, both rams or ewe replacements, are virgins.

Vesicular stomatitis

This *Rhabdovirus* is very rare. It is really only of relevance as it may cause confusion with FMD. It mainly occurs in other species but has been reported in goats although not in sheep. There are only small vesicular lesions in the mouth causing excess salivation, and no foot lesions. The disease is self-limiting. It may occur worldwide but the main reports have been from the Americas.

Bacterial Skin Diseases

Actinobacillosis

This condition occurs in small ruminants. It is normally associated with the head and neck but in Norfolk (UK) it has been reported on the body (Fig. 16.1). It is characterized by thickening of the skin with multiple granulomatous swellings often associated with the lymphatics. These swellings are unrewarding to lance as the pus is only in small pockets. The actual organism is *Actinobacillosis lignieresi*. This is thought to gain entry either through wounds in the skin or the mucosa of the mouth. Treatment with penicillin is unsatisfactory, although prolonged daily dosing with streptomycin is normally effective. A minimum of 10mg/kg for 10 days is suggested.

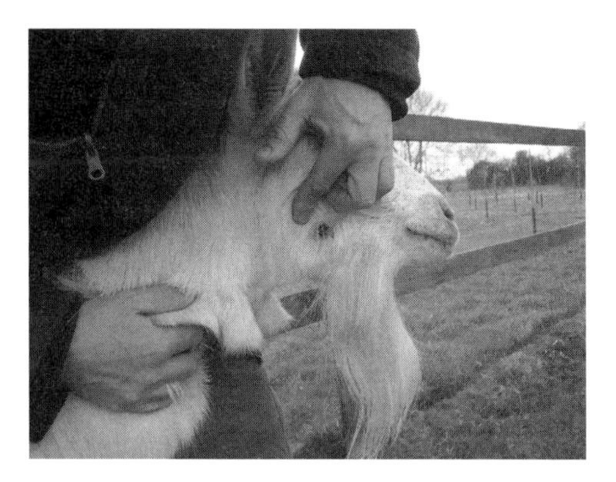

Fig. 16.1. Actinobacillosis.

Actinomycetic mycetoma

This is a very rare condition found in sheep and goats in Central Asia. Two organisms have been isolated: *Actinomadura madurae* and *A. pelletierii*. The lesions are very similar to those caused by *Actinobacillosis lignieresi*. Diagnosis is by culture and treatment is similar.

Actinomycosis

This condition is really a disease of cattle called 'lumpy jaw' or, if it occurs in the soft tissues of the mouth, it is called 'wooden tongue'. The syndrome is very rarely seen in sheep but frequently in goats. *Actinomyces* spp. form firm nodules on the face. Lancing is unrewarding as they are granulomatous and only release small amounts of yellowish-white granules. Treatment with penicillin is unsatisfactory, but prolonged daily dosing with streptomycin is normally effective. A minimum of 10mg/kg for 10 days is suggested.

Anthrax

This is normally a systemic disease in small ruminants, although sheep can get a cutaneous form similar to that seen in humans (see Chapter 19). In sheep it takes the form of a malignant pustule, normally on the face but the author has seen it in the groin. Smears made from the lesion will reveal the bacteria on staining with old methylene blue (see Chapter 4). The disease is notifiable in the UK and is extremely unlikely to be seen. However the author has treated cases in Africa which have responded well to 5 days of procaine penicillin.

Caseous lymphadenitis

CLA is caused by *Corynebacterium pseudotuberculosis* and occurs in sheep and goats throughout the world. It was first isolated in the UK in 1990 (Baird, 2003) from an importation from Germany. Studies have revealed that all cases in the UK have come directly from that case. There has been no official action as control was thought not to be feasible.

Rams tend to show a much higher prevalence of clinical disease than ewes, although there is no evidence to suggest that males are more susceptible to infection than females. However, it does seem clear that factors in ram management make the spread of infection within these groups more likely.

Abscesses usually develop in the lymph nodes under the skin but can also occur in internal organs, most commonly in the lungs. It will then be manifest as a respiratory condition (see Chapter 11). Swollen abscessed lymph nodes are easy to see. If incised they take on an onion-like appearance in sheep with concentric rings of fibrous tissue and inspissated pus. In goats they are just filled with soft pasty pus. They are very obvious on meat inspection. Although the condition is not zoonotic, carcasses will be destroyed if there are multiple active abscesses. Normally the animals have lost a considerable amount of condition and so there is little flesh on the carcass. The main spread is from the rupture of abscesses into the environment where the organism can survive for a very long time. If there are abscesses in the lungs the disease can spread by the respiratory route. The flock or herd can contract the disease by importation of infected animals, but also from contaminated fomites such as clipper blades, sheep hurdles and lorries.

Diagnosis can be made on clinical grounds and confirmed by culture of the organism from an abscess. There is a useful blood test in sheep but this has not yet been validated in goats. This is an ELISA test with a mean specificity of 99% and sensitivity of 79%. The advantage of the blood test is that it can identify sheep lacking obvious abscesses or respiratory signs so that they can be removed from the flock. Culling is the only course of action as there is no effective treatment. Total eradication can be achieved (Baird and Malone, 2010). In theory the organism is sensitive to several antibiotics but penetration into the abscesses is impossible. A vaccine is available (see Chapter 7) but it is not licensed in the UK.

Clostridial cellulitis

This is often called malignant oedema and can occur in sheep and goats, but it is most common in rams as a result of fighting wounds; it has been called big head disease. A variety of *Clostridial* spp. have been isolated, namely *Cl. chauvoei*, *Cl. oedematiens*, *Cl. perfringens*, *Cl. septicum* and *Cl. sordellii*. All these organisms are now covered by a licensed vaccine for sheep. This same vaccine is licensed for cattle at double the dose. It can be used in goats but it should be used at the sheep dose. The higher cattle dose causes adverse reactions in the form of cold abscesses.

It is a very serious condition. The area of swelling is initially hot and painful with crepitus. This then turns cold and gangrenous. Initially the animal has a fever but this rapidly abates before death. Diagnosis should be made on clinical grounds, but confirmation is difficult as there is rapid autolysis after death. However if smears are obtained promptly they will confirm the diagnosis using the fluorescent antibody test (FAT).

Treatment may be attempted if the disease is caught in the febrile stage. High doses of crystalline penicillin should be given intravenously, together with NSAID.

Dermatophilosis

Textbooks often call this condition mycotic dermatitis; this is a misnomer as it is caused by a bacterium, *Dermatophilus congolensis*. It is also called 'lumpy wool' and when found on the lower limbs in sheep is known as 'strawberry foot rot'. The disease is manifest as an exudative dermatitis affecting the ears, face and lower limbs of lambs, and the back and flanks of adult sheep. In rams the scrotum may be affected and in ewes the udder. The disease is progressive: it starts with exudation, which then crusts and scabs. The initial penetration is facilitated by prolonged wetting of the fleece during periods of prolonged wet weather. Diagnosis may be made on clinical grounds and confirmed by Giemsa stain of the scabs.

Treatment in severe cases is parenteral antibiotics and antibiotic cream on the raw areas. Most mild cases will heal spontaneously. Dips of 0.5% zinc sulfate or 1% alum have been advocated, although there is no evidence for their efficacy.

Fleece rot

This condition is correctly termed necrotic dermatitis, and is caused by *Pseudomonas aeruginosa*. It results in downgrading of the fleece. However, more importantly, it predisposes the animal to myiasis. Preventive measures need to be stepped up. It appears to follow prolonged rainy conditions, particularly within 6 weeks of shearing, but the exact trigger mechanism is not known. Animals can become very ill if the area of the affected skin is large. The local lymph nodes will become swollen. The diagnosis can be confirmed on culture.

Morel's disease

This disease is clinically very similar to CLA, but the causal organism is *Staphylococcus aureus* subsp. *aerobius*. It has a shorter incubation period of 3 weeks, rather than the months of incubation with CLA. The abscesses are not as closely related to the lymphatics as in CLA. The initial morbidity is 70–90%. This falls to 10–20% as it becomes endemic. It has not been seen in sheep, but only in goats in Europe (Poland, Germany and France), and in Africa and Asia. Antibiotic treatment appears to be ineffective. Autogenous vaccines do not offer protection.

Nocardiosis

This disease was first reported by Peter Jackson at Cambridge, UK (Jackson, 1986). It is very rare in the UK, but seems to be widespread in Central Asia. Abscesses are common in Central Asia but the actual bacteria involved appear to be similar to those seen in the UK. There is a very rare bacterium, *Actinomadura madurae*, that causes granular pus in similar abscesses all over the body. This condition is also called Actinomycetic mycetoma.

Periorbital eczema

This condition is thought to be bacterial and is likely to be caused by a *Staphylococcus*. Occasionally contagious pustular dermatitis virus has been isolated, but other contagious pustular dermatitis infections look very different clinically. The condition characteristically affects the ewe in the final 4–8 weeks of pregnancy; it also occurs in trough-fed goats. The early lesion is seen as a small inflamed and scabbed area on one or other of the bony prominences of the face, or less commonly on the nose. This extends, usually around the eye, hence the name, and develops into an alarming scabbed, discharging sore. The condition is not serious except on the rare occasions when the infection actually spreads to the eye. Most cases are self-limiting and do not require treatment, although severe cases may require aggressive antibiotic treatment. The author recommends daily injections for 3 days with amoxicillin with clavulinic acid and local treatment with the same antibiotic, which is available as an intra-mammary preparation for cows.

Scald

This is also called benign foot rot in lambs. It mainly occurs in warm moist conditions with animals on lush pastures. The interdigital skin becomes inflamed and painful, but normally there is no separation of the horn or suppuration, and no smell like typical foot rot. The bacteriology is not straightforward; certain strains of *Bacteriodes nodosus* are involved, but normally *Fusibacterium necrophorum* is not present.

Individual cases respond well to antibiotic aerosols. If large numbers are affected then foot bathing in 0.5% zinc sulfate is helpful.

Staphylococcal dermatitis

This may actually be the same condition as periorbital eczema, as it occurs on the face and nasal bones in sheep and goats; however it also occurs on the limbs, vulva and prepuce. It is a suppurative condition which takes 4–6 weeks to resolve. The causal organism is a beta-haemolytic *S. aureus*.

Staphylococcal folliculitis

This is a benign condition which affects young lambs and kids and is normally associated with housed animals. Occasionally it will affect the udders of ewes and does. In does it is called 'mammary impetigo'. The clinical signs are normally mild with small pustules on the lips, muzzle and nostrils. Diagnosis should be made on clinical grounds, although it can be confirmed on the isolation of a beta-haemolytic *S. aureus* or histologically as a pyogenic folliculitis with ulceration of the epidermis. The condition will normally resolve without treatment in a few days. It should not be confused with contagious pustular dermatitis or *Staphylococcus* dermatitis. Induced folliculitis has been recorded in goat kids in Spain, caused by *S. chromogenes* (Ortin *et al.*, 2010), and the lesions resolved without treatment in 10 days. *S. hyicus* and *S. intermedius* will also cause skin disease in goats, as will *S. xylosus* in lambs.

Fungal Skin Diseases

Aspergillosis

This is a rare disease of goats caused by *Aspergillus fumigates*. It is found sporadically in east Africa. Sheep running with the goats do not seem to become infected. The condition takes the form of ulcerating nodules in the groin. It is refractive to treatment. As the disease may be contagious, slaughter should be advised. The disease may be diagnosed by culture but false negatives will occur. Histopathology is a safer method of diagnosis.

Cryptococcosis

This is an extremely rare skin disease of goats. Nodules, which may become ulcerated, are seen on the head. *Cryptococcus neoformans* can be isolated on culture. The disease is seen in Central Asia.

Malassezia dermatitis

Malassezia spp. may be isolated from the skins of normal sheep and goats. They can be seen on impression smears stained with a modified Wright's stain such as Dif-Quik. If very large numbers of peanut-shaped yeast organisms are found on diseased skin they may well be significant. Swab samples may be cultured on ordinary Sabouraud's medium. The clinical signs will include erythema, scale, hyperpigmentation and malodour. Workers (Uzal *et al.*, 2007) have reported infection with *M. sloofiae* which was associated with generalized trunkal alopecia. Various baths seem effective, such as chlorhexidine, enilconazole, miconazole, or selenium sulfide 1% w/v in a mild detergent base can be used twice weekly for a minimum of 3 weeks and then regularly at weekly intervals until the condition resolves. However if there is a trigger factor involved this will need to be treated at the same time.

Phaeohyphomycosis

These infections are seen in goats in Central Asia but are similar to the fungal diseases seen in the UK. However, one is of particular interest, the opportunist free-living fungus *Peyronellaea glomerata*, which forms papules and aural plaques on the ears. The goatherds think that it is spread by the new EU regulation ear tags. It appears to be self-limiting.

Pythiosis

This rare fungal disease is seen in South America in wool sheep. It seems that the causal organism, *Pythium insidiosum*, can only affect the skin of wool animals exposed to total immersion in water for some hours. The ulcerated plaques will heal if the animals can be kept dry for 3–4 weeks.

Ringworm

This is a rare condition in wool sheep and fibre goats and is normally seen on the non-fibre covered areas. On hair sheep and goats it may be found all over the body. The most common organism is *Trichophyton verrucosum* and it is normally caught from cattle. It must be remembered that it is a zoonotic condition (see Chapter 19), so the practitioner should warn the owner to take normal hygienic precautions. Washing carefully with soap and water or dilute chlorhexidine is worthwhile. Owners should avoid rigorous scrubbing or strong disinfectants as the skin barrier will be breached allowing the fungi to penetrate. The other organism caught from another species is *Microsporum canis* from dogs. The species actually linked to goats is *Trichophyton mentagrophytes*, an organism which has also been found in sheep. The clinical picture of round crusting lesions is the same for all three species of fungi. Pruritus is more marked with *T. verrucosum* infection. Obviously several animals are likely to be infected.

The areas most commonly affected include the face, ears and back. In very rare instances the legs and tail head are affected. The lesions are first seen as firm raised plaques attached to the underlying skin, which then become detached to reveal circular raised crusts with local thickening of the skin. Thickening of the stratum spinosum with hyperkeratosis and proliferative dermatitis will be seen on histological sections; however histology is not normally required to confirm a diagnosis. The organism is readily grown on proprietary plates and will be identified by changing to a red colour within 10 days. Often there will be secondary bacterial infection. Only debilitated animals will get a bad infection. In normal animals the infection is self-limiting in a few months. If treatment is required for special animals (e.g. showing animals), topical fungicides such as natamycin and oral antibiotics like griseofulvin may be used. The latter is very effective against *T. verrucosum* and *T. mentagrophytes* but not so effective against *M. canis*. Griseofulvin must not be used in food-producing animals in the UK.

Protozoal Skin Diseases

Besnoitosis

This is a disease of goats in South America, and does not seem to affect sheep. It is caused by the protozoa *Besnoitia caprae*. Diagnosis is difficult as it causes large areas of thickened skin, which appears very similar to scabies. Diagnosis can only be made from skin biopsies. The condition is refractory to treatment, and euthanasia is advised.

Leishmaniosis

This disease is seen in sheep in South Africa and is seen as crusty lesions all over the head. The organism can be seen on Giemsa-stained deep skin scrapings. The method of spread is not known but it is likely to be biting flies (e.g. the 'horn fly'). The condition is refractory to treatment and slaughter is recommended.

Sarcocystis capricanis

This condition has been reported in Central Asia although in fact it occurs throughout the world. The author found the organism in goats with severe alopecia in Mombasa, Kenya. However, demodectic mange was present at the same time and so the cause of the alopecia was in doubt.

Parasitic Skin Diseases of Sheep

Sheep scab

This well-known, highly contagious ectoparasitic disease affects all ages of sheep (Bisdorff *et al.*, 2006). It is caused by a mite, *Psoroptes ovis*. It is highly pruritic and will cause serous exudation and severe debilitation. If neglected it may affect the whole flock and if untreated it can become a serious welfare problem.

The incubation period of sheep scab varies from 2–8 weeks, depending on the ambient temperature. It is primarily a condition of wool sheep but will occur in hair sheep and goats. In temperate climates mite populations on sheep are small in the spring and summer, when the mite resides in body folds and fossae. Most sheep scab outbreaks are diagnosed during the autumn, which corresponds with the natural increase in the activity of the mite, although rapid spread of the infestation can occur during the seasonal latent phase (Sargison, 1995). In ideal conditions, the life cycle of the mite through five instars to the point of oviposition takes between 10 and 14 days. Eggs are laid on the edges of the lesions and hatch in 1–3 days. The mites can continue laying 1 or 2 eggs a day for 40 days and are capable of surviving away from the host for 15 days. There are several strains of mite, but all can live in the ears and travel all along the back.

Diagnosis can actually be made with a magnifying glass, although normally skin scrapings from the edge of the lesions are examined under the low power of the microscope. Recently an ELISA test has been developed, so sheep scab can be detected before signs of infection are shown by the sheep.

It is vital that treatment of the whole flock is carried out, together with disinfection of sheep-handling equipment. The drug of choice is a single intramuscular injection of doramectin at 33 mg/kg. Ivomectin can be used at 200 μg/kg but needs to be given subcutaneously and repeated in 7 days.

Blowfly strike in sheep

Fly strike (cutaneous myiasis) is a debilitating and sometimes fatal condition of humans and animals caused by the feeding and development of fly larvae on the host's dead or living tissues, usually at the skin surface or a body orifice.

As with many of the conditions seen in sheep, this is largely preventable. It is our duty to educate our clients on how to do this, for the benefit of their animals, as well as their pockets.

An average of 1.4% of ewes and 2.8% of lambs in the UK are infested per annum and around 2% of infestations lead to death. Some farms will have up to 60% of a flock infested, however, which is clearly unacceptable. The prevalence is highest in the south-west of England.

The first strikes of the season have been shown to occur equally in both ewes, which will have long fleeces at this time, and lambs. With each subsequent generation of blowflies, a greater proportion of strike occurs on lambs. This is due to the seasonal increase in lamb faecal soiling with rising helminth infection and fleece growth, and because ewes will have been sheared.

In the UK the primary fly involved is *Lucilia sericata* (the green bottle), which favours warm wet conditions with low wind speeds. Therefore if it is dry during the spring when both lambs and ewes have short fleeces, eggs become desiccated, resulting in suppression of the fly population and a subsequent lower incidence of strike.

The most commonly infested area is the breech. This is predisposed to infestation by faecal soiling due to diarrhoea, tipping sheep up on unsuitable ground or contamination with fetal fluids or urine in inadequately dagged ewes. Body strike is the second most common type of strike, followed by foot strike. The former can occur when the wool is soiled from foot rot lesions when sheep lie down or dermatophilosis lesions. The latter occurs in feet with conditions such as scald, foot rot and contagious ovine digital dermatitis. Poll strike is seen in rams wounded whilst fighting, or due to an accumulation of sweat at the base of the horns. Other areas less commonly involved are the preputial orifice called 'pizzle strike', shearing wounds, damaged horn shafts in horned breeds and discharging abscesses. The condition may occur around the mouth in neglect cases suffering from orf.

Diagnosis is usually very easy following a thorough clinical examination. The sheep are restless in the early stages, and then become separated from the rest of the flock. With breech strike they will wag their tails and try to chew at the affected area or rub it on the nearest available solid object due to the intense pruritic nature of the lesions. Sheep with poll strike will shake their heads, which they carry low. On closer inspection the infested area will appear moist, discoloured and have a characteristic putrid smell. Maggots may not be obvious on a brief inspection if they have burrowed into the skin. In later stages of the infestation animals become toxaemic, depressed and recumbent, and death soon follows. If greater than one-third of the skin area is involved the prognosis is hopeless.

To treat the condition the area around the lesion should be clipped to gain access to the wound. Care should be taken not to be too bold, in order to avoid subsequent sunburn. The demarcation between brown, moist, infested fleece and normal, white, dry fleece is obvious. The margins of these areas often contain clusters of unhatched yellow eggs, which should also be removed. The clipping will disturb the maggots which can then be scraped away using dagging shears or similar. A cream containing acriflavin and BHC is then applied. This seems to cause less discomfort to the sheep than organophosphate or high-cis cypermethrin dressings, and is easily carried in the back of the car. The latter should be applied to the surrounding area as soon as possible to prevent secondary strike. Deltamethrin (Coopers™ spot-on insecticide 1% w/v cutaneous solution; Pfizer Ltd, Sandwich, UK) is also licensed for the treatment of established strike.

Broad-spectrum antibiotics and NSAID are given prior to maggot removal, and continued for 3–5 days as necessary. The hydration status of the patient should be considered too, as the sheep may have been too distracted by the strike to drink, so oral fluids may be required. Unfortunately once the animal is recumbent and toxic, the prognosis is hopeless so euthanasia is necessary on welfare grounds.

The condition should be prevented by good farm management, which is just as important as the use of chemicals in the prevention of strike. Flock health plans should be drawn up with this in mind. Strike prevention should be integrated into an overall ectoparasite control strategy and, if possible, products specific to blowfly control (insect growth regulators) should be used to spare the other products (organophosphates and synthetic pyrethroids).

Good husbandry to prevent concurrent diseases such as scab, diarrhoea and lameness will also prevent strike. Ideally, weaned lambs should be turned out onto silage or hay aftermaths to reduce helminth larval challenge, diarrhoea and anthelmintic usage during the fly season. The flock should be inspected closely (not from inside a vehicle) at least daily. Ewes require dagging before lambing and 'cleaning up' if necessary afterwards. Lambs will need dagging if their wool becomes contaminated with faeces following an episode of diarrhoea. Tail docking of lowland lambs reduces the incidence of strike. Adult sheep should be sheared as soon as weather conditions permit, and should have received adequate nutrition during lactation to encourage the fleece to rise. Shearing will cause fly eggs to dry out, preventing hatching. During dry weather this will allow the application of chemicals to be delayed for a month, giving up to 20 weeks' protection. Rubbish and muck heaps which act as fly breeding grounds should be disposed of promptly. Blowflies can travel for several miles so unfortunately cannot be eradicated from the farm.

There is some evidence that susceptibility to strike may be hereditary. Farmers may cull breeding ewes and rams with repeated breech strike for this reason.

The use of chemicals needs to be carefully timed. Manufacturers of insecticides provide websites that forecast the incidence of blowfly strike in particular areas and we should make our clients aware that such facilities are available. Alternatively, baited traps can be used to monitor fly activity on a particular farm so that chemicals are applied before the first case of strike. With warmer winters and wetter autumns strike will occur earlier and disappear later in the year in temperate countries. Therefore if weather conditions favour heavy challenges, chemicals may need applying several times over the strike season. In the future fly traps may help to control fly numbers (Broughan and Wall, 2006). There are several chemical products currently available for the prevention of strike (see Chapter 6).

The choice of ectoparasiticide depends on several factors including manpower and facilities; required duration of efficacy; economics; sheep condition; other parasites in the flock; operator competence and qualifications; the environment; disposal facilities; weather; withdrawal periods for meat and fleece; and husbandry, including the use of concurrent medicines and need for handling after treatment.

Care has to be taken if choosing a product which is effective against more than one parasite. Widespread, routine, prophylactic use of synthetic pyrethroids against strike may contribute to the spread of resistance in mites and lice.

The insect growth regulators are very safe, and to date are not associated with resistance problems. They can be used in organic flocks too but are about twice the price of the other pour-on products.

To summarize: prevention is better than cure for this condition, which can cause very serious welfare problems, and clinicians should help their clients to achieve this goal.

Blowfly strike is not so important in hair sheep and so preventive measures similar to those for non-fibre-producing goats can be recommended.

Lice in sheep

Sheep can be infested with biting lice, *Damalinia ovis* and sucking lice *Linognathus ovillus* and *L. pedalis* (Bisdorff *et al.*, 2006). Biting lice are more commonly found on the fleece areas. Sucking lice are usually confined to the hairy areas and are more commonly found in hair sheep. Lice will cause intense pruritus especially in the cold months of the year.

Sheep keds

These are the wingless flies *Melophagus ovinus*, which are 5–7 mm long with six legs. They cause irritation in a similar manner to lice.

Ticks in sheep in the UK

Hard ticks are distributed throughout the UK and there are concerns that their numbers are increasing and their distribution and competency to transmit disease are changing, due partly to changes in climate and in land management (Sargison and Edwards, 2009). In the UK ticks transmit louping ill virus, resulting in significant production losses and welfare problems in sheep flocks. The louping ill virus is also an important cause of high mortality in red grouse, which underpin the economy of many hill and upland areas of the UK. Control of louping ill virus in these birds often depends on control of the disease in sheep, which is becoming increasingly difficult due to the decreasing number of acaricides available for tick control. Only three species of tick readily infest sheep in the UK, and these are all hard ticks. They are *Ixodes ricinus*, often called the sheep tick; the hard bean tick; the castor bean tick and the pasture tick. These ticks are found in many heath and hill areas of the UK. *Haemaphysalis punctate*, often called the coastal red tick, is found in southern England and coastal Wales. *Dermacentor reticulatus*, often called the marsh tick, is found in coastal southern England and throughout Wales. There have also been reports of non-endemic ticks imported from abroad. The three species mentioned above feed indiscriminately on the blood and tissue fluids of three hosts, which may be reptilian, avian or mammalian, for a total period of less than 4 weeks during their 3-year life span. The sheep may be host to any of them. The life span depends on environmental conditions during the long free-living periods during which the ticks develop and moult. The ideal environment of adequate warmth and humidity is provided by a dense mat of vegetation in an area of high rainfall (i.e. hill, upland and rough pasture), although other habitats may hold tick populations, for example in field margins and hedgerows, woodlands, heath areas, conservation areas and the banks of drainage ditches and streams.

The adult male and female tick mate while the female is still attached to the third host. After leaving the third host, the females lay several thousand eggs in the matted vegetation over a period of about 1 month before they die. The eggs lie dormant for 1 year before the life cycle starts again. In sheep the ticks usually attach to the head, particularly the ears, neck, axillae and groin. Many thousands may attach themselves to one sheep and cause anaemia. The three-host life cycle of these ticks means they are ideal vectors of disease. Tick control depends on the use of acaricides to prevent infestation. Organophosphate dips are very effective and are used throughout the world but they are banned in the UK. Diazinon as a plunge dip is licensed in the UK, and affords protection for 3–6 weeks. Three pour-on treatments can be used: deltamethrin, to give 6 weeks' protection; high-ciscypermethrin, to give 8 weeks' protection; and alphacypermethrin, to give 12 weeks' protection.

As mentioned earlier, ticks transmit louping ill and tick-borne fever (see Chapter 14), babesiosis and theileriosis (see Chapter 11). They also cause a disease in their own right, tick pyaemia. Ticks inoculate staphylococcal bacteria, which cause abscessation on the skin or the internal organs and most commonly in the joints. Clinical cases occur about 2 weeks after exposure to ticks. Sometimes up to 5% of the lambs may be affected. Treatment is rarely successful and the condition is a welfare problem.

Parasitic Diseases of Goats

Blowfly strike in goats

This is not as common as in wool sheep, but it is very common in Angora goats and other fibre-producing goats (Bisdorff *et al.*, 2006). In these breeds it is vital that preventive measures as described for wool sheep are carried out.

Fly strike will occur in goats normally when there is a wound, although primary strike has been reported in temperate countries and commonly occurs with screw-worms in tropical and sub-tropical countries.

The flies belong to the sub-order Calliphoridae. *Lucilia sericata*, the green bottle (Fenton *et al.*, 1998) and the blue bottle, *Protophormia terrae-novae* cause problems in the UK. *P. regina* causes problems in North America. They all require a primary wound. A primary wound can be a very small puncture in the flesh between the digits or elsewhere. They are both very common in temperate and subtropical areas. *Wohlfahrtia magnifica*, the flesh fly, is rare but can act as a primary striker in these areas. *Chrysomyia bezziana* and *C. megalacephala* are called 'Old World screw-worms' and can both cause a very unpleasant myiasis. The flies attack goats and do not require a wound, although if there is a wound this is their main target. They lay thousands of eggs around a wound or around the anus and vulva. These hatch into larvae which attack not just diseased tissue but also healthy tissue, and the goats die of toxaemia within 12 h. Unlike in temperate areas, fly strike is restricted to the summer and the screw-worm has a much longer strike period. The goatherds are aware of the bad geographical areas and tend to avoid them. There is some use of pour-on treatments when they are forced by their nomadic habits to move through bad areas in warm weather. They can avoid fly strike by staying at altitude during the very hot weather. The infestation in goats occurs in all breeds and resembles fly strike in sheep. A similar problem occurs in the tropical and sub-tropical areas of the Americas caused by the screw-worms *Cochliomyia hominovorax* and *C. macellaria*.

Lice in goats

There have been alterations in the naming of biting lice of the order Mallophaga in goats. The genus name historically was *Damalinia*, but this has been changed to *Bovicola*. *B. caprae* is very common in all goats worldwide. The species is host specific and causes pruritus and major hair loss. It normally resides in the dorsal areas (i.e. neck, withers and tail root) and is not killed by injectable or oral ivomectins. Pour-on preparations are not advisable, and animals should be washed in synthetic pyrethrins such as deltamethrin, cypermethrin and permethrin. Modern 'louse powers' are rarely effective unless applied weekly for several applications. Angora goats are affected by *B. limbata* and *B. crassiceps*. These biting lice cause severe fleece damage and are very common, but control is not easy because of the length of fleece. The manufacturer's recommendations should be followed. Amitraz preparations may be used in short-fleeced goats but their use should be avoided in Angora goats for toxicological reasons. Fipronil is very effective as a spray, but its use is normally restricted to pygmy goats on account of the high cost.

Goats also suffer from infestations of sucking lice of the order Anoplura. *Linognathus stenopsis* is found in temperate areas and *L. africanus* in Africa and other tropical areas. Sucking lice suck blood so in large numbers they can cause severe anaemia. However, on account of this behaviour control is much easier with injectable ivomectins. The lice can be found all over the body and the legs and they cause pruritus and fleece loss in Angora goats.

Nematocera insects infesting goats

In the UK these are restricted to *Culicoides* spp. and *Culex* spp. Apart from causing severe irritation and the risk of self trauma, they may cause a hypersensitivity reaction. Repellents are not very effective; diethyl toluadine (DEET) is effective but only lasts for 6h. Keeping the goats inside is not effective unless very fine mesh is used over all the doors and windows, as the gnats will enter buildings. They are poor fliers so fans are effective. Oily creams help to prevent the gnats biting and corticosteroids can be used in severe cases. These gnats are found worldwide, and in tropical and subtropical areas. *Simulium* spp. (black flies and sand flies) and *Anopheles* spp. (mosquitoes) cause similar problems. The mesh has to be even finer to prevent sand fly attack.

Muscidae flies infesting goats

There are many species found in the UK, including *Musca domestica* (the house fly), *M. autumnalis* (the face fly), *Morellia simplex* (also called the face fly), *Haematobia irritans* (the horn fly), *Hydrotoea irritans* (the head fly) and *Stomoxys calcitrans* (the stable fly). They all attack the head, neck and perineal areas causing severe irritation. They will transmit mastitis-causing organisms in both lactating and dry goats. The stable fly will cause large inflamed plaques and sometime an urticarial reaction. This can be treated with corticosteroids except in pregnant animals. All these flies can be controlled with synthetic pyrethrums. Muck heaps where the larvae develop should be kept well away from goat houses.

Tabanidae flies infesting goats

Worldwide, there are three genera with species which bite goats. They are *Tabanus* spp. (the horse fly), *Chrysops* spp. (the deer fly) and *Haematopota* (the cleg). They often cause small swellings and annoyance but do not transmit disease and can be repelled by synthetic pyrethrums.

Glossinidae flies infesting goats

These are the tsetse flies which only occur in Africa south of the Sahara and north of the Limpopo River. They will bite goats and spread the protozoal disease trypanosomiasis (see Chapter 11). The organism has to develop inside the tsetse fly before infectivity but the disease is not passed from pregnant female flies to their eggs. They prefer female goats to male goats and pregnant goats to non-pregnant goats. They cannot fly more than 400m, but can be carried in vehicles and in the vortex of vehicles, and by animals. There are 23 species divided into three groups: the savannah species (e.g. *Glossina morsitans*), the forest species (e.g. *G. fusca*) and the riverine species (e.g. *G. palpalis*). Tsetse flies are very sensitive to environmental conditions and will not survive in areas that are too hot, too dry or too high.

Mites parasitic in goats

Psoroptes cuniculi

This is the rabbit mite; however it will infest goats and pass from goat to goat. There may actually be a specific goat mite, which certain authors have named *P. caprae*. Both live mainly in the ears and cause chronic irritation. This may lead to aural haematomata in floppy-eared species. The mites also cause excoriation of the pinna and otitis externa. They are very sensitive to doramectin; ivomectins are also effective. Both need to be given by injection. A single drop of the solution is useful actually in the ear.

Psoroptes ovis

This is the sheep scab mite, however it will infest goats, particularly Angora goats. It is highly contagious and will cause acute irritation resulting in hair or wool loss. Self-mutilation will result in open wounds. These should be dressed with a cream containing acriflavin and BHC. A single injection of doramectin is effective treatment, or two injections of ivomectins separated by 7 days. In the UK there are no licensed dips for goats, although they are available in other parts of the world.

Sarcoptes scabiei

This mite causes very serious mange in goats. It is contagious between goats, and between sheep (normally hair sheep) and goats. It does not appear to be contagious between goats and other species, except man, and is therefore a zoonotic disease (see Chapter 19). There is acute irritation and papule formation turning into crusts. The excoriations affect the eyelids, prepuce and vulva, as well as the skin generally. Ivomectin is more effective than doramectin. Both should be repeated at weekly intervals for four injections. Antibiotics may need to be injected in serious cases, together with cream containing acriflavin and BHC applied daily to the sore areas.

Chorioptes caprae

There is some doubt as to whether this mite is a different species to the cattle mite *C. bovis*, which may in turn be the same species as the equine mite *C. equi*. Prudent clinicians will assume that these mites are contagious to all species of ruminants and pseudo-ruminants. Pygmy goats seem to be particularly sensitive to infestations, and housed goats are more likely to suffer from the condition than goats which are always kept outside. This condition seems to be more common in the winter months in temperate climates. The mite tends to affect the feet, perineum, udder and scrotum with alopecia, erythema and crusting. Some individual goats are particularly susceptible to infestation and develop a severe hypersensitivity response leading to significant self-trauma and clinical signs. Injectable doramectin or ivomectins do not seem to be very effective. Regular topical treatment with fipronil or pour-on ivomectins painted onto affected areas seem to be the treatment of choice. Some clinicians dilute the pour-on products 50:50 with dimethylsulfoxide (DMSO) to try to aid penetration. The mites can survive off the host for many weeks in the environment, and many infested animals are not severely affected and so act as a major reservoir. Consequently it is very important to treat the herd as a whole. Used bedding must be destroyed. Selenium sulfide shampoos applied every other week are useful. Lime sulfur dips have an unpleasant smell and stain surfaces but they are safe and, if used weekly, offer a good method of overall control.

Demodex caprae

This infestation is very rare but when it does occur it is difficult to cure. It often occurs in immune-incompetent individuals. The mite affects the hair follicles and sebaceous glands and there is alopecia on the face, ears, neck and legs. Secondary bacterial infection occurs. Treatment should include antibiotics by injection for several days and topical treatment with amitraz. Amitraz can be toxic so it may be prudent to treat only 25% of the goat's body on one day, then the next 25% and so on a 4-day cycle until there is some resolution. Unlike the other mites that will appear in a deep skin scrape, *D. caprae* may require a skin biopsy to make a definitive diagnosis.

Raillietia caprae

This mite should not be confused with *Raillietina*, which is a tapeworm genus found in chickens in Iran. *Raillietia caprae* are mites found in the ears of goats in Turkmenistan. They are larger than the chorioptic mites found in the UK and can actually be seen with the naked eye as small pin-head sized dots. They do not appear to cause much irritation but goatherds report that some animals develop painful ears which become infected with otitis externa. Goats with floppy ears are likely to get aural haematomas. It is important that the underlying cause (i.e. the mites) is dealt with before the haematomas are treated with antibiotics and surgery.

Free-living mites that will infest goats

Several species of these infest goats; the most common in the UK is the harvest mite *Thombicula autumnalis*. These mites attack the legs, ventral abdomen, face and ears in the autumn, and cause irritation. Species from three other genera, namely *Cheyletiella* spp., *Dermanyssus* spp. (from poultry) and *Tyroglyphus* spp. (the forage mites) have all been recorded as causing dermatitis in goats.

Ticks in goats

Ixodes ricinus, I. hexagonus and *Haemaphysalis punctate*, the so-called hard ticks, all occur in the UK and in goats in mainland Europe. They commonly affect the pinnae, axillae and inguinal regions of the goat. As one moves eastwards into the Middle East and Central Asia other ticks are found, namely *Boophilus microplus, Dermacentor marginatus, Haemaphysalis punctata, Hyalomma anatolicum* and *Rhipicephalus bursa*. They all infest sheep, particularly hair sheep, as well, and can become a serious problem if they occur in very large numbers. They will then cause debilitation and wasting. More importantly they are the vectors of life-threatening diseases (see Table 16.1). The control of these ticks is not only expensive but also time consuming. Many goats in Central Asia are kept by nomads with no permanent farms and so dipping is not an option. They have to resort to pour-on products or spraying, treatments which are even more expensive.

Ticks are the scourge of Africa south of the Sahara, where many species are found, including *Ixodes pilosus, I. rubicundus* (these two are restricted to South Africa). *Boophilus decoloratus* is restricted to Ethiopia but *B. microplus* is found throughout tropical Africa. *Rhipicephalus* is found throughout Africa and *R. bursa* is found in southern Europe as well. *Ambylomma hebraeum* is confined to Africa but *A. variegateum* is also found in the Caribbean. *A. cajennense* is found in Brazil.

Soft ticks also attack goats. *Otobius megnini* is found in the Americas, southern Africa and India. *Ornithodorus* spp. are found throughout Asia and in the USA. Many diseases are spread by ticks (see Table 16.1).

Oestridae flies in goats

Hypoderma diana

This is the deer warble fly, which has been eradicated in the UK but is found in central Europe. It is sensitive to ivomectins. It rarely attacks goats and has never been reported in sheep. The eggs are laid on the legs of goats. The larvae hatch and when still very small burrow into the skin, migrating through the body but dying on the dorsal surface. They form hard calcified small nodules. The goat is an end host; the deer is the normal host and is required to complete the life cycle.

Oestrus ovis

This parasite does occur in goats but is more commonly seen in sheep. The fly lays its eggs on the nostrils of the goat. These hatch into small larvae, which migrate up the nasal cavity, growing in size. After some weeks they are sneezed out by the goat. They then pupate, normally over winter, and hatch out in the warmer weather in late spring. The signs of

Table 16.1. Diseases spread by different species of tick.

Disease spread by ticks	Area	Species of tick
Anaplasmosis	Asia, USA	*Ornithodorus* spp.
Anaplasmosis	Africa	*Rhipicephalus appendiculatus*
Babesiosis	Africa	*Rhipicephalus bursa*
Babesiosis	Asia, N. Africa, S. Europe	*Haemaphysalis punctata*
Borreliosis	Ethiopia	*Boophilus decoloratus*
Heartwater	Africa	*Ambylomma hebraeum*
Heartwater	Africa, Caribbean	*Ambylomma variegatum*
Louping Ill	Europe	*Ixodes ricinus*
Nairobi sheep disease	Africa	*Rhipicephalus appendiculatus*
Q fever	Asia, USA	*Ornithodorus* spp.
Theileriosis	Asia, USA	*Ornithodorus* spp.
Theileriosis	Africa, S. Europe	*Rhipicephalus bursa*
Theileriosis	Europe, N. Africa	*Haemaphysalis punctata*
Tick-borne fever	Europe	*Ixodes ricinus*
Tick-borne fever	India	*Rhipicephalus haemaphysaloides*
Tick paralysis	Brazil	*Ambylomma cajennense*
Tick paralysis	Europe	*Ixodes ricinus*
Tick paralysis	S. Africa	*Ixodes rubicundus*
Tick paralysis	Worldwide	*Dermacentor* spp.

infection shown by the goat will be sneezing and a copious nasal discharge. This may be unilateral, so clinicians will have maxillary molar cheek teeth apical abscessation on their differential list. The larvae can often be found on the ground near the sneezing goat.

Przhevalskiana silenus

This is the goat warble fly. It only attacks goats, and not sheep or cattle. It is found in Central Asia but is no longer common as it is sensitive to ivomectins. The eggs are laid on the legs of goats; the larvae hatch and when still very small burrow into the skin, migrating through the goat and increasing in size before emerging through the skin on the back. They ruin the hide but do not spread disease.

Fleas in goats

Pulex irritans

This flea attacks humans in the UK. When humans live in very close proximity to goats this flea can be a problem not only to man but also to goats. It can cause severe anaemia with chronic hair loss in goats. It is found in east Africa and in Central Asia but is rare in the latter because of the very dry conditions and the truly nomadic lifestyle of the goatherds. In east Africa, although the Masai are technically nomads, they tend to stay in Manyattas for considerable periods. Goats can develop a sensitivity to fleas. These should be removed from the goat with synthetic pyrethrums and also from the environment. The goat should be treated with antibiotics by injection and with corticosteroid injections if the skin is very inflamed. The skin should be treated with cream containing acriflavin and BHC to aid healing and prevent fly strike.

Helminths causing skin disease in goats

Stephanofilaria spp.

These worms are spread by biting flies and cause a pruritic crusting dermatitis on the face and necks of goats. They are very rare. *S. kaeli* is reported in Malaysia, *S. assamensis* in India and *S. dedoesi* in Indonesia. Ivomectins by injection are effective treatments.

Elaphostrongylus rangiferi

This worm will affect goats kept in close proximity to reindeer. It is spread by tabanin flies and causes chronic irritation. Neurological signs have been reported, particularly after ivomectin treatment; however the animals normally recover.

Parelaphostrongylus tenuis

This worm requires the goat to ingest an infected slug or snail, the intermediate hosts. The main primary host in North America is the white-tailed deer. The deer passes the larvae out in its faeces, which is eaten by the snails. Goats may show neurological signs as well as linear crusty lesions in the thorax or abdomen. The skin lesions are cleared with avermectins but the neurological signs are normally fatal.

Vitamin- and Mineral-related Skin Diseases

Cobalt deficiency

Deficient animals will have a rough, brittle hair-coat or wool. Other deficiency signs are more severe (see Chapter 9).

Copper deficiency

Black sheep and goats will show a lack of pigment, and fibre animals will show a lack of crimp. The other signs of copper deficiency are much more important (see Chapter 9).

Iodism

Alopecia and scaling will be seen in sheep and goats if they are fed foods very rich in iodine such as seaweed, over long periods of time.

Sulfur deficiency

This is extremely rare but it has been reported in sheep and goats. It is more marked in fleece animals as there is fleece biting and alopecia. Diagnosis can be made from serum or liver samples.

Vitamin A deficiency

It is extremely rare for sheep and goats to be fed a diet deficient in vitamin A. The coat will show a generalized seborrhoea. However the main sign is an irreversible retinal atrophy causing blindness.

Vitamin E deficiency

This condition is seen in goats. It is not a real deficiency but rather a vitamin E/selenium-responsive dermatosis. The goats appear healthy and are non-pruritic but losing their hair.

Zinc deficiency

This is rarely a zinc deficiency but usually a zinc-responsive condition. There is marked scaling and crusting. Clinicians should remember that any blood samples for zinc levels must be taken into bottles without rubber stoppers or erroneous results will be obtained.

Physical Causes of Skin Disease

General

Clinicians should never forget commonplace trauma. Air-gun pellets will cause abscesses, normally on the flank. They may be found when lanced or confirmed quite simply with a rectal linear scanner. Tethered goats will develop tether galls or bell strap galls (Fig. 16.2). These are welfare issues and owners should be counselled carefully. Chronic foot lameness in the front legs will result in excessive kneeling and the formation of hygromas on the carpi in all species. Burn cases will often result in keloids and crusty nodules.

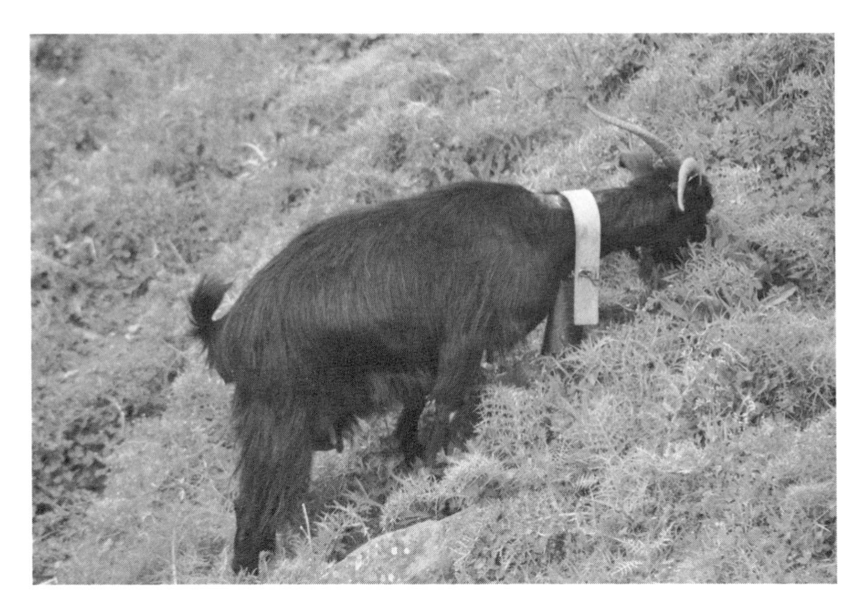

Fig. 16.2. Bell strap gall.

Frostbite

This condition has been seen in sheep and goats when outside in extreme weather conditions. The ears are normally affected and the skin will slough. The animals should be given antibiotics to prevent secondary bacterial infection and NSAID to lessen the pain. Obviously they should be brought inside until the weather improves.

Photosensitization

Sunburn will cause crusting in photosensitized animals. This condition occurs because of the presence of photodynamic substances in the skin capable of causing severe dermatitis in the presence of sunlight. Such agents release energy obtained from the light in hyperoxidative processes harmful to the skin. This may be primary, as a result of a photodynamic agent such as a plant (e.g. *Hypericum perforatum*, St John's Wort) (see Chapter 17), or to a photosensitizing drug (e.g. phenothiazine). The condition may however be secondary, due to impairment of liver function resulting in failure to denature chlorophyll and consequent build-up of the photodynamic agent phylloerythrin in tissues. The plant *Narthrecium ossifragum* (Bog asphodel) has been implicated in this secondary type.

The clinical signs typically occur in non-pigmented areas of the animals free from wool in sheep and anywhere on hair sheep and goats. Diagnosis may be made on clinical grounds with confirmation by showing raised serum levels of phylloerythrin and, in the case of hepatogenous disease, raised levels of serum liver enzymes. Animals should be housed and any severely affected areas treated with oily creams. The condition is often first seen when animals are turned out on to lush green pastures such as silage aftermaths having been on poor pasture. The liver is unable to cope with the increased amounts of dietary chlorophyll.

Sunburn

The harmful effects of ultraviolet radiation from direct sunlight in shorn sheep or shorn fibre goats should not be forgotten as a potential cause of skin damage, particularly in areas where there is no shade. Encrustment of the non-pigmented skin with ultimate necrosis of the epidermis, upper dermis and superficial sebaceous glands may occur. Animals should be housed and oily creams applied to the affected areas. Antibiotics and NSAID may be required in severe cases.

Trauma

Sheep can obviously be burnt by either a naked flame or a hot piece of metal. There are some more unusual forms of trauma, for example attacks by magpies. Shearing wounds are sadly rather common.

Toxic Causes of Skin Disease

Hyalomma toxicosis

This occurs sporadically in east Africa. The tick *Hyalomma truncatum* produces a toxin which causes a systemic disease in wool sheep. All the wool falls off leaving a thickened, reddened skin. Sheep will recover if kept out of sunlight and given antibiotics parenterally to prevent secondary infection. The sheep should have all the sore areas covered with oily cream before dipping.

Milk toxicity

Lambs will develop a toxicity similar to photosensitization when suckling ewes suffering from hepatic toxicity from eating certain poisonous plants such as sacahuista or beargrass (see Chapter 17).

Neoplastic Conditions

These are rare in goats but are more often reported than in sheep, mainly because goats tend to be kept to greater ages. The more common neoplastic skin nodules tend to be benign. The thyroid gland can become enlarged and will appear as a benign growth. This is not goitre and has no relationship to iodine deficiency. Further down the neck the thymus can become enlarged in young goats. This is a thymoma and it is also normally benign. Benign cysts may occur in the wattles or in the salivary glands. Tetragenic dental cysts may be seen on the faces of goats.

The malignant tumours which may occur in the skin anywhere on the body are histiocytomas, lymphosarcomas, malignant melanomas and squamous cell carcinomas. The latter occur in the conjunctiva, on the third eyelid, the penis and the vulva. Melanomas are not restricted to white sheep or goats and can occur in animals of other colours. They are particularly malignant in the pigmented areas of Suffolk sheep.

Skin Diseases of Uncertain Aetiology

Pemphigus foliaceus

This condition causes a diagnostic challenge for the clinician. It is an autoimmune-mediated disease. Bacteria, fungi and even parasites may well be found as secondary invaders. If the skin condition persists after treatment for these conditions the practitioner should suspect pemphigus, and it can be confirmed by a biopsy. Pemphigus is very common in pygmy goats. The main presenting signs include a generalized severe pustular eruption involving most of the body. Treatment is difficult as all the secondary bacteria, fungi and parasites have to be removed before regular steroid treatment is carried out. Although in theory dexamethazone should not be effective if given orally that has not been the author's experience. The dose is 2 mg/kg given every other morning throughout the summer in temperate countries. Normally the condition calms down during the winter months, only to flare up again in the spring.

Wool slip

This condition is associated with winter shearing and seems to affect animals in poor conditions. There may be a link with either low copper levels or secondary low copper as a result of high molybdenum levels. This alopecia is non-pruritic and the underlying skin appears normal. There is no treatment. Prevention can be carried out by raising the nutritional level at times of stress, for example changing the time of shearing/housing.

The Horn

Introduction

Some sheep breeds have horns. They therefore have similarities with goats. All horned animals may be attacked by the horn fly. This fly will in fact attack non-horned animals. The practitioner may have problems with sheep with rudimentary horns or with goats which have not been dehorned properly. These small horns are best left alone unless they get caught, for example in wire, and start haemorrhaging. Normally there is no underlying bone tissue involved. The area can be anaesthetized with local anaesthetic and the horn, including a circumference of skin, can be removed (Fig. 16.3). The area must be treated with a cream containing acriflavin and BHC and allowed to heal by secondary intention. Special attention must be paid to the control of flies as well as to tetanus immunization.

Disbudding of kids

This must be performed during the first week of life but after the kids have received adequate colostrum. Great care should be taken with the surgery and the anaesthetic. The surgery should take place in a warm environment. The kid is masked down using a mixture of oxygen with halothane or isoflurane. The hair is clipped around the base of both horns. The kid should receive a subcutaneous injection of 1500 IU of TAT together with intramuscular injections of antibiotics and NSAID. The horn bud is removed with a scalpel. A specially prepared disbudding iron with a wide aperture (Fig. 16.4) is heated to red heat and applied to the horn after the oxygen has been turned off. The iron may have to be removed if the kid shows signs of movement, so that the mask with the anaesthetic mixture can be reapplied. It is vital that the iron is extremely hot and therefore will only need to be applied for bursts of 15 s. It is also important that all the horn-producing tissue is destroyed (Fig. 16.5).

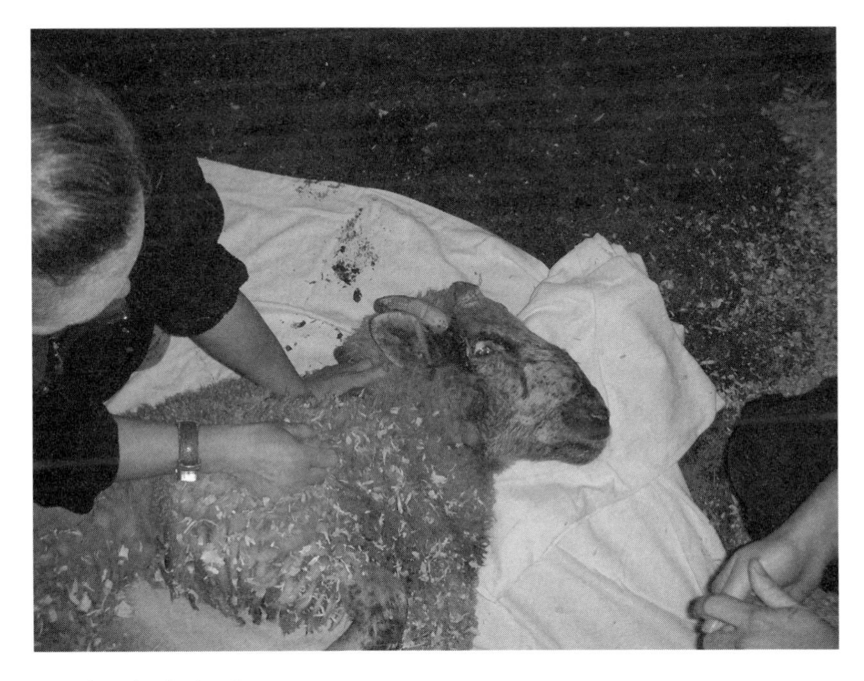

Fig. 16.3. Lamb with a broken horn.

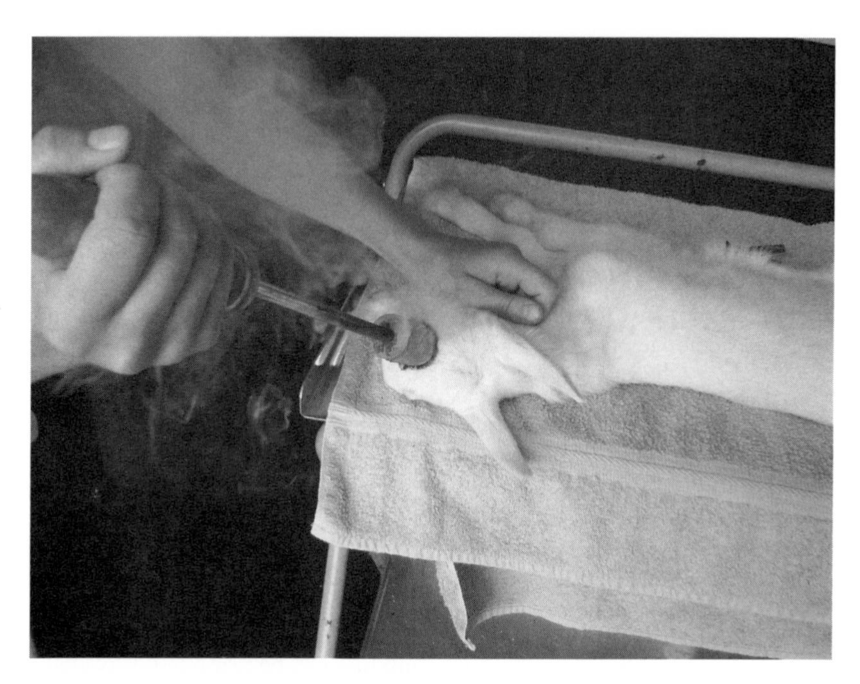

Fig. 16.4. Disbudding (1).

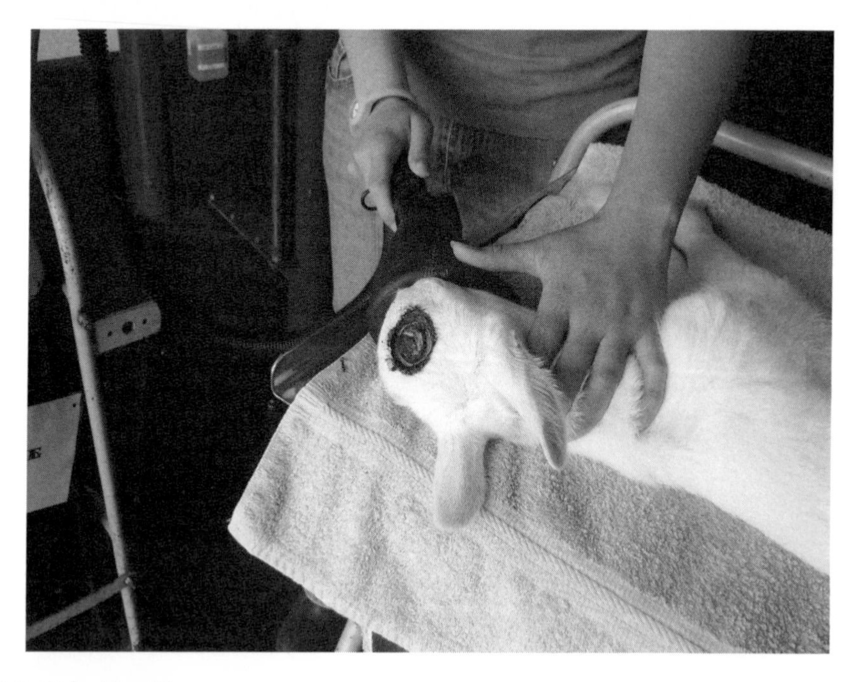

Fig. 16.5. Disbudding (2).

Dehorning of adult goats

This is major surgery and should only be undertaken after due consideration. It should not be performed for cosmetic reasons. If an adult horn has been fractured it needs to be removed. There is no reason why the good horn cannot be left *in situ*. If there is an ingrowing horn, the tip can be removed at regular intervals with a hacksaw or embryotomy wire. Provided only the tip is removed and the deeper structures are not involved, there is no pain and an anaesthetic is not required.

Certain individuals become aggressive to other animals or to humans and then, after due thought, dehorning can be undertaken. The goat should be given a combination of 0.1 mg/kg of xylazine and 0.1 mg/kg of butorphanol intravenously as a premedication after being starved for 12 h (see Chapter 8). This is followed in 5 min by intravenous ketamine at 0.2 mg/kg. This can be topped up if required, but with proper preparation and speed of action this can be avoided. The horn, including an area of skin at the base, is removed with embryotomy wire. There will be considerable haemorrhage, which should be controlled by pressure initially until both horns are removed. Any arteries which can then be picked up should be ligated. A cream containing acriflavin and BHC is applied, followed by two pads of folded gamgee. A pressure bandage is then applied in a figure-of-eight around the ears. Some bandage will have to be cut away so that the animal can see. These dressings will help to absorb the blood and they need to be replaced every 2 days. The author finds manuka honey very effective after the initial dressing, to aid healing. Great care should be taken with bandaging so that the larynx and the trachea are not constricted. It should be stressed that the goat should be fully immunized against tetanus (see Chapter 7). Antibiotics should be given daily by injection together with NSAID for pain relief. Flies must be controlled. The goat should be separated from other goats to prevent head butting, which might restart the bleeding.

17

Poisons

Introduction

The first problem with poisoning cases is establishing a diagnosis. If the poison is definitely known that is obviously very helpful. However, owners are often very keen to wrongly blame farmers for suspected poisonous sprays! So any history needs to be taken with caution. If a chemical has definitely been spilled, then make sure this fact is used immediately so that any antidote can be obtained while the patient is being brought in. Equally, if a plant has been eaten, make sure the owners pass on the name of the plant so the toxicity can be checked and treatment prepared as they are coming in (Forsyth, 1954; Harwood *et al.*, 2010a). If a plant has definitely been eaten but they do not know what it is, make sure they bring some of it in with them. It needs to be stressed that the leaves, fruit and maybe even the roots are required to help identification. Clinicians should also remember to tell the owner to move any other animals away from the toxic plant or substance. Where common names are given for plants in this chapter, these are generally the names that are used in the UK, but some relate to plants from the USA or Australia.

If the small ruminant is seriously ill a full clinical examination should be carried out. If there are no helpful diagnostic signs and the poison is unknown, a drip of normal isotonic saline with a 16G catheter should be set up. Clinicians should remember that the saline must be warm. Efforts should be made to ensure that the animal itself is warmed up, not only by being in a warm place but also by having hot water bottles around it. The large dog coats or foal coats as shown in the picture of the goat with radial paralysis are very useful (Fig. 17.1). Obviously if the poison is known and there is a specific treatment available, this should be given as a priority, otherwise the clinician should carry out symptomatic treatment. She needs to make a careful clinical judgement if the animal is *in extremis*. Welfare, and possible euthanasia, must be considered. If several animals are affected it may be kinder to put the really badly affected animals to sleep and to concentrate on treating the animals which could possibly survive.

Remember to take notes, as poisoning cases often lead to litigation or to insurance claims. It is likely that any animals that have died or are put to sleep will require a post-mortem. Once again, careful notes should be taken, with a full identification of the animal. Obviously careful samples will need to be collected (see Chapter 3).

It is important to try to establish a time of death for animals found dead. The owner may be convinced that it has been sudden but in reality it may be that he has not looked at the animals for a length of time (see Chapter 18).

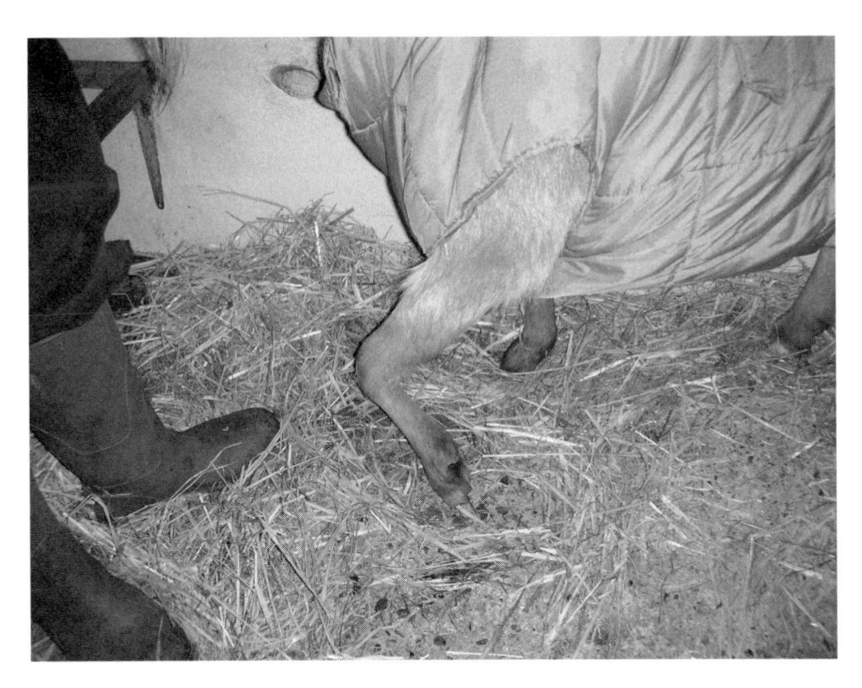

Fig. 17.1. Goat with radial paralysis.

Treatment

The first effort must be to try to prevent further absorption of the toxin. Should the clinician carry out a rumenotomy? If the animal is very ill and a specific treatment is not being given, the practitioner has very little to lose. A GA will not be given, as a local block is to be used. A rumenotomy may well make a diagnosis by finding the plant in the rumen. It is advisable to stitch the rumen to the peritoneum of the abdomen (Goetz's method) so there will be very little contamination. Any remaining plant toxins can be disposed of by removing the ingesta and flushing the rumen. The animal can be rehydrated by half filling the rumen with electrolytes. A proprietary antacid preparation containing some bicarbonate can be used. If there is a specific treatment then that must be carried out, and in all cases symptomatic treatment will be useful.

Plant Poisons

Plant poisoning is liable to occur under a variety of circumstances. Obviously if goats are allowed to escape they are not only in danger of being hit on a road but also of gaining access to toxic plants. Sheep or goats are at risk if they are allowed to escape into woods or gardens (Fig. 17.2). Tethered goats are at risk if they are short of food and only have access to a plant which they normally would not eat but that is toxic. Obviously all small ruminants are at risk from access to garden rubbish or, indeed, by being fed cut toxic plants. These may be presented as browse or dried in hay or haylage. Small ruminants will find it particularly difficult to reject plants in silage. It is very important to remember that it is a complete myth that small ruminants will not eat plants that are bad for them.

A logical approach to treating plant poisoning in small ruminants in the UK

Classification of plants requiring the same specific treatment

1. Plants which contain a cyanogenic glycoside:

Laurus spp. (laurel; large amounts need to be ingested so poisoning is very rare except in

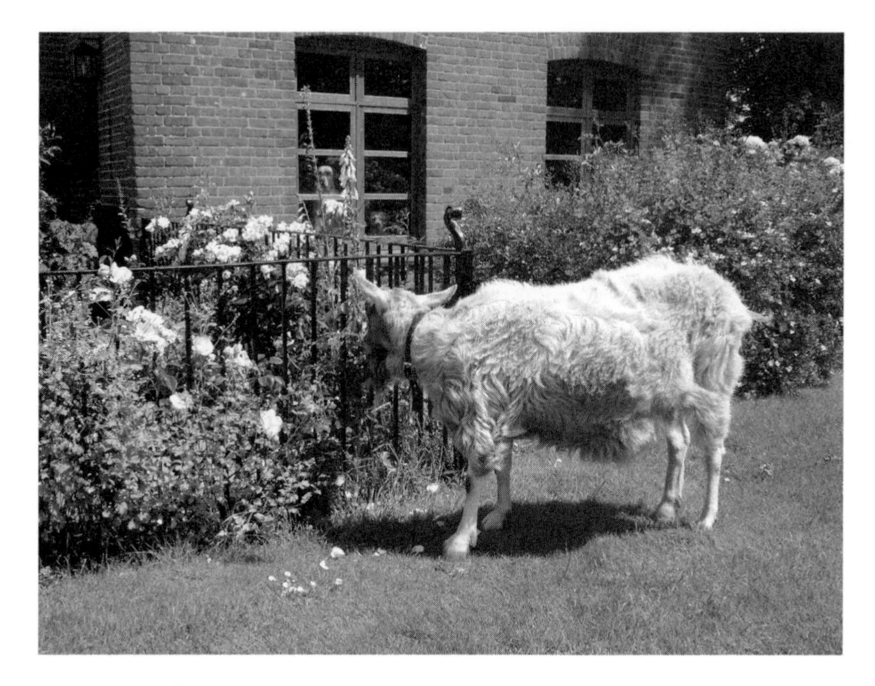

Fig. 17.2. Goat in a garden.

pet animals given access to the dried leaves on rubbish dumps).

Lotus corniculatus (birdsfoot trefoil; commonly found in cleared woodland).

Nandina domestica (Chinese sacred bamboo; found in gardens but imported from China).

Photinia fraseri (Chinese photinia; found in gardens but imported from China).

Prunus spp. (wild cherry; found in gardens and woodland).

Triglochin maritima (arrowgrass; found in gardens but imported from the USA).

Specific treatment is 30/kg i/v sodium thiosulfate, together with 1 g/20 kg by mouth to detoxicate the remaining hydrogen cyanide (HCN) in the rumen. This can be repeated in 1 h.

2. Plants which contain oxalic acid:

Beta vulgaris (sugarbeet; only causes problems if animals are suddenly fed large quantities).

Chenopodium album (fat hen; commonly found on waste ground and in cultivated areas between fruit trees. Large amounts are required so poisoning is very rare except in tethered animals).

Mesembryanthemum spp. (ice plants; only found in gardens, originated in S. Africa).

Rheum rhaponticum (rhubarb; found in the vegetable garden but poisoning normally from leaves thrown to goats).

Rumex acetosa (sorrel; a weed found in certain pastures and a relative of *R. acetosella* (sheep sorrel). Poisoning is very rare).

Salsola kali (soft roly-poly; a weed found in open areas of woodland).

Specific treatment is vitamin B preparations and 20% calcium borogluconate, both given slowly and intravenously. The dose of the 20% calcium borogluconate is 30 ml for a small sheep or pygmy goat, and 60 ml for a normal-sized sheep or goat.

3. Plants which contain nitrate/nitrite:

Silybum marianum (variegated thistle; originated in Australia but is now a garden plant).

Zea mays (maize; a cultivated crop which is highly palatable and can easily be eaten to excess).

Specific treatment is methylene blue. This should be given i/v at 10 mg/kg very slowly.

4. Plants which contain hyoscamine and/or atropine and solanine:

Adonis microcarpa (pheasant's eye; originally from Australia but now commonly found in gardens; see Woods *et al.*, 2011).
Atropa belladonna (deadly nightshade; found in hedgerows. Normally animals will not touch this very toxic plant except when it is in hay; see Hubbs, 1947).
Datura stramonium (thorn apple; a very toxic woodland plant).
Hyoscyamus niger (henbane; a very toxic, ubiquitous garden plant).
Solanum dulcamara (woody nightshade; a trailing woodland plant not normally eaten).
Solanum nigrum (black nightshade; found in gardens, and not as toxic as the deadly nightshade, *Atropa belladonna*).
Specific treatment is neostigmine. This should be given at 0.01 mg/kg subcutaneously. Flunixin is useful to control the ileus.

5. Plants which cause acute gastritis:

Kalmia spp. (kalmia; a common flowering plant found in gardens).
Nerium oleander (oleander; a pink-flowered garden plant from Morocco. Eaten when cut).
Pieris japonica variegata (pieris; a common garden plant from Japan).
Rhododendron occidentale (azalea; found in gardens and ornamental woods. Animals show marked salivation and projectile vomiting) (Fig. 17.3).
Rhododendron ponticum (rhododendron; originating in Nepal, this shrub is very common in gardens and woodlands. It is particularly dangerous as it is readily ingested by sheep and goats).
Viburnum spp. (viburnum; there are many different species of this genus growing as shrubs, bushes or small trees. They are readily eaten).
Specific treatment is 1 ml twice daily of a 5% wt/vol solution of morphine sulfate and 1 ml twice daily of a 0.5% wt/vol solution of atropine sulfate. Pygmy goats should be given 50% of this dose.

6. Plants toxic to the liver:

Anabena spp. (blue-green algae, found in inland lakes such as the Norfolk Broads).
Aphanizomenon spp. (blue-green algae, found in inland lakes such as the Norfolk Broads).
Echium plantagineum (Patterson's curse; an annual garden herb with blue flowers).
Galega officinalis (goat's rue; large herb with purple flowers. Large amounts are required for toxic symptoms).
Heliotropium amplexicaule (blue heliotrope; an annual flower commonly found in gardens).
Heliotropium europaeum (common heliotrope; annual herb with white flowers).
Hypericum perforatum (St John's wort; a common marshland plant).
Lantana camara (lantana; found in the wild as well as in gardens).
Microcystis spp. (blue-green algae, found in inland lakes such as the Norfolk Broads).
Narthecium ossifragum (bog asphodel; found on marshy ground. The main danger is when it is cut in hay).
Panicum spp. (panicum; grown as a fodder crop. Large quantities required to cause ill effects).
Senecio jacobea (ragwort; an annual plant with yellow flowers. Found in large quantities on wayside verges and horse pastures).
Tribulus terrestris (caltrop; creeping herb with yellow flowers).
Specific treatment is high doses of vitamin B and a low-protein diet.

7. Plants which cause blood clotting deficiency:

Melilotus officinalis (sweet clover; only causes poisoning when crushed, i.e. spoilt or made into hay).
Specific treatment is vitamin K by injection at 3 mg/kg.

Classification of plants requiring no specific treatment

1. Plants which contain cardiac glycosides and therefore cause vasodilatation with signs of acute shock:

Daubentonia punicea (purple sesbane; garden varieties have purple flowers; the wild plants may have white flowers).
Digitalis purpurea (foxglove; an erect herb with purple flowers).

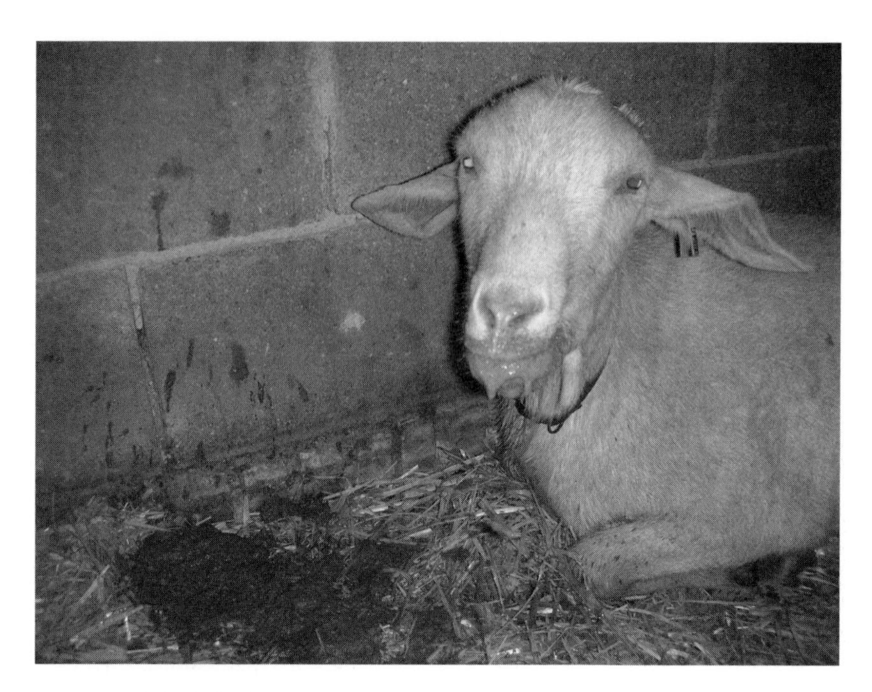

Fig. 17.3. A goat with rhododendron poisoning.

Helleborus niger (Christmas rose; common garden flower. Very bitter so only a danger when cut).

Homeria spp. (cape tulip; the varieties with one leaf and two leaves are both toxic).

Symptomatic treatment should be given for shock.

2. Plants which contain taxine:

Taxus baccata (yew; a very common evergreen tree found in churchyards and as hedges in gardens).

There is no realistic treatment. However recent observations (Stevenson, 2010; Swarbrick, 2010) indicate that although yew is extremely toxic to cattle it may not be so toxic to small ruminants.

3. Plants which cause acute respiratory signs:

Anabena spp. (blue-green algae; found in inland lakes and ponds).

Aphanizomenon spp. (blue-green algae; found in inland lakes and ponds).

Ipomoea batatus (sweet potatoes; large quantities required. Usually fed by mistake).

Microcystis spp. (blue-green algae; found in inland lakes and ponds)

Perilla frutescens (perilla mint; found in gardens. Normally not eaten on account of unpleasant smell. Symptomatic treatment rarely successful).

Verbesina encelioides (crown beard; common herb with yellow daisy-like flowers).

Zantedeschia aethiopica (arum lily; found in gardens, actually causes laryngeal oedema with frothing at the mouth. The condition soon subsides).

Treatment is symptomatic, steroids and antibiotics (Fig. 17.4).

4. Plants which cause neurological signs:

Aconitum napellus (aconite, monkshood; a small flower found in gardens).

Aethusa cynapium (fool's parsley; a herbaceous plant with white flowers found as a weed in gardens).

Cannabis sativa (marijuana; a problem when escaped animals find the plant being grown illegally in the UK).

Cicuta virosa (water hemlock; the roots are very poisonous and are eaten after ditch dredging; see Stratton, 1919).

Conium maculatum (hemlock; plant with a white flower found in ditches. A danger

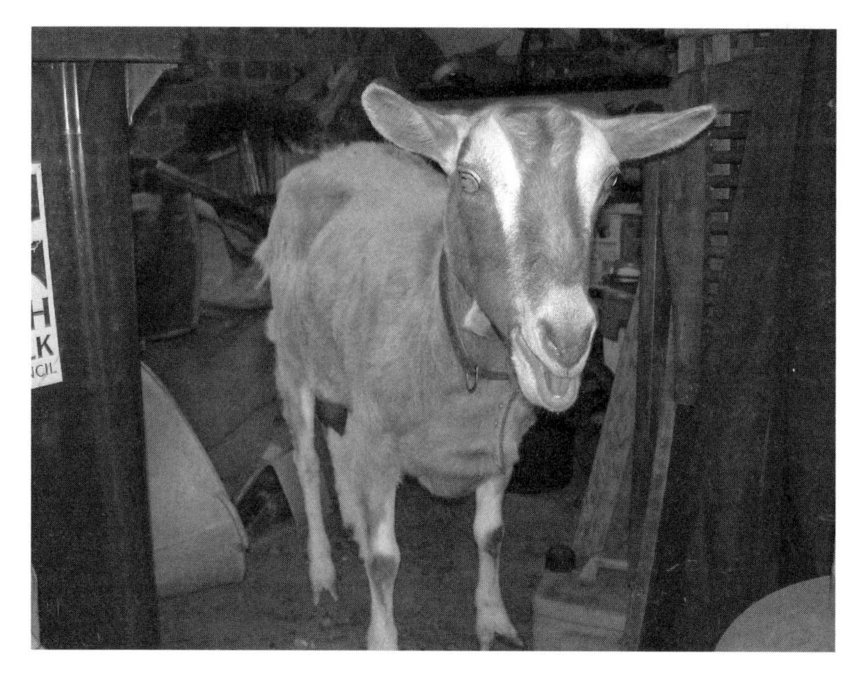

Fig. 17.4. Goat in respiratory distress.

after ditch clearance; see Copithorne, 1937).

Dryopteris filix-mas (male fern; unlikely to be consumed in sufficient quantity. The roots are very toxic.

Equisetum spp. (mare's tail; a very common pasture plant. Only eaten if starving).

Haplopappus heterophyllius (golden rod; this garden flower affects suckling offspring).

Ipomoea muelleri (poison morning glory; a vine grown in gardens, with pink trumpet flowers).

Juncus spp. (rushes; a marshland plant only eaten if starving).

Laburnum anagyroides (laburnum; a very toxic tree with yellow, hanging flowers).

Lolium spp. (rye grass; poisoning caused by two saprophytic fungi living on the rye grass).

Lupinus spp. (lupins; found in gardens and hedgerows. The seedpods are toxic; see Brash, 1943).

Malva parviflora (marsh mallow; a common wasteland plant, which only causes problems to suckling young).

Nicotiana tabacum (tobacco; not normally eaten as a plant but as cigarettes).

Oenanthe crocata (water dropwort; the roots are very poisonous and are eaten after ditch dredging).

Pteridium aquilinum (bracken; a very common plant found on hills and common throughout the UK. It is not toxic in small amounts).

Stypandra glauca (blind grass; not a grass but a small blue-flowering perennial).

Trachyandra divaricata (branched onion weed; originally from south-west Australia. A perennial plant with a white flower and a rhizome).

Treatment is symptomatic to control the neurological signs.

5. Plants which cause colic:

Bryonia dioica (white bryony; a hedge-climbing weed which is very toxic).

Phytolacca americana (pokeweed; originally from the USA, now common in gardens in the UK).

Tamus communis (black bryony; a common hedge-climbing plant with white–green flowers. Only the berries are toxic).

Treatment is symptomatic to control the colic signs.

6. Plants which cause bloat:

Allium spp. (onions; large quantities need to be ingested).
Trifolium spp. (clover; an excess in pastures causes problems).
Treatment is symptomatic to control the bloat, trocarization and/or surfactants.

7. Plants which cause gastroenteric signs with diarrhoea:

Arum maculatum (cuckoo-pint, lords and ladies; very bitter but young animals attracted to the very toxic red berries).
Buxus sempervirens (box; a common evergreen hedge plant in gardens. Not touched when growing but toxicity occurs when animals are fed trimmings).
Clematis vitalba (wild clematis, old man's beard; very irritant and rarely eaten).
Colchicum autumnale (autumn crocus, meadow saffron; mainly affects kids as the toxin colchicine is excreted in the milk).
Delphinium spp. (delphinium; not eaten except when cut and dried).
Ligustrum spp. (privet; a common hedge plant in gardens. Large quantities will cause mild toxic signs).
Linum spp. (linseed; often included in animal feed. Purgative in large quantities).
Mercurialis perennis (dog's mercury; only mildly toxic).
Narcissus spp. (daffodil bulbs are mildly toxic).
Persea americana (avocado; the skins are often consumed from compost heaps. The toxin persin affects the udder and causes mastitis).
Ricinus communis (castor oil plant; its seed (the 'bean') is often included in animal feed. Only a problem in large quantities).
Sambucus ebulus (dwarf elder; a common garden weed only mildly toxic).
Sinapis arvensis (charlock; a common weed with yellow flowers seen in cornfields. A brassica).
Solanum tuberosum (potatoes; only a problem when fed to excess).
Treatment is symptomatic and includes demulcents, NSAID to treat the pain and antibiotics to treat any secondary bacteria.

8. Plants which cause gastroenteric signs with constipation:

Pinus spp. (pine needles; various trees found throughout the UK).
Quercus spp. (acorns; acorns are much more toxic than the oak leaves which are often browsed by goats. Problems occur in dry autumns when there are high winds when the acorns are green; individual animals seem to develop a craving for them).
Stellaria media (chickweed; a small, white-flowering plant traditionally grown to be fed to chickens).
Treatment is symptomatic and includes liquid paraffin and NSAID to treat the pain and toxicity.

9. Plants which cause haematuria:

Brassica napus (rape; a brassica field crop).
Brassica oleracea (marrowstem kale; a brassica grown worldwide as a fodder crop and often eaten to excess).
Raphanus raphanistrum (wild radish; found in all temperate climates and contains S-methylcysteine sulfoxide (SMCO).
Rapistrum rugosum (Turnip weed; this herb contains SMCO and is not very palatable but requires only small amounts to cause toxicity).
There is no realistic treatment except to remove the animals from the plants.

10. Plants which cause irritation of the oral mucous membranes:

Euphorbia spp. (Spurges; found as hedges or on wasteland).
Treatment is symptomatic and involves copious flushing with cold water.

Plants that Taint the Milk

Milking sheep and goats are very susceptible to the plants and poisons listed above that alter the smell, taste and consistency of their milk. All of the above will render the milk and flesh of the animal unsuitable for human consumption. However, this is the least of the practitioner's problems, as they will all markedly reduce milk production and most are life-threatening for the animal. On the other hand there are a large number of plants which will taint the milk and render it at best unpleasant and at worse repulsive. The list of the most common plants known to taint milk but not known to be poisonous is shown below. The active principles of some plants (e.g. ragwort, hemlock, horseradish and lupins), not toxic in small quantities to the milking goat or sheep, are secreted in their milk, but it is very doubtful if they are actually in sufficient quantities in the milk to be a hazard to human health.

Achillea millefolium (yarrow)
Aethusa cynapium (fool's parsley)
Allium spp. (garlics)
Anemone spp. (anemone species)
Anthemis spp. and *Matricaria* spp. (chamomiles)
Beta vulgaris (sugarbeet tops)
Brassica spp. (turnips)
Caltha palustris (marsh marigold)
Chrysanthemum spp. (ox-eye daisy)
Coronopus didymus (lesser watercress)
Equisetum spp. (horsetails)
Hedera helix (ivy)
Melampyrum spp. (cow-wheat)
Mentha spp. (mints)
Narthecium ossifragum (bog asphodel)
Oxalis spp. (wood sorrels)
Pinguicula vulgaris (butterwort)
Polygonum aviculare (knotgrass)
Ranunculus spp. (buttercup)
Raphanus raphanistrum (wild radish)
Rhamnus spp. (buckthorn)
Salvia spp. (sages)
Silaum silaus (pepper saxifrage)
Sisymbrium officinale (hedge mustard)
Sium erectum (lesser sium)
Sium latifolium (water parsnip)
Tanacetum vulgare (tansy)
Thlaspi arvense (pennycress)

Chemical Poisons

Alphachloralose

Alphachloralose is the active ingredient of mouse bait and causes death in mice through coma and hypothermia. Adult sheep or goats are unlikely to consume enough to cause problems but it is possible that lambs or kids might be affected. They should be warmed in a hot box to raise their core temperature. There are no references in the literature of incidents of toxicity.

Aluminium

Although this metal is potentially toxic because it binds up phosphorus, it does not appear to be toxic to small ruminants.

Amitraz

This acaricide, used for dipping and spraying cattle, is toxic to small ruminants. Goats may drink the solution. Sheep and fibre goats may absorb a toxic dose from massive fleece contamination. It normally causes rumen atony and constipation, with resulting colic. Treatment is NSAID and oral liquid paraffin. Obviously the animal should be bathed to remove further chemical contamination.

Antimony

This metal is not found free in nature but may cause toxicity from wastes associated with mining or indeed by discarded alloys containing antimony. Acute poisoning causes diarrhoea. Treatment is with oral magnesium oxide to precipitate the antimony and other demulcents to protect the mucous membranes. Chronic poisoning causes liver damage. The animals should be removed from further ingestion and treated with B vitamins by injection.

Arsenic

Poisoning from arsenic can come from an inorganic source or organic source. The source for inorganic poisoning is usually rat bait or acaricides. The principal sign is severe dysentery. The diagnosis can be confirmed by analysis of the ingesta, liver or kidney. Low doses of arsenic were once included in tonics for horses to improve their coats. These should not be given to sheep or goats. The specific treatment is sodium thiosulfate at the rate of 30 mg/kg twice daily, ideally given by very slow intravenous injection. If a very dilute solution is used it can be given subcutaneously but it may cause a severe reaction and damage the fleece. Oral administration is not effective. Obvious supportive therapy should be put in place.

Historically, arsenic used to be included in pig food to prevent swine dysentery and as a growth promoter. This is the usual source of organic arsenic. Organic poisoning has a slower onset compared with the acute inorganic poisoning and shows neurological signs. There may also be diarrhoea, which should be controlled symptomatically as there is no specific treatment.

Battery acid

If animals lick the acid from batteries they will get ulcers on their tongues reminiscent of FMD lesions. The condition is not life threatening.

Cadmium

Direct toxicity in small ruminants has not been recorded, although rams in Asia had reduced fertility when exposed to high levels of contamination.

Caesium

Radioactive caesium was recorded in sheep in the UK after the Chernobyl disaster in 1986 but no toxic effects were observed.

Cantharidin

Blister beetles of the *Epicauta* genus swarm onto alfalfa during harvesting. The beetles contain cantharidin, which is very toxic to all animals, causing acute abdominal pain with diarrhoea. Shreds of mucosa will be seen in the faeces. It also causes haematuria. Animals will die unless stabilized by an isotonic saline drip. The toxicity of canthanaridin does not diminish in stored hay.

Carbamate

These substances, which are herbicides and insecticides, will cause poisoning in all animals. The signs and treatment are the same as for organophosphorus poisoning.

Chlorinated hydrocarbons

These insecticides and acaricides are very potent poisons in all animals. They cause nervous signs from over-stimulation of the CNS. There are no specific antidotes and supportive treatment is rarely effective.

Closantel

Closantel is a salicylanilide drug used for the treatment and control of fasciolosis in sheep. It is also active against *Haemonchus contortus* and the nasal bot, *Oestrus ovis* (Barlow *et al.*, 2002). When is was given at four times the recommended dose rate it caused blindness 2 weeks later on account of retinal degeneration.

Copper

There is a very fine margin of safety with copper in sheep and goats. They all require some, particularly on the rare copper-deficient land. What is more likely is land that is high in molybdenum or sulfur. These two elements bind up the copper so it is not available for the animals, and copper supplementation is then required. However copper is very toxic to sheep and goats, and so supplementation has to be carried out with care. With sheep there is a variation between breeds. Down sheep (e.g. Suffolks and Texels) are very sensitive to copper poisoning but Scottish Blackface are more resistant (Sargison, 2001). Copper ingestion can be cumulative. Historically pigs used to be fed diets high in copper to act as a growth promoter, and if such pig food is fed to sheep or goats it will cause copper toxicity. The main sign is jaundice, mirrored by an increase in liver enzymes (e.g. GLDH, AST and GGT). The sheep or goat will be ataxic and if this is evident then the outcome is death. For a definitive diagnosis at post-mortem, liver copper levels need to be above 8000 μM/kg dry matter (DM) or kidney levels higher than 650 μM/kg DM. Kidney samples are more reliable as there is not the same interference by iron as in the liver. There is no reliable antidote when the disease has developed that far, but a subcutaneous injection of 3.4 mg/kg ammonium tetrathiomolybdate on 3 alternate days has been used successfully for treatment of copper poisoning in sheep (Sargison, 2001). This author suggests treating the entire in-contact group. Young animals of all species are more susceptible to toxicity and deficiency. Soil ingestion may account for up to 305 of DM intake of copper.

The availability of dietary copper varies between different feeds. Those with high concentrations of available copper, which are liable to cause toxicity, include:

- Pasture, silage and root crops grown on ground to which large quantities of pig or poultry manure have been applied.
- Distillery by-products feeds such as dark grains produced from copper stills.
- Concentrate feeds containing palm oil or molassed sugarbeet pulp. (Whole grain cereals are relatively poor sources of copper.)
- Milk provides a highly available source of copper and copper absorption is very efficient in young animals, hence lambs and kids suckling dams fed on copper-rich diets are at risk of copper poisoning.
- Other potential sources of copper include access to cattle minerals, copper sulfate foot baths and fungicide-treated timber or vines.
- The concentrations of copper antagonists are often low in preserved rations fed to housed animals.

Polyuria-polydipsia (PUPD) is very unusual in sheep and there are few reports of it occurring naturally, only in experimental studies. However some authors in Greece (Giadinis *et al.*, 2010) found several dairy sheep affected with PUPD linked with nephrogenic diabetes insipidus secondary to chronic copper hepatotoxicity.

Cyanide

Although this poison could potentially be ingested by sheep and goats when used in the inorganic form as a rodenticide, this is not the normal type of poisoning seen. Many plants, such as *Linum* spp. (linseed, flax), *Prunus* spp. (wild black cherry), *Sorghum* spp. (sorghum) and *Sorghum vulgare* (Sudan grass) contain cyanogenetic glycosides. These glycosides can be released by damage to the plants by herbicides or wilting. Ruminants are very susceptible; the main sign is bright red mucous membranes, severe asphyxia and convulsions followed by death. The blood will appear bright red on post-mortem. Tests for hydrocyanic acid can be performed on the stomach contents to confirm the diagnosis, although the smell of bitter almonds is strongly indicative of poisoning. Treatment is specific: 30 mg/kg i/v of sodium thiosulfate should be given. At the same time 3–5 g should be given by mouth hourly to detoxify any remaining HCN in the rumen.

Fluoride

This element has been reported to cause chronic poisoning in sheep from factory contamination. There is marked excessive wearing of the teeth, together with some enlargement of the long bones including the mandible. There are increased levels of fluorine in the urine and plasma. Obviously the animals should be removed from the contaminated pasture. Feeding of calcium carbonate will reduce the fluoride in the gut contents. If pastures may contain toxic levels of fluorine, animals should be fed rock phosphate to lower the danger of toxicity. The provision of salt licks will help prevent animals licking the soil. They should be moved off contaminated land at least 16 weeks before slaughter. Provision of uncontaminated water is important. Any ponds or other sources of water should be fenced off.

Acute fluorosis is extremely rare and will only occur if there are several millimetres of ash on a pasture. The initial signs are gastroenteric, quickly leading on to collapse and death.

Formaldehyde

This is used in a diluted form in foot baths. It is normally stored in a concentrated form and would not be attractive to animals. It is therefore unlikely to cause severe toxicity with nervous signs but is more likely to cause mild signs of abdominal discomfort and salivation if animals eat contaminated straw. Symptomatic treatment would be indicated.

Lead

Historically, lead poisoning was mainly recorded in artificially reared lambs and kids kept in an enclosure constructed of very old farm gates with flaking lead paint. This cause of poisoning is relatively rare nowadays as lead paint has been banned in the UK for over 50 years. However other sources are available, such as lead–acid batteries, burned building materials and contaminated soil from mining or even clay pigeon shooting (Payne and Liversey, 2010). Most cases will be seen when animals are out on pasture, or in the case of goats, on waste ground.

Animals may be found dead, although more often they will be showing advanced neurological signs. Death is caused by convulsions leading to respiratory failure. There is a raised temperature, which may confuse the practitioner into thinking an infection is involved. Pregnant animals will abort. There is ruminant atony. There is blindness, as in cases of CCN, which is the main differential, but the high temperature is absent in CCN. Diagnosis can be made from whole blood in a lithium heparin tube (which normally has a green top). There is marked anaemia but no jaundice, unlike in copper poisoning. Haemonchosis must be ruled out. Chelation therapy with sodium calciumedetate will give rapid improvement. The dose is 75 mg/kg dissolved in normal saline given intravenously. This dose can be repeated several times. A daily injection of thiamine is helpful to reduce the deposition of lead in the tissues; the dose is 20 mg/kg. The use of thiamine will also reassure the practitioner that CCN is being treated, in case the diagnosis is in doubt.

For prevention, farmers are urged to dispose of all waste carefully, particularly batteries and building materials. Goat owners are strongly advised to check all over any waste ground, especially old bonfire sites, before turn out. If land to be used is likely to have high levels of geochemical lead, farmers are advised to make sure the grass is not grazed too short. Payne and Liversey (2010) have suggested that animals are removed from the pasture when the grass has been grazed to a height of 3 cm. It is vital that good water is supplied in troughs and that sheep are not allowed to drink from run-off water.

Levamisole

Goats have a very small safety margin with this useful anthelmintic. Mild signs of diarrhoea will be seen when dosages are doubled as recommended by some authorities (see Chapter 6). Greater overdosing will cause neurological signs and even death. There is no specific antidote. Treatment is supportive.

Metaldehyde

This lethal poison is found in slug and snail bait, which is normally a blue-green colour. It can be spread on the ground surrounding crops. Animals are liable to be poisoned by spillage. It is very palatable and small ruminants will actively seek it out, but it is very toxic causing neurological signs. There is no specific antidote but 2 ml of diazepam i/v for an adult goat or sheep will help to control the convulsions. Give 1 ml of acetylpromazine (ACP) 10 mg/ml i/m first to help to control the animal for the intravenous injection, although this is not easy in a woolly sheep that is convulsing. B vitamins will aid the liver in detoxicating the poison and will help to prevent liver damage, which has been reported. Sadly, in the author's experience death has resulted if convulsions have occurred, even if they are controlled with medication.

Mercury

Organic mercury compounds were once used as a dressing for seed. Small ruminants having access to a bag of such old corn will show neurological signs. These may have a delayed onset. There are two recommended treatments. Sodium thiosulfate can be given at the rate of 30 mg per kg i/v, well diluted in normal saline; or the easy option is to give British Anti Lewisite by mouth at the rate of 6.5 mg per kg. Both of these are a one-off treatment and cannot be repeated.

Ionophores

This poisoning only occurs if cattle feed containing ionophores (used as a growth promoter) is fed to sheep or goats in high doses. They are extremely toxic and will cause total collapse and death from cardiac failure. Treatment is unrealistic but oral vitamin E has been recommended. Ionophores are used in some parts of the world as coccidiostats. They are not licensed in the UK.

Mycotoxins

Poisoning results from the ingestion of food contaminated with toxins produced by moulds, which occur throughout the environment and may be found in a variety of foodstuffs. Mycototoxins affect animals in a wide variety of ways and as there are also many different types, diagnosis and identification are inherently difficult. In fact animals are rarely poisoned. Mycotoxins are an increasing problem as higher-milk-producing sheep and goats are more susceptible to challenge. Great use is being made of higher dry matter forages and increased storage of feeds on farms. There are three common moulds and mycotoxins which affect sheep and goats. They are *Fusarium*, *Penicillium* and *Aspergillus*. *Aspergillus* is typically associated with warm climates, whereas the other two are common in the UK. Specific toxins are also found in plants such as ergot, perennial ryegrass, sweet clover and fescue grass. However the majority are found when there is poor harvesting and storage of feed (e.g. slow clamp filling and poor clamp consolidation leading to poor fermentation). They may also be a problem when feeding out with poor face management.

Nitrate

This is a fertilizer. It rarely causes poisoning although it is advisable not to put sheep onto a treated pasture until after a shower of rain. It is bitter and sheep will not willingly eat it. The signs are those of vasodilatation similar to shock (i.e. a weak, rapid pulse and low rectal temperature). There may be haemoglobinuria and petechial haemorrhages. The blood is said to be chocolate brown. The treatment is specific: a slow injection of 1% methylene blue at the rate of 5 mg/kg i/v.

Organochlorine pesticides

These are very potent poisons. They cause peracute neurological signs, quickly followed by collapse and death. There is no antidote.

Organophosphate insecticides

These insecticides are very potent poisons. Their acute toxicity is due to cholinergic overstimulation. Poisoned animals will show neurological signs. Initially they will be ataxic with continuous attempts to urinate. This will lead on to convulsions and death. In theory an adult sheep or goat should be given 5 mg of i/v atropine sulfate and a further 20 mg sub/cut, however the prognosis is extremely grave. There is also a danger of a delayed neurotoxicity. Suffolk sheep are believed to be more susceptible.

Paraquat

This common weedkiller is very toxic to animals and there is no antidote. Death is relatively rapid in 6–8 h and is the result of massive pulmonary oedema. It is likely to contaminate the water, as recorded in Australia (Philbey and Morton, 2001).

Propylene glycol

This oily chemical is used as antifreeze in cars as well as being given to cattle with ketosis. It can also be given to ewes with twin lamb disease but is toxic if overdosed. Practitioners should read instructions carefully on any twin lamb drenches.

Prostaglandins

Great care with these medicines should be taken in all small ruminants. Acute pulmonary oedema has been reported in all species and there is no antidote. Oxygen may be helpful but normally they are found dead 12 h after the injection.

Salt

Goats and sheep can be remarkably stupid when offered large quantities of salt. Obviously they become very thirsty, then have diarrhoea and then start to stagger. Severe nervous signs will follow. Water should be given little and often, as large amounts seem to make the symptoms worse. Dexamethazone by i/v injection is helpful, although fluid therapy must be the treatment of choice.

Selenium

Selenium normally causes chronic poisoning in grazing animals, particularly sheep, which ingest herbage containing very high levels of selenium. The first signs are loss of hair with cracking of the feet. Animals will totally recover when removed from the diet high in selenium. However, if the animals are left on these pastures they will be found dead. Liver and kidney should be sent to the laboratory to confirm the diagnosis.

Sodium chlorate

This is an old-fashioned weed killer. Its modern equivalent is sodium monochloroacetate. Sodium chlorate is palatable to sheep and causes convulsions and death. There is no specific treatment but diazepam should be used to control the convulsions. Fluid therapy will be helpful.

Urea

This can cause poisoning when animals manage to break up molasses blocks containing urea. If they eat chunks of these blocks rather than licking them, they will suffer urea poisoning. This will be manifest as neurological signs, mainly of hyper-excitement. Treatment with tranquillizers (e.g. acetylpromazine or diazepam) is recommended followed by intravenous fluids.

Warfarin

This is found in rat bait and is an anticoagulant. Ruminants appear to detoxicate them in the rumen, and there are no reports of poisoning in the literature. If sheep or goats are found to have consumed some quantity, their mucous membranes should be checked regularly for pallor. If that occurs injections of vitamin K should be administered.

Wood preservatives

These substances contain phenol. They are very corrosive and unlikely to be drunk. The author understands that creosote has been banned in the UK but the modern compounds are still toxic. The only likely problem would be a sheep knocking over a large container and getting its wool soaked. The phenol can be absorbed through the skin. The animal will show depression, diarrhoea and a very subnormal rectal temperature. Shearing may be the best course of action so that the substance can be washed off with warm soapy water. The animal should be kept warm.

Zinc

Zinc is much less toxic than copper and so it has replaced copper in sheep foot baths. However it is toxic and will cause diarrhoea and weight loss in sheep.

Other Toxic Products

Cloth

This is mainly a problem in goats kept as pets in gardens and around houses. They may ingest anything from string to washing off the line. Certain goats do seem to have strange picas. The problem arises if the cloth or string balls up in the rumen, when the animal will become inappetant. Diagnosis is difficult. Removal by rumenotomy is the only treatment as liquid paraffin will be ineffective (Fig. 17.5).

Stale concentrate feed

This is likely to be attractive to sheep and goats and can cause many problems. First of all, excessive hard feed will cause acute acidosis. Treatment will consist of fluids by mouth and intravenous fluids spiked with bicarbonate. Vitamin B injections will be useful. Stale food also is liable to contain aflatoxins. This will result in ataxia, convulsions and hyperammonaemia leading to hepatic encephalopathy. There is no helpful treatment and therefore euthanasia must be advised.

Stored fruit

This is normally a problem in goats which break into food stores. If they ingest large quantities of fruit, particularly if is fermenting, they will get alcoholic poisoning and diarrhoea. Treatment is with large doses of vitamin B by injection.

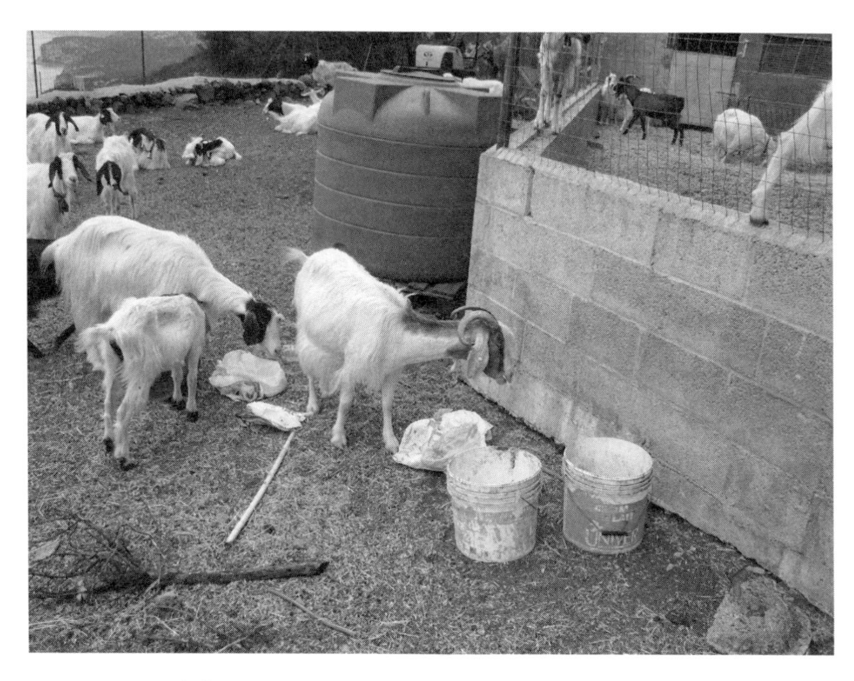

Fig. 17.5. A goat eating polythene.

18

Sudden Death and Post-mortem Techniques

Iatrogenic Causes of Sudden Death

'Sudden death' is a misnomer. In reality it is 'found dead since last seen'. The owner will very rarely see an animal die and it is even rarer for the clinician to see death. Sadly, when such deaths occur it is usually at the time of veterinary treatment. A list of iatrogenic causes is shown in Box 18.1.

Anaphylaxis from Administration of Medicines

This must be a very rare event but has been reported following the use of prostaglandin injections in goats. The antibiotic tilmicosin Micotil™ (Elanco Animal Health, Basingstoke, UK), which is licensed in sheep, has been associated with sudden deaths in goats and should not be used in this species. On account of dangers of toxicity in humans, Micotil may only be injected by veterinary surgeons. This means that its use in sheep is much curtailed, which is a pity as it is a very useful antibiotic in this species.

Dehorning

Dehorning of adult goats is a very risky procedure. Not only is the use of sedatives and anaesthetics dangerous in itself, but these products are even more dangerous when such radical surgery is attempted. Equally, if they are not used, there are other risks associated with large volumes of local anaesthetics. These include the toxicity of the local anaesthetic itself and the danger of shock from the pain. Therefore dehorning should only be performed if there is a clinical reason to do it, for example if the horn has been fractured at its base.

Disbudding

Disbudding kids less than 7 days of age is not nearly as dangerous as dehorning older kids and adults. A general anaesthetic should be used because of the difficulty in getting adequate anaesthesia by local infiltration. This is a much safer procedure in young kids than adults. GA can be accomplished by the use of intravenous anaesthetics or by the use of a mask and inhalation anaesthetics. With the latter great care should be taken to turn off the oxygen and the anaesthetic mixture when a naked flame or a red hot iron is near.

General Anaesthesia

GA in adult animals is bound to carry a high risk, particularly if the surgery is likely to be

Box 18.1. Possible iatrogenic causes of sudden death.

- Anaphylaxis from administration of medicines.
- Dehorning.
- Disbudding.
- General anaesthesia.
- Lumbar/sacral epidural.
- Massive haemorrhage (this could occur at parturition where there is no human involvement).
- Intra-arterial injection.
- Intra-venous injection.
- Sedation.

long and gaseous anaesthesia is required. The risk can be minimized by careful monitoring and supervision of recovery.

Lumbar/Sacral Epidural

This technique has been perfected by workers at Edinburgh Veterinary School and in their hands it is not a hazardous procedure. However, unless clinicians have been adequately trained, it is a procedure which does have risks as the spinal cord is present at this site.

Massive Haemorrhage

This can occur at parturition without human interference. However, it is extremely rare unless there has been trauma caused by rough parturition techniques. Very great care should be taken by clinicians when assisting the parturition of small breeds of sheep and pygmy goats. Haemorrhage occurs from the middle uterine artery. This artery may also be ruptured at the time of uterine prolapse.

Intra-arterial Injection

This type of injection is always an error. However it is relatively common, with most clinicians admitting that it has occurred when they have been attempting an intravenous injection. The carotid artery lies just deep to the jugular vein in the caudal third of the neck.

Intravenous Injection

In the UK, there are few licensed medicines for sheep and very few for goats. Most medicines can be used in small ruminants using the cascade principle. Certain licensed medicines anecdotally cause collapse and death in cattle and horses when given intravenously, the most notable being potentiated sulfonamides and vitamin B complexes. It is not suggested that these medicines are never given intravenously, but clinicians should consider carefully before using them by this route and should always inject them extremely slowly. It is well known that magnesium sulfate, which is supplied in a 25% solution, should never be given intravenously but subcutaneously. Even the 5% solution should be injected very slowly if given intravenously.

Sedation

Although xylazine is widely used as a sedative it should be used with caution. The safety margin is not large. It is prudent to dilute the 2% solution, as this is manufactured for cattle and small ruminants are lighter in weight. Weights can be deceptive, particularly in fleece-covered animals. Very small doses are required.

Reasons for Animals to be Found Dead

True sudden deaths are very rare. The reasons are shown in Box 18.2.

Anthrax

This is not easy to diagnose from gross pathology in small ruminants. As it is so rare

Box 18.2. Causes of sudden death.

- Anthrax.
- Cast on the back.
- Chemical poisons.
- Clostridial disease.
- Drowning (may occur at dipping or in deep water).
- Electrocution.
- Hypomagnesaemia.
- Lightning strike.
- Poisonous plants.
- Ruptured aneurysm.
- Ruptured uterine artery.
- Snake bite.
- Trauma (mainly road traffic accidents or fighting in rams).

clinicians are unlikely to take a blood smear and find the classical encapsulated bacteria. Obviously if an enlarged spleen is found in any of these species then anthrax should be suspected. This feature is not often seen in goats, although enlarged lymph nodes with echymoses and petechiae will be seen on the mucosal surfaces in this species.

Cast on the back

This is only a problem in over-fat sheep, heavy in the wool. It is a sad condition and actually with good shepherding is very unlikely to occur. Sheep can survive for many hours and will recover when righted. However, it is vital that the individual is shorn without delay, as it will often be cast again in the next 48 h.

Chemical poisons

There are very few chemicals which will actually cause sudden death, as normally quite large quantities need to be consumed. Metaldehyde in 'slug bait' is a possibility, as is nicotine from a pipe smoker's pouch full of tobacco. Both these poisons will be found in the rumen. Normally lead poisoning is a chronic toxicity but acute deaths with neurological signs have been reported.

Clostridial disease

This is the most likely cause of sudden death in sheep. *Clostridium perfringens* type C, the cause of 'struck' is specific to sheep but is only found in certain areas of the UK (e.g. in Kent). *Cl. perfringens* type D, which causes 'pulpy kidney' in fast growing lambs, will also cause sudden death in goats. In all species there will be rapid autolysis. There will be an excess of abdominal fluid and pericardial fluid. The small intestine will be hyperaemic and ulcerated. Diagnosis can be confirmed by toxin neutralization tests. Glucosuria is only seen in sheep and not in goats. *Cl. chauvoei* will cause black leg in all small ruminants and there will be an area of crepitus felt on one of the large muscle areas. Smears should be taken for testing for fluorescent antibodies. *Cl. septicum* will cause 'Black's disease' in small ruminants. The muscles have a distinctive smell of rancid butter. The disease can be confirmed by testing for fluorescent antibodies.

Drowning

The diagnosis is likely to be obvious, with the lungs being full of water or dip. Inhalation pneumonia from incorrect drenching technique will not cause sudden death.

Electrocution

This is an extremely rare cause of death. It is only likely to occur if an animal gets tangled up in an electric fence powered from the mains. Goats have been known to chew through electric leads, resulting in electrocution.

Hypomagnesaemia

This condition can occur in both sheep and goats, although it is extremely rare in goats.

The classic situation for sheep to be affected is in orchards where the grass has been very heavily fertilized. Actual sudden death is unusual. The area around the carcass should be examined carefully, as often the signs of the convulsions before death will be seen. Normally the sheep will be recumbent and showing severe neurological signs, which even with magnesium treatment are irreversible. A serum blood test from an animal which is still alive will be diagnostic, and testing the aqueous humour from a carcass will be helpful. Haemorrhages may be seen on the endocardium but these are not actually diagnostic, only indicating that the sheep has died after having convulsions. The history will, however, indicate that hypomagnesaemia is the most likely cause.

Lightning strike

Diagnosis is likely to be circumstantial – there has to have been a thunder storm in the last 24 h! The whole body should be examined for signs of burning, and then careful skinning should be performed so that lines of subcuticular haemorrhages are not missed.

Poisonous plants

There are poisonous plants which will cause sudden death in small ruminants, but these are rarely consumed in large enough quantities to bring about almost instant death. Diagnosis of plant poisoning can be made by examination of the contents of the rumen. The plant most often quoted in the textbooks is Yew. This certainly causes sudden death in cattle, which require very little to cause rapid death. Nevertheless, there is considerable doubt now if yew is as toxic to small ruminants as previously thought (Angus, 2010; Scott, W.A., 2010; Stevenson, 2010; Swarbrick, 2010). These authors indicate that certain breeds of sheep and deer are relatively resistant, however herd and flock owners should still be vigilant particularly when other feeds are not available (e.g. in snowy conditions).

Goats are particularly at risk from plant poisoning when tethered. In this scenario normal feed will be eaten first and then the animals may consume a large volume of a toxic plant. Obviously both sheep and goats are at risk if they escape from their normal habitat or if they are presented with cut toxic plants on rubbish dumps or compost heaps.

If plant poisoning is suspected then the mouth should be checked to see if any parts of the plant are still present. Some plants containing alkaloids which directly affect the heart are so toxic that death will occur instantly. Sheep and goats will die very rapidly if they consume laburnum seed pods. The area around the body should be checked for evidence of browsing.

Ruptured aneurysm

Aneurysms can occur anywhere in the animal and if they occur in the brain the animal will be found dead. Diagnosis without multiple histological sections will be very difficult. If the rupture occurs in the mesenteric vessels then the abdomen will be full of blood. This is seen in horses on account of the damage done to mesenteric blood vessels by the migration of large strongyle larvae. This does not happen in small ruminants so such a rupture is extremely rare.

Ruptured uterine artery

This is a very rare occurrence in small ruminants and is seldom seen. It may occur while there is an assisted parturition but more commonly the parturient animal is found dead, with the lamb or kid alive and well. Obviously on post-mortem the abdomen will be full of blood.

Snake bite

The author doubts that an adder would have sufficient venom to kill an adult sheep or goat in the UK, but in countries where there are more venomous snakes this is certainly a possibility. Normally sheep and goats are bitten on the face and so the small puncture wounds should be looked for if the head is swollen.

Trauma

The signs shown from road traffic accidents will be broken bones, subcutaneous haemorrhage and rupture of internal organs (Fig. 18.1). Trauma from fighting in rams may not be obvious externally, but careful skinning of the head will reveal localized subcutaneous haemorrhages and close examination of the neck may reveal a fracture. Very great care will be required when opening the cranium and neck vertebrae to examine the brain and spinal cord. Samples should be taken for histology.

Post-mortem Examinations

Equipment required

- large plastic bucket with disinfectant, warm water, soap and towel;
- butcher's knife and flaying knife;
- scalpel and blades that fit;
- rat-toothed forceps (15 cm);
- fine forceps (15 cm);
- blunt-nosed straight scissors (20 cm);
- bowel scissors;
- bone cutters, saw and hedge loppers;
- sampling materials;
- plastic trays (50 × 30 × 5 cm);
- plastic bags of various sizes;
- sterile universal bottles;
- plastic jars (1 l);
- bottles of formalin (kept separate from other equipment);
- pots containing 50% glycerol for virus isolation;
- swabs (plain, transport media and specialized for respiratory pathogens);
- vacutainers:
  - red top (serum) for routine serology and biochemistry;
  - green top (heparin) for glutathione peroxidise (selenium)-isolation of louping ill virus;
  - lilac top (EDTA) for haematology;
  - grey top (oxidase/fluoride) for glucose;
  - blue top (acid wash) for special ions e.g. Zn.

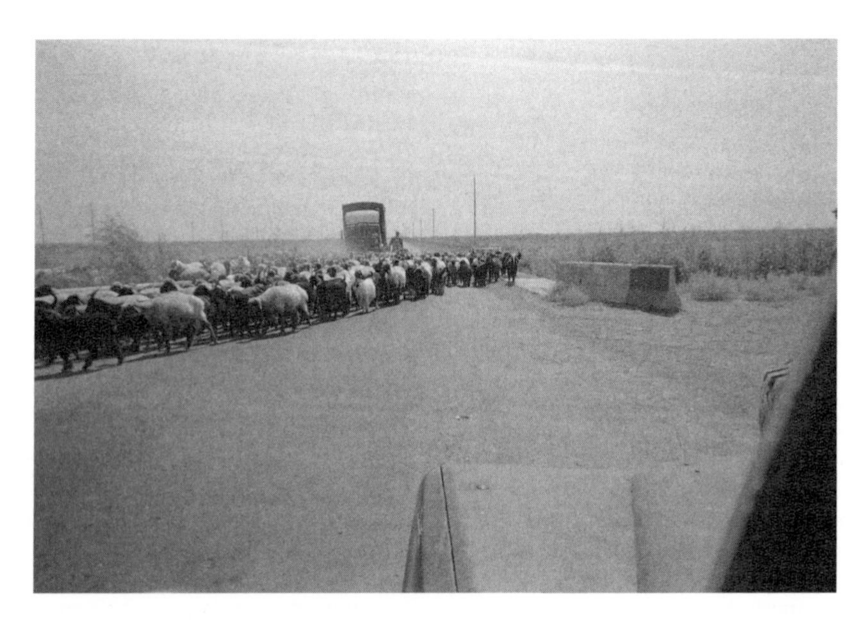

Fig. 18.1. Sheep on road.

- pasteur pipettes and rubber sucker;
- clipboard;
- post-mortem report form, laboratory submission form.

Sampling

1. If the animal is presented alive and blood is required for examination, then it is better to take it before the animal is killed.
2. If you require examination of the brain then it is better to use chemicals for euthanasia, rather than a humane killer or free bullet.
3. Before sampling it must be decided if swabs are to be taken and/or bacteriological plates are to be prepared immediately.
4. Abnormal lymph nodes should be transected and put into two universal bottles. These must be labelled. One will be kept fresh and at a later stage the other will be filled with 10% formalin.
5. As a general rule there should be 10 parts of formalin to 1 part of tissue.
6. Impression smears should be taken from the cut surfaces of any malignant oedema seen in the subcutaneous tissues and muscles. The smears should then be air dried.
7. Individual samples can be put into plastic bags or universal bottles. 10% formalin can be added if histology is required at a later date.
8. Urine can be collected into a universal bottle (testing for glucose is useful).
9. Milk can be collected into a universal bottle.
10. Faeces can be collected from the rectum.
11. Blood samples can be taken from the heart blood. These are not useful for biochemistry or haematology, but certain serological examinations are useful and a zinc sulfate turbidity test is meaningful.
12. The entire thyroid gland should be dissected out for later weighing.
13. Samples of diseased lung should be taken from the edge of the lesions after swabs have been taken, as antibiotics do not penetrate consolidated lung tissue. Samples for bacteriology can be taken from such a site.
14. Samples from abscesses should include scrapings from the interior of the abscess wall.
15. Abnormal heart lesions are often best examined microscopically after swabs have been taken of the heart blood.
16. Swabs should be taken from joint cavities.
17. Muscles can be stored fresh in plastic bags or bottles and some should have 10% formalin added later.
18. Smears can be made from bone marrow and some can be retained to have an addition of 10% formalin later.
19. Swabs should be taken from liver, spleen and kidney.
20. 100 g of both liver and kidney should be retained for toxicology.

Only after these samples have been taken are the intestines examined and opened.

1. Bezoars should be preserved in universal bottles.
2. 1 kg of rumen contents should be placed in a plastic bag for toxicology.
3. The rumen contents should be examined carefully for the presence of poisonous plants. If they are found they should be stored in plastic bags for identification.
4. Rumen contents can be tested for thiaminase to diagnose CCN.
5. For helminthological studies, the entire contents of the abomasum and/or the small intestine should be collected into a large jar for washing and sieving later.
6. The contents of affected parts of the small intestine should be collected into universal bottles (minimum 20 ml) to examine for clostridial toxins.
7. 30 g of caecal contents or faeces should be placed in a plastic bag for worm egg counts and bacterial culture.
8. Histological samples are only worthwhile from the intestines if the carcass is absolutely fresh.

Technique for single-handed post-mortem without a trough to hold the animal in dorsal recumbency

1. Examine the external surfaces and feel the superficial lymph nodes. Record the breed and sex.
2. Weigh the animal and note its condition score.
3. Examine its incisor teeth and eyes. Take a sample of the aqueous humour into a red vacutainer.

4. Look at its feet and feel its peripheral leg joints for swellings.
5. Examine the udder/scrotum.
6. Place the animal in lateral recumbency with its right side uppermost.
7. With a knife cut through the skin in the axilla and the muscles of the shoulder so that the whole of the right foreleg can be reflected back to lie on the floor.
8. With a knife make a bold cut through the skin in the groin. Cut through the muscles into the hip joint, cutting the femoral ligament and lay the right hind leg on the floor.
9. Flay the skin from the front leg caudally along the midline to the incision near the hind leg so the skin can be laid back over the backbone. The inside surface can be used to lay out visceral organs.
10. Flay the skin from the front leg rostrally up to the head so the teeth and mandible are exposed.
11. At the xiphisternum carefully open the abdomen with a pair of blunt-nosed scissors and make an incision along the midline caudally to the pelvis.
12. Make a second incision through the body wall from the xiphisternum along the line of the last rib to the backbone, so that the abdominal muscles can be reflected.
13. Examine the abdominal organs *in situ*. The abomasum and the ventral sac of the rumen will be visible ventrally along the midline. The bulk of the abdomen will be taken up by the small intestine, with the caecum dorsally. The descending duodenum is dorsal to the caecum, overlying the sigmoid colon. The right kidney will just be visible caudally to the last (13th) rib.
14. Cut the diaphragm under the ribs with a pair of blunt-nosed scissors.
15. With the garden loppers cut the ribs either side of the sternum so it can be removed.
16. Cut the intercostal muscles with a knife between every other rib and then break them back over the backbone.
17. The right lung will now be visible cranially, with the liver caudal to it.
18. Starting under the mandible elevate the tongue with a knife so that the whole 'pluck' (i.e. larynx, trachea, lungs and heart) can be removed for examination later after the oesophagus has been tied. Examine the cheek teeth at this time.
19. Examine the lungs having cut down the trachea. Sample the heart blood and examine the heart.
20. After tying off the rectum, the rumen, reticulum, omasum, abomasum, intestines and liver can be removed.
21. Examine the whole of the gastroenteric tract and the lymph nodes from the outside.
22. Take samples after examining the liver and spleen.
23. Away from the carcass open up the gastroenteric tract after taking samples and even milking out the small and large intestines separately for parasite examination. Examine the contents and the mucosal surface.
24. The bladder can be examined and a urine sample can be taken.
25. The female or male genital organs can be examined.
26. The kidneys can be removed and examined.
27. After this the head can be removed from the neck and the brain can be removed.
28. The brain should be examined for CNN.
29. A sample of the brain should be stored in 50% glycerol for virus isolation of the Louping ill virus.

If there is a proper post-mortem table available, the post-mortem can be performed with the sheep in dorsal recumbency (Fig. 18.2).

Removal of the brain in sheep and goats

This is not an easy procedure, and clinicians should take special care for health and safety reasons. Rubber gloves should be worn, as for all post-mortem examinations, and goggles and face masks should also be worn. The skin over the head including the ears should be flayed away from the bones of the skull. If the animal is horned the skin should be removed from around the two horn bases. Using a meat saw two parallel cuts are made through the skull in a rostral–caudal direction laterally to the eyes. A third saw cut is made across the nasal bone just caudal to the eye sockets joining the two lateral cuts. A final fourth saw cut is made across the caudal aspect of the cranium linking the caudal ends of the two lateral saw cuts. The skull, including the horns, can

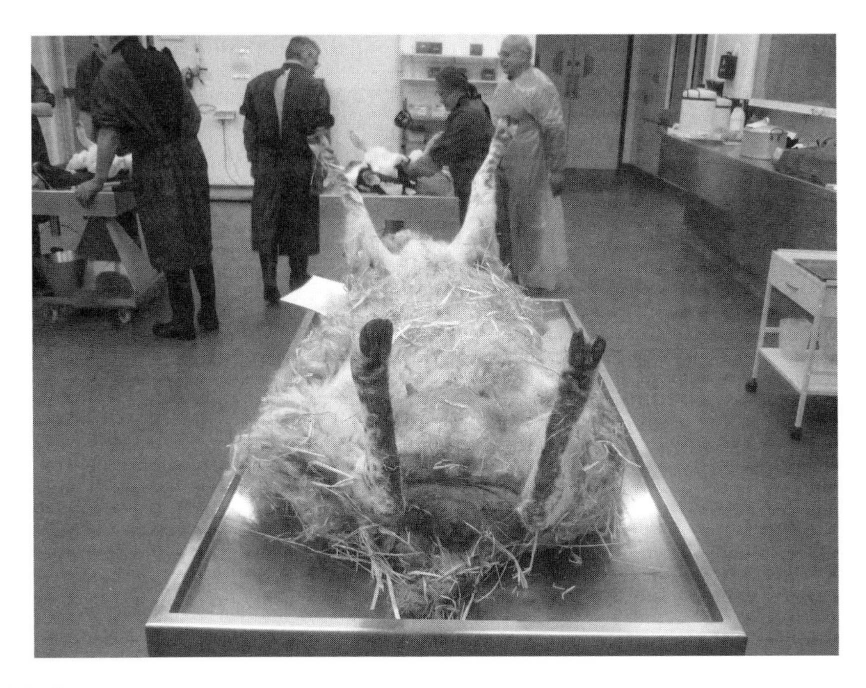

Fig. 18.2. Sheep post-mortem.

then be lifted off revealing the brain underneath. This should be examined for gross pathology and then examined under fluorescent light to diagnose CCN. The brain can then be removed to take histological samples after any bacterial samples have been collected.

Post-mortem examinations of neonatal lambs, kids and aborted fetuses

1. It should be remembered that mummified fetuses are useless for diagnostic purposes.

2. Cotyledons and placenta are vital for referral to laboratories. Over 80% of diagnoses are made from them compared from 20% from fetuses.

3. If fetuses cannot be sent then fresh peritoneal fluid, pleural fluid and abomasal contents are useful. Fresh liver, and liver in formalin should also be sent.

The laboratory staff will look for *Brucella*, but as practitioners you will be aware that this does not occur in the UK. They will also look for *Toxoplasma*, *Chlamydophila*, *Listeria* and *Salmonella* as well as carrying out general bacteriology.

19

Zoonotic Diseases

Introduction

Zoonotic diseases have always been important. However they are even more important now as the number of emerging diseases with zoonotic implications is increasing rapidly. Veterinarians have a large role to play in controlling these diseases and in advising their medical colleagues on the real risks that they pose to man. Zoonotic diseases can be viral, bacterial, fungal, protozoal and parasitic in origin. Veterinarians are uniquely qualified to advise on prevention and reduce the chances of transmission to humans by proper education and management techniques. Veterinarians have a duty of care to the general populace, the owners and carers of the animals concerned, their own staff, and of course to themselves. Washable protective clothing should be worn if possible.

Some very simple measures can be taken to protect yourself, your family and your staff from zoonotic diseases. You can also advise your clients on how to protect themselves and their families as well as visitors to their farms:

- Never drink unpasteurized goat's milk.
- Never eat undercooked goat's meat.
- Never cuddle goats or give newly born kids mouth-to-mouth resuscitation.
- Always wash your hands thoroughly after handling goats.
- Always wash your hands before handling food.
- Always wash your hands after handling fresh meat and milk before eating or handling cooked food.
- Remove dirty clothes before entering the kitchen.
- Pay particular attention to the hygiene of children.

Goat farmers, particularly if supplying milk or meat or have an open farm, have an obligation to:

- Keep the farm clean.
- Keep animals, their feed and water clean.
- Handle dung, manure, slurry and sewage safely.
- Protect water supplies and watercourses.
- Practice 'clean milk production'.
- Reduce transport stress of animals.
- Keep transport vehicles clean.

Viral Zoonotic Diseases Common to Small Ruminants Categorized by their Human Medical Names

Contagious pustular dermatitis

This viral sheep disease is extremely common and is also is seen in goats. Animals do build up immunity and the vaccines available are quite effective if used properly. However, the virus is very hard to eradicate and survives for a considerable length of time in organic matter, whether inside or out on the pasture (Gallina and Scagliarini, 2010). It is very contagious to man and only requires a small abrasion to infect the skin, normally on the hands or forearm. The lesions tend to develop into what used to be called a 'cold abscess'. These should not be lanced as the open wound will take weeks to heal.

Crimean–Congo haemorrhagic fever

This disease occurs in sheep and is mainly asymptomatic or causes a mild illness. Ticks are the vector: the larvae and first nymph stages live on rodents and the adult tick will feed on man or sheep, so the sheep is not an actual carrier. It occurs in Central Asia, Bulgaria and in the Congo, and the original virus was thought to have come from monkeys in central west Africa. There are 19 species of tick involved in Eurasia and nine in Africa. Most of the ticks belong to the genera *Hylomma, Dermacentor, Rhipicephalus* and *Boophilus*. The human disease occurs in rural areas and is mainly restricted to people involved with livestock. Man acquires the infection from the bite of infected ticks, and also through an abrasion on the hands if an infected tick is crushed. This can occur when animals are skinned. The disease is invariably fatal in man. An inactivated vaccine is now available.

Foot and mouth disease

This is obviously a very important livestock disease infecting sheep and goats. Man is very resistant to the disease. It is therefore a very rare zoonotic disease. Transmission of the virus either between humans or from humans back to animals has never been confirmed. The disease in man is primarily found in people in close contact with infected animals. The incubation period is 2–4 days. Normally there is a skin wound or wound on the oral mucosa where the primary vesicle appears. Other vesicles may appear in the mouth or on the hands and feet. Normally, after brief pyrexia, the person is fully recovered in 1 week.

Goat pox

This is caused by a *Capripox* virus and as far as the author is aware has not been recorded in the UK. The virus will infect sheep. This was first recorded in Kenya by Glynn Davies (Davies and Otema, 1978). In goats and sheep the disease has an incubation period of 1–2 weeks and starts with a fever. The skin lesions are painful circular papules which appear on parts of the body not covered by hair. The disease occurs in Africa, the Middle East, Central Asia, India and the Far East. The disease in man occurs in personnel looking after infected animals. They develop vesicles on various parts of the body. These do not form pustules and clear up in 10 days.

Louping ill

This disease of sheep is caused by a *Flavivirus* and is spread by the sheep tick *Ixodes ricinus*. In sheep the disease is manifest as biphasic pyrexia. Most animals recover rapidly but a few develop neurological signs of an encephalitis. Some pregnant animals will abort or produce live lambs which show neurological sign. These lambs are known as 'hairy shakers'. Sheep in an endemic area have immunity, but incoming sheep are affected. The disease in man is extremely rare, and as in sheep, is biphasic. Following the bite of the tick there is an incubation period of 2–8 days, with the first few days of fever; next comes 5 days where there are no symptoms; and then in the occasional case there will be neurological signs resembling poliomyelitis. These cases may need a long convalescence but all will recover.

Rabies

This dreaded disease is caused by a *Lyssavirus*. Sheep and goats are the end host and do not exhibit the furious form and so they are not a real danger to man. Nevertheless it is possible for there to be virus particles in the saliva in certain cases, and so clinicians should take care when carrying out examinations on any suspect animals. The signs of disease shown by small ruminants are at first nondescript.

They normally contract the disease from the bite of an infected carnivore or an infected bat. They move away from the others and appear to be depressed, with dilated pupils. Often the clinician will be drawn to the place of the bite wound as the animal will show a hypersensitivity reaction at that site. They will generally develop progressive neurological signs starting with muscle tremors and slight incoordination, progressing to collapse, convulsions and death. The disease is invariably fatal in these animals, as it is in man once there are severe neurological signs. There is no treatment but very good vaccines are available for humans and small ruminants.

Rift Valley fever

In man this disease is often called enzootic hepatitis. It is caused by a *Phlebovirus* and is spread by mosquitoes. It was first isolated from sheep on a ranch in Kenya in 1931, and has been found throughout Africa south of the Sahara and also in Egypt. It mainly attacks lambs and kids but can occur in adult animals. Mortality is very high in young animals but drops to 20% in adults. It will cause abortions in pregnant animals. Adult sheep and goats show excessive lacrimation and may even vomit. Lambs and kids may have jaundice; they show a high fever and progress to rapid death. There is focal necrosis of the liver. The incubation period in man is 4–6 days followed initially by fever, nausea, myalgia and photophobia. These signs only last a few days but the fever may reoccur around the 6th day. Normally there is complete recovery unless jaundice is seen and then mortality is a possibility. A vaccine is available for humans. Sheep and goats have a very high viraemia and so the mosquitoes are likely to pick up an infective dose. A good vaccine is available. Pregnant sheep and goats should not be vaccinated as there is a risk of abortion; ideally females should be vaccinated before service.

Russian and central European spring–summer encephalitis

This is a tick-borne disease caused by a *Flavivirus*. The main vectors are ticks found on sheep and goats, such as *Ixodes ricinus*, *I. persulcatus*, *Haemaphysalis concinna* and *H. japonicadouglasi*. Several species of *Dermacentor* spp. also transmit the disease. Both trans-stadial and transovarial transmission of the virus can occur in the ticks. Infected adult sheep normally survive after a brief illness but lambs die in 5 or 6 days after an encephalitis. Goats can also become viraemic. It is thought that man can become infected by drinking infected milk. This should be avoided by boiling the milk from sheep and goats as the disease is very serious in man, causing neurological signs with a very slow recovery. There is a 20% chance of mortality. There is a vaccine available for humans.

Scrapie

This disease has a very slow onset and has been known in sheep for over two centuries. It has risen to prominence in the last 20 years on account of the emergence of 'Mad cow disease' in the UK. This latter disease appears very similar to CJD in man and is thought to have occurred in cattle fed offal from sheep, particularly the brain and spinal cord. The histological findings in the brain link all the conditions together. The infective agent seems to be even smaller than a virus and is called a prion. These agents have a very long incubation period extending for months or even years. They are very resistant to heat, formalin, ultraviolet rays, ionizing radiation and pH changes. Goats will also contract the condition, which initially is manifest as lumbar prurigo. There is a genetic susceptibility. Lambs and kids become infected from the colostrum. There is no treatment. The disease is found in Europe and North America; however the link with CJD is not straightforward as this latter condition is found worldwide.

Vesicular stomatitis

The disease known as 'sore mouth' mainly affects horses and cattle but has been seen in sheep and goats. It is of little importance except that it resembles FMD and causes problems with diagnosis. The disease in sheep is characterized by a short pyrexia after an incubation period of 2–4days. Small papules and vesicles appear on the mouth, teats and interdigital areas. They very quickly regress. In man the disease resembles a mild infection of influenza with a few vesicles in the mouth.

Wesselsbron disease

This disease is mosquito-borne and caused by a *Flavivirus*. It affects sheep and goats mainly in South Africa but antibodies have been found further north. The incubation period is as short as 1 day and the disease leads to abortions and a high neonatal mortality. In adults there is brief pyrexia with some animals showing jaundice. The disease is similar to RVF and a combined vaccine is available for both diseases. In man the disease is less severe than RVF and the pyrexia usually only lasts for 2 days.

West Nile fever

This disease has risen to prominence as although it is a *Flavivirus* and spread by mosquitoes, it is very prevalent in veterinary surgeons, particularly those dealing with horses. The main reservoir for the virus is wild birds. The horse and to a much lesser extent the sheep are just incidental hosts. Man also is an incidental host but the virus can cause fatal encephalitis. The disease can also be severe in horses and in sheep. A vaccine is still in the experimental stage. Controlling the vector is difficult as the mosquitoes are ornithophilic but are not always anthropophilic.

Bacterial Zoonotic Diseases Common to Small Ruminants Categorized by their Human Medical Name

Actinomycosis

Although it is just possible that this is a zoonosis, in reality it is extremely unlikely. Actinomycosis in man is normally caused by *Actinomyces israelii*. This bacterium is found in the normal flora of the human buccal cavity. It invades the soft tissue and bones when teeth are extracted. It also invades the genital tract of women using intrauterine contraceptive devices. This organism has never been isolated from animals. However, *A. bovis* is a common pathogen in cattle, causing the condition of 'lumpy jaw'. *Actinobacillus ligniersii* causes the condition called 'wooden tongue' and has been isolated in sheep and goats. It causes granulomatous lesions in the soft tissues of the oral cavity and in the mandible. In Norfolk (UK) it is responsible for skin lesions in small ruminants. *Actinomyces bovis* has been found in oral lesions in man but it is extremely rare. Treatments in animals rely on high doses of streptomycin given over long periods if the organism has invaded the bone, but for shorter periods if just soft tissue is involved. Both organisms are found worldwide.

Animal erysipelas (human erysipeloid)

There is considerable confusion concerning this condition as a zoonosis. The zoonosis is caused by the bacteria *Erysipelothrix rhusiopathiae*. This organism is found in the soil all over the world. It commonly causes disease in pigs and will also cause a joint infection in lambs. This normally occurs when lambs are dipped in a very dirty dip solution. In man *E. rhusiopathiae* is a skin disease found in persons working in close proximity to pigs. The organism needs an abrasion to cause the infection, which is known as human erysipeloid. The disease is readily cured by penicillin in both man and animals except when there is long-term damage to the joints in lambs.

The confusion arises as there is a condition in man termed erysipelas or 'fish sorters' disease' which is not caused by *E. rhusiopathiae* but by a streptococcus. This organism is found in fish and in marine mammals. It is a systemic disease as well as a skin disease and so is a more serious condition in man, however it too is sensitive to penicillin.

Anthrax

This disease is perhaps the most notorious zoonosis. The organism *Bacillus anthracis* occurs in all mammals. It has three manifestations in man. 'Wool-sorters' disease' is the invariably fatal pneumonic form caught from the skins of sheep and goats. There is also an enteric form from eating carcasses contaminated with *Bacillus anthracis*. Although this is an acute form, liaison between veterinary surgeons and doctors can prevent deaths by prompt treatment with penicillin. The third, and most common, is the skin form. This occurs in slaughterhouse workers, knackermen and even veterinary surgeons who handle diseased carcasses. Although it has a slower onset, it is still a very serious disease. It starts as a malignant pustule; the bacteria then rapidly move up the lymphatics. Once again prompt penicillin treatment will prevent deaths.

Anthrax is renowned for causing sudden death in cattle and it can do this in sheep and goats if they eat large numbers of spores in contaminated feed. This has normally occurred by feed being transported in containers which previously have contained contaminated hides and skins. The very resistant spores are only formed when carcasses are opened and the bacteria are in an oxygen-rich environment. This should be avoided as the soil, or even worse a watercourse, will become contaminated. Small ruminants may get an acute form; they will have a high fever with bloody diarrhoea and even haematuria. The organisms in their chains with their distinctive staining capsules can be found on a blood smear. After heat fixing, these smears need to be stained for 30 s in old methylene blue stain (MacFadyen's stain). This is then washed off with tap water and the slide is examined under oil immersion. Treatment in these cases can be successful with intravenous crystalline penicillin in high doses. Treating an animal in this way does not lead to contamination of the environment.

Botulism

This disease is caused by the toxin produced by the anaerobic spore-forming bacterium *Clostridium botulinum*. All warm-blooded animals can be affected and there is a high mortality both in animals and in man. The picture is confusing as there are four groups of organism which produce seven antigenic types of toxin. Most human deaths are caused by eating contaminated food. There is a form that can affect infants, where the organism colonizes the intestine and produces toxin, and a third form where the organism can enter the skin through an abrasion and then produce toxin in an anaerobic environment.

Botulism is normally not an actual zoonosis as man is poisoned by eating food in which the bacteria has produced toxin (e.g. in contaminated fish). Cases have been recorded worldwide. However if bovine carcasses contaminated by the toxin (normally type D) are consumed, they will cause death. Sheep die from a type C toxin. This has only been confirmed in South Africa, where the disease is called 'lamzieke', and in Western Australia. Type C toxin has never been known to cause human fatalities. Cattle in Europe become infected by eating contaminated silage but this mode of infection has not been recorded in sheep. Goats will be affected by type D toxin like cattle and therefore are a zoonotic risk. They have only been infected with type C toxin experimentally.

Most human cases are associated with toxins A, B and E.

Brucellosis

Brucella melitensis

World-wide this is the most common *Brucella* spp. to cause brucellosis in man. Its geographical prevalence exactly mirrors the incidence in goats. It is not found in the UK but is common in the Mediterranean basin, the Middle East and in Central Asia. *B. melitensis* is a very serious disease in man causing high fever which may undulate over 24 h and in attacks separated by several days. It causes severe headaches, depression and splenomegaly, and therefore may be confused with malaria. Attacks may keep recurring for several years. It is picked up by drinking milk or water infected by the organism from products of abortion. The main symptom in goats is abortion in the 3rd or 4th months of pregnancy, and it will also cause arthritis and orchitis in males. The disease will also affect sheep but the disease is not as important as a zoonosis in sheep, as milking of sheep is less common worldwide than milking of goats. However, it will cause abortion in ewes and epididymitis in rams.

Brucella ovis

This condition is much rarer than *B. melitensis* in both sheep and goats and hence it is rare in humans. However it is a very serious disease in man and may be fatal. In sheep the principal symptom is epididymitis in rams but it will also cause abortion. In mixed groups of sheep and goats it tends to target sheep. Mastitis is seen in sheep but not in goats. The distribution of the organism is much more limited than *B. melitensis*; it is really restricted to tropical Africa and Latin America.

Campylobacteriosis

This is caused by *Campylobacter jejuni* and is the main cause of acute bacterial enteritis in the UK. The most common animal host to be a danger to man is the chicken. However, lamb carcasses have recently been implicated and therefore hygiene standards for any person handling sheep, particularly diarrhoeic sheep, should be high (Garcia *et al.*, 2010). In humans the organism causes acute, self-limiting diarrhoea. Care should be taken to protect children if they are vomiting, as severe dehydration has very serious consequences. It is extremely rare in goats.

Clostridial food poisoning

Although there are many species of clostridial bacteria that are very important and prevalent in sheep and goats, it is not an important zoonosis. The organism is found in soil and dust and so animals are not the main cause of infection. The *Clostridium* spp. that occurs in sheep and goats cause a very mild enteritis in man which is self-limiting and rarely lasts more than 24h. The important pathogen in man is *Cl. difficile*, which is not pathogenic, or found in sheep and goats.

Clostridial wound infections

The most important bacterium in this group is *Clostridium tetani* and this receives a large amount of media attention. Tetanus is a very serious disease in man causing neurological signs but an animal is not required for the infection, which normally comes from a contaminated deep puncture wound. *Cl. tetani* is a ubiquitous organism in the soil throughout the world, requiring anaerobic conditions to multiply and release its sometimes fatal toxin. Tetanus is a very serious disease in small ruminants but these are not contagious to man. Other *Clostridium* spp. will infect wounds in man or in small ruminants causing serious gangrene and death but man cannot become infected from animals. The main organisms are *Cl. novyi*, *Cl. septicum* and *Cl. sordellii*. These organisms may infect man, sheep and goats by injections with contaminated needles.

Colibacillosis

This is a significant and life-threatening zoonotic disease, particularly serious in the old and in children. The most important highly pathogenic *Escherichia coli* is the verocytotoxigenic strain *E. coli* O157. In other countries there are other verocytotoxigenic strains, such as O26; the latter does occur in sheep and goats but is not pathogenic to them. Investigations by the Veterinary Laboratory Agency (VLA) over a 10-year period indicated that cattle were the most likely to be positive, with 59% positive samples. There were 29% positive samples in sheep and 10% positive samples in goats. It should be noted that the strain is O157 not 0157 (i.e. a somatic (O) antigen is present, not a zero antigen). Hygiene for humans when handling animals is very important particularly in children who are really at risk on open recreational farms. The greatest danger to man is from cattle. However, sheep and goats are well recognized as animals harbouring the organism and therefore are a risk to humans. Verocytotoxigenic (VTEC) O157 is carried asymptomatically by animals and owners of animals should be aware of the potential for zoonotic transmission of VTECO157 even from healthy animals. Avoiding contact with animal faeces and adopting principles of good hygiene following animal contact is crucial in reducing the risk of zoonotic infections. O157 infection can be acquired directly or indirectly from animals. The organism colonizes the rectal–anal junction, with certain individuals being super-shedders. The routes of infection in man are contaminated food or water, direct animal contact, indirect animal contact through the environment and person-to-person spread (Keen and Elder, 2002; Griffin, 2010).

Corynebacteriosis

Corynebacterium diphtheria is a very serious condition in humans but it does not occur in animals. *C. pseudotuberculosis* is a very important pathogen in sheep and goats and although some cases are reported in man, they are extremely rare. The disease causes caseous lymphadenitis in animals and this is seen in man but only in immune-suppressed individuals.

Dermatophilosis

This is an important skin condition in sheep and goats. It causes extensive mycotic dermatitis called 'lumpy wool' in sheep and Angora goats. However there have been very few cases recorded in man and so it is not an important zoonosis.

Leptospirosis

There is considerable confusion about this zoonotic disease. *Leptospira icterohaemorrhagiae*, also known as Weil's disease, is a very serious and often fatal disease in man. It manifests as jaundice, fever and vomiting. Sometimes jaundice is not a feature but the condition remains just as serious. This disease is passed to man from rodents, which are normally symptomless carriers. Pigs can get the disease and infect man. This serovar is not a known pathogen of small ruminants but these species can become infected with *L. harjo*. This infection is rare, unlike in cattle where it is a very common pathogen. In fact sheep and goats are likely to be symptomless carriers, as often certain flocks or goat herds have a high prevalence of animals showing raised antibody levels. If sheep or goats do show symptoms it is usually a widespread, short-term malaise but sometimes abortions will occur. *L. harjo* is not a serious disease in man. It is caught from drinking contaminated fresh milk, or, more commonly in farmers, from cattle urine. Sheep and goats are rarely a zoonotic focus as they are rarely affected. In man the disease is similar to a short influenza attack, often over in 48 h.

Listeriosis

This disease is caused by *Listeria monocytogenes*. It is an extremely serious infection in very young babies and will cause abortion in man, and can also cause fatalities in elderly patients. It is found throughout the world. Man becomes infected by eating contaminated food, such as cheese made from contaminated milk. Neonates can become infected in late pregnancy. In sheep and goats the disease causes encephalitis, neonatal mortality and septicaemia; mortality can be high, up to 30%. It is particularly common in animals eating poor quality silage.

Meliodosis

This disease is caused by *Pseudomonas pseudomallei* and is also called rodent glanders. The organism is very similar to *P. mallei*, the agent which causes glanders in horses and man. It is mainly confined to the tropics, particularly South-east Asia, where it can survive in hot, humid, muddy conditions for over 2 years. Often the disease is not serious in man, but if there is a septicaemia or a pneumonia it is likely to be fatal. In sheep and goats it causes pneumonia or peritonitis with abscesses throughout the chest and abdomen. Epidemics are rare, but mortality may then be as high as 20%. Treatment with antibiotics is rarely effective if the disease is in an advanced state.

Necrobacillosis

This condition is caused by *Fusobacterium necrophorum* which is an extremely common pathogen in sheep worldwide, causing foot rot. This is an annoying disease with welfare implications but does not cause systemic disease in sheep. It is an extremely rare disease in man but can be very serious, particularly in children, leading to tonsillitis and septicaemia.

Pasteurellosis

There is confusion in the nomenclature of the two agents causing this disease, which used to be called *Pasteurella multocida* and *P. haemolytica*. The species have now been transferred to the genus *Mannheimia*. These are common pathogens in sheep and goats, where they cause severe pneumonia. The disease in man is extremely rare and even more rarely related to sheep or goats, normally being transferred by bites or scratches from dogs and cats, as the organism lives asymptomatically in their mouths. It is not found in the mouths of herbivores.

Salmonellosis

Salmonella abortus ovis

Although, as the name implies, this organism will cause abortion in sheep, it has never been associated with abortion in women or enteric disease in humans generally.

Salmonella typhimurium

This organism has been recorded in sheep but has never been recorded as a zoonosis from sheep, although it is a common cause of enteritis in man. *Salmonella enteritidis* is a very common cause of enteritis in man but is caught from chickens and does not occur in small ruminants. Other causes of salmonellosis are ever-present on farms, namely *S. enterica* subsp. *diarizonae*, *S. montevideo* and S. *dublin*.

These organisms are not renowned for being present in sheep and goats and are more commonly found in other farm animals.

Most human *Salmonella* infections are acquired as a result of eating contaminated food. Infection on farms is more commonly acquired by mouth from hands contaminated by infected animals, their bedding and surroundings. People who are ill with salmonellosis often have diarrhoea, vomiting or a flu-like illness. Children, pregnant women, the elderly and occasionally healthy adults may become seriously ill and require hospital treatment.

These simple precautions will go a long way to prevent people associated with livestock from becoming infected with salmonellosis:

- Do observe high standards of personal hygiene; wear rubber boots and protective over-garments when working with animals.
- Do change and launder overalls frequently and disinfect boots to avoid spreading the infection to other animals and people.
- Do wash your hands using hot water and soap immediately after working with infected animals.
- Do wash hands before eating, drinking or smoking.
- Do ensure that anyone with diarrhoea, vomiting or flu-like illness consults a doctor, and informs the doctor if *Salmonella* spp. have been isolated from livestock.
- Don't take or wear dirty clothing and boots into the home.
- Don't allow vulnerable people, including children, the elderly and pregnant women to come into contact with infected animals.
- Don't drink raw milk or eat undercooked eggs from the herd/flock when *Salmonella* spp. have been isolated – even healthy animals may excrete the bacteria.
- Don't bring infected animals into any room where food is prepared or eaten.

- Don't allow pets to come into contact with infected animals.

Tularemia

This disease is caused by *Francisella tularensis*. It is mainly found in North America and Russia. It used to be relatively common in man but now it is rare. It is usually spread by ticks and is seen commonly as infected tick bites which spread to the local lymph node. There will then be a fever and general malaise; however, high-mortality outbreaks have been reported in Canada, the USA and Russia. The tick involved is *Dermacentor andersoni*. This tick has a predilection site in sheep's ears. Normally the other host is a rodent.

Yersiniosis

Yersinia pseudotuberculosis causes Parinaud's oculoglandular syndrome in man and a similar syndrome in goats. Goats develop a sudden-onset mucopurulent ocular discharge, blepharospasm, corneal opacity and neovascularization. The disease spreads to the parotid and submandibular lymph nodes. Morbidity can be as high as 5% in some goat herds but there is no mortality. Obviously any person handling the goats is at risk.

Zoonotic tuberculosis

Tuberculosis in man is normally caused by the human pathogen *Mycobacterium tuberculosis* but man can also become infected by *M. bovis*. This is primarily a disease affecting cattle and badgers and is a chronic condition eventually leading to severe caseous pneumonia and death in both cattle and badgers. Man becomes infected by drinking unpasteurized contaminated milk. In sheep *M. bovis* is extremely rare. This is not so in goats. They will quite readily become infected either from badgers, cattle or other goats. It is a real zoonotic problem as man can easily become infected by close contact or by drinking unpasteurized goat's milk. The intradermal skin test is not very reliable in cattle and even worse in goats. At the time of writing the blood test is little better. In goats the disease can be of a very chronic nature and therefore very difficult to recognize clinically. There is no suitable treatment.

Chlamydioses and Rickettsioses Common to Small Ruminants Categorized by their Human Medical Names

Chlamydiosis

This is caused by *Chlamydophila abortus*, which is found in sheep and goats. The medical profession is very aware of the disease and its zoonotic implications and the general public is also alarmed. A large amount of investigation into the condition in man has been carried out and it is now thought that the organism is not nearly as dangerous as had been suggested. The organism is a very common specific ovine pathogen causing abortion and it is rare that it infects humans. Only three cases had been recorded over the last 20 years in the UK but it is advisable for pregnant women not to have close contact with sheep at lambing time.

Q fever

Coxiella burnetti causes Q fever. It can be spread between sheep and goats, and to man through drinking water. It can also be spread by ticks. There has been a recent Q fever epidemic in the Netherlands, which is the largest epidemic ever reported globally. The source of infection was aerosol transmission from a very high concentration of large, infected dairy goat units located close to human populations. However, it is unlikely that a similar outbreak would occur in the UK, due to a smaller national goat population and less association with urban areas (Harwood *et al.*, 2010). The disease is an influenza-type condition in humans and does respond to oxytetracyclines in high doses. It causes abortion in sheep and goats, and the results of abortion are contagious to man.

C. burnetti is shed in large numbers from the reproductive tracts in a spore-like form, which is very resistant in the environment.

Fungal Zoonotic Diseases Common to Small Ruminants Categorized by their Human Medical Names

Dermatophytosis

Compared to cattle, ringworm in sheep and goats is extremely rare, but they can contract *Trichophyton verrucosum* from cattle. The lesions are normally around the face in wool sheep but will occur elsewhere in hair sheep and goats. The organism is very contagious to man. Prevention by thorough washing with soap and water must be recommended. Violent scrubbing and very strong disinfectants should be avoided as these will damage the skin. *Microsporum canis* has been recorded following bite wounds from dogs on the hind legs and rump, and *M. gypseum* has been recorded in lambs and kids. However neither of the *Microsporum* spp. is very contagious to man.

Protozoal Zoonotic Diseases Common to Small Ruminants Categorized by their Human Medical Names

Babesiosis

Although this protozoan has a worldwide incidence it is not an important zoonosis. It is spread by ticks, but man seems resistant to the disease so infections are extremely rare. It is also rare in sheep and goats, being primarily a cattle parasite. The disease in man is characterized by a severe illness with jaundice and haemoglobinuria.

Cryptosporidiosis

This protozoan has a worldwide distribution. It can cause a very serious disease, either meningitis or pneumonia, in man. However, such extremes are very rare and the normal manifestation is acute diarrhoea which is unpleasant but normally self-limiting. Sheep and goats, particularly young animals, will become infected by the organism. They may show quite severe diarrhoea or they may be symptomless carriers. Bottle-fed animals are very often symptomless carriers. The main human danger is from children visiting open, educational farms. The disease can be well contained by strict hygiene involving/including hand washing and not allowing eating and drinking near the animals.

Toxoplasmosis

The causal organism is *Toxoplasma gondii*. There is no doubt that this organism is pathogenic to man. Equally there is no doubt that it causes abortion in sheep but the level of infection in aborted fetuses and their membranes is extremely low. On the other hand the level of infection in the faeces of certain cats is very high, and cats and rodents need to be controlled to prevent this dangerous disease. The sheep is innocent in the spread of this unpleasant zoonosis.

Parasitic Zoonotic Diseases Common to Small Ruminants Categorized by their Human Medical Names

Coenurosis

This disease is caused by *Coenurus cerebralis*, the larval stage of the tapeworm *Taenia multiceps*. The normal life cycle occurs in the dog or wild canids (e.g. fox, jackals and coyotes). As definitive hosts, they harbour the tapeworm in their intestines. The life cycle starts with the expulsion of gravid proglottids or eggs within the faeces of the definitive host. Intermediate hosts are affected by ingesting the eggs with grass or water. The normal intermediate host is the sheep, or rarely the goat. The oncospheres penetrate the wall of the small intestine and, via the blood vessels, are distributed to different tissues and organs. The cycle is completed when a dog or wild canid ingests tissue or an organ containing the coenuri. In the case of *C. cerebralis* the organ is the brain. In sheep the cystic *C. cerebralis* will reach a size of 5 cm in 6 months and cause neurological signs, the disease called gid. Man is not the normal intermediate host although rare cases have been recorded. The tapeworm is found worldwide in temperate areas.

Dicroceliasis

Dicrocoelium dendriticum is a lancet-shaped trematode that lives in the bile ducts of sheep and goats as well as other domestic and wild herbivores. It requires two intermediate hosts for its development, the first being a land snail and the second an ant. The adult trematodes deposit their eggs in the bile ducts of the definitive host; the eggs move with the bile and are eventually carried by the faecal matter to the exterior. The eggs contain a miracidium and can survive for many months. This is released when the egg is ingested by the mollusc. In the snail's tissues, the miracidium gives rise to two generations of sporocysts, the second of which produces large numbers of cercariae. These are eaten by the ant, which in turn is eaten by the herbivore. The parasite is found in North and South America, Europe, Asia and North Africa. The disease is rare in man as it relies on a human ingesting an infected ant. The disease in man is not serious, causing dyspepsia and flatulence, or it may be asymptomatic. In sheep and goats the disease is not nearly as serious as fascioliasis, but anaemia and diarrhoea have been reported. It can be treated with flukicides.

Fascioliasis

This is a very serious disease in sheep and goats (see Chapter 10) caused by *Fasciola hepatica* throughout the world and also by *F. gigantic* in Africa and Asia. The herbivore is the main host. The flukes live in the liver and lay eggs. The amphibious snail *Lymnaea truncatula* is the main intermediate host and sheds metacercaria onto the vegetation. In some areas other *Lymnaea* spp. are also involved. Man is a rare host but normally becomes infected by consuming contaminated watercress. The severity of the disease in man is related to the number of metacercaria ingested. Normally there is some transitory liver disease; some cases develop anaemia and serious liver disease. It can be treated with flukicides.

Hydatidosis

The normal life cycle for this tapeworm is between the sheep and the dog but man can become infected. The adult tape worm *Echinococcus granulosus* infects dogs and wild canids. It lives in the small intestine and sheds gravid proglottids which contain several hundred eggs. These are then ingested by the intermediate host which is commonly the sheep but can also be the goat; other herbivores or omnivores which also can be the intermediate host. Man is in this last group. In man the ingested egg may take years to become a cyst. The symptoms caused by the cyst vary with its location. It may be asymptomatic but normally the large amount of fluid will cause some mild malaise. The normal site is the abdomen. It can attach to the liver or any other organ and abdominal swelling will be observed. If it occurs in the lungs it will be walled off by fibrous tissue. The main danger to the patient is rupture of the cyst. This will cause an anaphylactic reaction in many cases, which may be fatal. It may also cause seeding of eggs to multiple other sites.

In the sheep and the goat the disease is often only diagnosed on post-mortem, although it could be diagnosed on abdominal ultrasonography or thoracosonography. If the cyst or cysts are in the lung, respiratory symptoms may be observed. These will be chronic. The life cycle is complete if the sheep or goat is eaten by a dog, when the tapeworm develops in the dog's intestine. Treatment of dogs is very effective. Obviously, unlike the sheep or goat, man is an end host. The disease is found worldwide and used to be common in New Zealand until radical public hygiene measures were taken.

Linguatuliasis

This disease is caused by *Linguatula serrata*. The female of this linguiform parasite measures

10 cm and the male 2 cm. It is found in the nasal passages and frontal sinuses of dogs and cats. Eggs are laid and pass to the environment by sneezing or spitting. They need to be eaten by a small ruminant, the secondary host. These eggs develop into larvae which penetrate the wall of the intestine. After 6 months and a series of moults the larvae in the abdominal cavity penetrate into various tissues. These are taken in by the carnivore, the tertiary host, when it consumes the secondary host. The nymph travels up the oesophagus to the nasopharynx and the life cycle is complete.

This pentastomid worm is found in Europe, the Middle East, North Africa and throughout the Americas. The larvae are asymptomatic in sheep and goats. Man can become infected in two ways. The first is by ingesting eggs from vegetables or water. The larvae then may cause gastroenteric signs or the nymphs may cause ocular infection by invading the anterior chamber of the eye. However, the second type of infection in man is more common, when humans ingest contaminated offal. The infection is immediate as the nymphs invade the nasopharynx and cause pain in the throat and a runny nose. This infection is called 'halzoun' in the Middle East and 'marrara' in North Africa and the Sudan. The disease is normally self-limiting.

Myiasis caused by larvae of *Oestrus ovis*

The adult of *Oestrus ovis*, a grey fly 12 mm in length, is larviparous, depositing larvae in the nostrils of sheep, goats and, occasionally, man. It is found throughout the world. The larvae enter the nasal fossae and feed on mucus, then penetrate the sinuses where they mature. After a period of months the mature larvae migrate again to the nasal fossae where they are expelled by sneezing, fall to the ground and pupate for 1 month. The flies that emerge can live for another month. The condition is easily controlled by ivermectins in sheep and goats.

Trichostrongyliasis

These short, slender nematodes inhabit the small intestine and abomasums of sheep and goats. They cause severe problems and have become resistant to several anthelmintics. Man is only very rarely infected by chance ingestion of the eggs. On the whole the disease is asymptomatic. It should not be confused with the specific human parasite, *Trichostrongylus orientalis*, which is passed indirectly from human to human via the faeces. This pathogen has very rarely been seen, only in small numbers in sheep. It does not cause disease in this species. In man the signs are variable with low-grade gut pain being a feature. Control with anthelmintics is easy as this species is not resistant. The nematode is found in Central Asia and the Far East and is particularly prevalent in central Iran.

Zoonotic scabies

Whether this is a zoonotic disease found in sheep and goats is contentious. *Sarcoptes scabiei* is definitely a mite which can cause severe skin disease in man. Some authorities suggest that this mite can infest animals, but most think that the *Sarcoptes* spp. which infect sheep and goats are a different species. There was only one definitive animal linked to human infestation and that involved pigs. There has been no proven link with small ruminants. *S. scabiei* does cause serious disease in sheep and goats.

20

Herd and Flock Health Plans

Assessing the Risks of Disease Introduction in Imports

Before practitioners can prepare realistic herd and flock health plans they need to be aware of the relative disease risk in their country or larger region. In the UK, DEFRA is constantly monitoring the international disease risk with the help of OIE, the European Commission, the UK's Foreign and Commonwealth Office, scientific articles and personal contact with reference laboratories.

There is a continual low risk of the introduction of an exotic disease into the UK and the EU from an affected region such as Africa, the Middle East and Central/East Asia, but occasionally that risk level can be raised when a particularly high-risk route becomes prominent (Roberts *et al.*, 2011). Likewise, an outbreak of disease in domestic livestock in a country from which the UK imports that species will trigger an increase in risk.

If the approved certification and inspection process is carried out there is a negligible risk of introduction of an exotic disease. However, there would be an increased risk of disease introduction if for some reason the certification process failed, either due to fraud or to the certification of an infected consignment in good faith before the disease was detected in the country of origin.

Sheep Flock Plan

General considerations

The vital part of this concept is the establishment of a team to help the welfare and productivity of a sheep flock. The team may be just the shepherd and the veterinary surgeon or it may be very large if the flock is owned by government, but the key members will be the head shepherd and the practitioner. They may well co-opt other interested parties who can be split into different groups:

- The financial team, e.g. the owner of the sheep, the owner of the land, the bank manager, the accountant and the prospective buyers of the lambs and the wool.
- The management team, e.g. the head shepherd, the subordinate shepherds and the farm manager.
- The health team, e.g. the veterinary surgeon, the nutritionist and the veterinary medicine supplier.

However, the impetus must come from the flock owner with encouragement from the practitioner and the full support of the shepherd. The flock owner may have read the practitioner's newsletter suggesting the value of flock health plans and pointing out that veterinary surgeons are not allowed to prescribe prescription-only medicines unless they are happy that the flock is under their care. The Royal College of Veterinary Surgeons (RCVS) in the UK does not require a rigid timetable of flock visits but leaves this to the discretion of the practitioner. The flock owner, who is likely to have to pay the veterinary bills, may have attended a farmer's meeting where the costs and benefits of disease control and health plans have been pointed out. These meetings will have been advertised on posters in the veterinary practice or in monthly newsletters. After holding meetings, many practitioners will specifically target flock owners by letter or telephone call to offer further encouragement to develop a flock health plan. Practitioners may link up with medicine suppliers and diagnostic laboratories to obtain better terms for flock owners who join flock health schemes. The flock may have experienced a disease outbreak which has galvanized both the practitioner and the flock owner to take a more proactive role in disease prevention. Finally, there could have been a chance meeting of the shepherd and the practitioner at the local agricultural show.

Regardless of how the concept has been broached, the veterinary surgeon will need to gather some basic facts about the flock. The practitioner may well know the farm already. The farm account can be viewed on the practice computer to ascertain what is spent annually on professional fees and medicines. The practitioner needs to know the numbers of ewes, replacements and rams. The lambing date is the most crucial fact to be recorded, as the whole flock annual calendar will be worked back from that date. The practitioner needs to seize the opportunity whenever it is presented and start from that point. The flock plan then needs to be built up from this date.

A specific example

We will consider a simple commercial flock first and then extras can be added. For example, the farmer has a large acreage of marsh land near to the Thames estuary in Kent (UK) where he keeps 1000 Kent (Romney Marsh) ewes. He keeps his 200 replacements and his rams at the home farm in mid Kent. The farmer meets the practitioner at a store lamb sale at the beginning of August. The shepherd has already persuaded the farmer of the value of a flock health plan. The setting up of a flock health plan is agreed and the practitioner arranges a visit the following day. The practitioner knows the home farm as the farmer keeps beef cattle there which he has already treated, but there is a dearth of information on the practice computer except for purchases of sheep clostridial vaccines and wormers. Armed with a loose-leaf notebook with a minimum of 52 pages marked out with one page for each week of the year, the practitioner arrives on the farm. Over the kitchen table and a cup of coffee the discussion begins with the lambing date. This is the beginning of the second week in March. This means the rams will have to go in at the beginning of the second week in October.

The rams

The farmer explains that he has Dorset Down rams. He likes to have three rams per 100 ewes and replacements with two rams spare. He therefore needs 38 in total. He buys replacement rams at a ram sale in Sussex at the beginning of September. The farmer and practitioner discuss the merits of having a full veterinary inspection of the rams with semen testing, which the farmer declines. They even discuss the merits of AI and embryo transfer for the farmer to breed his own rams. The farmer explains that he keeps them in a yard on arrival and has a protocol for clostridial vaccination and worming at that time. He has not used teasers in the past as the flock is a relatively late lambing flock but he will consider their use next year. He does use raddles. He does not worm his existing rams but does vaccinate them at the same time as the ewes in the spring. He will collect up his existing rams soon to check their feet and teeth, cull any with problems and replace them.

The ewes

The farmer has been farming Kent ewes on these marshes for decades and is well aware of the danger of over-fat ewes at tupping time; he says there is no need for the practitioner to come to condition score them. He has never had any real problems with large numbers of abortions and therefore does not carry out vaccination against enzootic abortion or toxoplasmosis, which would normally be carried out at this time. He normally buys his replacements as shearlings in the spring from known sources. The practitioner points out that there is always a risk with this procedure, as such animals may be at risk from contagious breeding disease and also there is a danger of bringing in bowel worms which are resistant to anthelmintics. The farmer agrees. He claims he is well aware of sustainable control of parasites in sheep (SCOPS) and tries to follow these principles. He knows that there is no need to give anthelmintics to his flock at tupping time. He has no lambs on either farm as they were sold in the store lamb sale in the first week of August.

The replacements

These have been on the home farm since the spring. They have been fully vaccinated against clostridial disease, with a double dose of a vaccine containing ten active ingredients to give protection against ten clostridial diseases. The farmer is well aware of the particular danger of 'struck' in his area. The tups will go in to the replacements at the same time as the ewes. However the ewes will remain on the home farm until after their lambs are weaned next year. Last year's replacements were transported up to the marshes on the same day as the August lamb sale.

Trace elements

The practitioner is well aware of the high levels of molybdenum on the Thames marshes. This will cause copper deficiency problems. The farmer says that he has been giving the ewes and the ewe replacements copper supplementation in January for many years, since his father's time. However he is not aware of any other problems with trace element deficiencies so he agrees for the practitioner to come to take some samples from the ewes in the near future. The practitioner explains he will take two blood samples from a sample of 12 ewes to get an understanding of the flock's trace element status. He will take a heparinized sample (green top) for copper, selenium, and iodine and a serum sample (red top) for cobalt. The practitioner feels this will be a useful visit as it will allow him to assess the management of the farm on the marshes and meet the shepherd there. It will give him a chance to prepare an initial report in the form of a flock health plan, which he can expand after the visit and if there are problems which the farmer thinks of after this meeting.

Home farm visit

After this sit-down discussion the farmer (who explains that he is his own shepherd on the home farm) and the practitioner take a walk around the farm seeing the orchards with the large apple trees. Only the rams are on the home farm at this time. The practitioner points out the danger of hypomagnesaemia for this group. The farmer is well aware of this problem and makes sure they are not on a lush pasture in the spring and that they have access to high-energy mineral blocks. In response to the practitioner's query the farmer explains why he uses high-energy blocks rather than high-magnesium blocks. The farm has read the labels and has found that they both have nearly the same level of magnesium. He has also found by careful observation that over one-third of the rams never touch the high magnesium blocks as they are not very palatable. On the other hand he claims that all the rams will lick the high-energy blocks. The farmer and practitioner also look at the lambing accommodation. There are over 40 small lambing pens, which the farmer explains are often nearly all used. This is not because the young shearling Kents have many sets of twins, but because they are all first-time mothers and the farmer likes them to be really bonded with their lambs before they are turned out onto the orchards. The whole shed is high roofed and well ventilated, so the practitioner agrees that *Pasteurella* vaccination is probably unnecessary with this set-up and can be carried out by the purchaser of the store lambs.

Pre-lambing visit

This visit will be particularly useful for the main flock on the marshes, as not only can the lambing facilities be discussed but also a nutritional profile can be carried out on the ewes. The only animals to be lambed at the home farm are the shearlings and so a nutritional profile on them would probably not be warranted. The most useful parameter to be measured is the beta-hydroxybutyrate level. Normally this will be measured in a serum sample. As the farmer has already had scanning carried out he will have four groups. Those not in lamb need not be blood sampled as they are likely to be culled. At least six samples should be taken from each of the other three groups, namely those carrying singles, twins and triplets. This parameter will reflect the energy status of each group and the feeding regime can be altered accordingly. A level of beta-hydroxybutyrate of <0.8 mmol/l is adequate. Those with a level of 0.8–1.6 mmol/l will need some extra energy; a level of >1.6 mmol/l indicates a severe deficiency and radical action needs to be taken. At the same time blood urea nitrogen (BUN) can be measured to look at short-term protein intake. On this farm only the ewes carrying twins or triplets are being fed hard feed. It is important that those tested are healthy ewes which have not been fed in the last 4 h or the results will be unreliable. Low levels e.g. <1.7 mmol/l will indicate a shortage of effective rumen degradable protein. This will require dietary adjustment.

At this time it will be worthwhile discussing bringing in aborted lambs **together with some fetal cotyledons** if these occur other than very spasmodically. Obviously the clinician will encourage the farmer to bring in any dead animals for post-mortem. Biosecurity should be discussed. The farmer and the shepherd should be encouraged to bring up any other conditions which are troublesome, such as foot conditions (foot rot and contagious ovine digital dermatitis), skin conditions (scab, lice, ticks, keds, orf, caseous lymphadenitis, etc.) and internal parasites (fluke, worms and coccidia).

Summary

Flock plans are rewarding to start and to maintain. Clinicians should always approach each holding with an open mind. Education is a two-way street and they may well learn a large amount from experienced farmers and shepherds. Practitioners should try to visit when routine tasks are being carried out on the farm. The joy of veterinary practice in general and flock plans in particular is that no two holdings are ever the same and there is a large amount of satisfaction to be gained by improving the lives of large numbers of animals and their keepers.

Goat Herd Health Plan

General considerations

Milk recording

This can be very useful in dairy herds so that individuals can have their milk recorded for quantity and quality. Quality can include cell counts. Does and their offspring can be selected for breeding for replacement does and bucks.

Organic Sheep Production in the UK

If prices for organic lambs are considerably higher than conventional lambs, producing organic lambs may be financially attractive. Changes in animal health management are not very arduous and with the resistance to many anthelmintics parasite control may not be as difficult as might be imagined. Conversion of the land, if it has been used before as farmland, takes a minimum of 2 years. However, if owners can show that land has been used for other purposes for the known past (e.g. forestry or parkland without farm animals), then a dispensation may be granted. If organic lambs are to be produced they must be born on organic land and from ewes which been managed organically from tupping. There are some strange anomalies. Replacement females should come from organic units, but if they are not available then conventional animals may be brought in before tupping, provided less than 20% of the flock are brought in. Rams may come from conventional farms provided they are managed organically after their arrival. There are no restrictions on buying or selling organic animals.

Lambs must not be weaned before 45 days of age. The author cannot imagine that creates any problems. A minimum of 60% of the dry matter fed to lambs must be forage. There are various rules regarding what constitutes organic forage and what constitutes organic hard food, however animals must receive minimal amounts of minerals and must not receive any genetically modified (GM) feed.

Indoor lambing, castrating and docking are allowed. Sick animals are allowed to be treated with any licensed products, but the withdrawal periods are doubled. Prophylactic use of vaccines is allowed if licensed and if justified on welfare grounds. Prophylactic use of anthelmintics is not permitted but if animals are clinically affected they are allowed to be treated on veterinary recommendation. However, ivermectins are not allowed unless a very strong case is made on welfare grounds and when resistance has been demonstrated to the other anthelmintics.

References

Angus, K.W. (2010) Apparent low toxicity of yew for roe deer (*Capreolus capreolus*). *Veterinary Record* 166, 216.

Baird, G. (2003) Current perspectives on caseous lymphadenitis. *In Practice* 25, 62–68.

Baird, G. and Malone, F.E. (2010) Control of caseous lymphadenitis in six sheep flocks using clinical examination and regular ELISA testing. *Veterinary Record* 166, 358.

Barlow, A.M., Sharpe, J.A.E. and Kincaid, E.A. (2002) Blindness in lambs due to inadvertent closantel overdose. *Veterinary Record* 151, 25–26.

Bates, P. (2004) Therapies for ectoparasiticism in sheep. *In Practice* 26, 538–547.

Bisdorff, B., Milnes, A. and Wall, R. (2006) Prevalence and regional distribution of scab, lice and blowfly in Great Britain. *The Veterinary Record* 158, 749–752.

Boundy, T. (1993) Collection and interpretation of ram semen under general practice conditions. *In Practice* 15, 219–223.

Brash, A.G. (1943) Lupinosis. *New Zealand Journal of Agriculture* 67, 83–84.

Broughan, J.M. and Wall, R. (2006) Control of sheep blowfly strike using fly-traps. *Veterinary Parasitology* 135, 57–63.

Buxton, D. (1989) Toxoplasmosis in sheep and other farm animals. *In Practice* 11, 9– 12.

Copithorne, B. (1937) Hemlock poisoning. *Veterinary Record* 49, 1018–1019.

Cubero, M.J., Gonzalez, M. and Leon, L. (2002) Enfermedades infecciosas de las poblaciones de cabra montes. In: Perez, J.M. (ed.) *Distribucion, genetica y estatus sanitaria de las poblaciones andaluzas de cabra montes*. Universidad de Jaen/Junta de Andulucia, Consejeria de Medio Ambiente, Jaén, pp. 199–253.

Davies, F.G. and Otema, C. (1978) The antibody response in sheep infected with a Kenyan sheep and goat poxvirus. *Journal of Comparative Pathology* 88, 205–210.

Dawson, M. and Del Rio Vilas, V. (2008) Control of classical scrapie in Great Britain. *In Practice* 30, 330–333.

DEFRA (2005) Ectoparasite control in sheep: a review of control strategies and recommendations to the industry for sustainable ectoparasite control. Proceedings of workshop, DEFRA, London, pp. 52.

Dzikiti, T.B., Stegmann, G.F., Dzikiti, L.N. and Hellebrekers, L.J. (2011) Effects of fentanyl on isoflurane minimum alveolar concentration and cardiovascular function in mechanically ventilated goats. *Veterinary Record* 168, 429.

Eichenberger, R.M., Karvountzis, S., Ziadinov, I. and Deplazes, P. (2011) Severe *Taenia ovis* outbreak in a sheep flock in south-west England. *Veterinary Record* 168, 619.

Erjavec, V. and Crossley, D. (2010) Initial observations of cheek tooth abnormalities in sheep in Slovenia. *Veterinary Record* 167, 134–137.

Fazili, M.R., Malik, H.U., Battacharyya, H.K., Buchoo, B.A., Moulvi, B.A. and Makhdoomi, D.M. (2010) Minimally invasive surgical tube cystotomy for treating obstructive urolithiasis in small ruminants with an intact urinary bladder. *Veterinary Record* 166, 528–532.

Fenton, A., Wall, R. and French, N. (1998) The incidence of sheep strike by *Lucilia sericata* on sheep farms in Britain: a simulation model. *Veterinary Parasitology* 76, 211–228.

Flanagan, A.M., Edgar, H.W.J., Foster, F., Gordon, A., Hanna, R.E.B., McCloy, M., Brennan, G.P. and Fairweather, I. (2011) Standardising a coproantigen reduction test for the diagnosis of triclabendazole resistance. *Veterinary Parasitology* 176, 34–42.

Forsyth, A.A. (1954) *British Poisonous Plants*. MAFF Bulletin 161, HMSO, London, pp. 42–43.

Foster, G., Hunter, L., Baird, G., Koylass, M.S. and Whatmore, A.M. (2010) *Streptococcus pluranimalium* in ovine reproductive material. *Veterinary Record* 166, 246.

Gallina, L. and Scagliarini, A. (2010) Virucidal efficacy of common disinfectants against orf virus. *Veterinary Record* 166, 725.

Garcia, A.B., Steele, W.B., Reid, S.W.J. and Taylor, D.J. (2010) Risk of contamination of lamb carcasses with *Campylobacter* species. *Preventive Veterinary Medicine* 95, 99–107.

Giadinis, N.D., Polizopoulou, Z., Roubies, N. and Karatzias, H. (2010) Presumed nephrogenic diabetes insipidus secondary to chronic copper hepatotoxicity in sheep. *Veterinary Record* 166, 433–434.

Griffin, G. (2010) Review of the major outbreak of *E. coli* O157 in Surrey 2009. Report of the Independent Investigation Committee, June 2010. Available at: www.griffininvestigation.org.uk.

Harwood, D. and Hepple, S. (2011) Drenching/bolus gun injuries in sheep. *Veterinary Record* 168, 308–309.

Harwood, D.G., Baird, G., Mearns, R. and Davies, I. (2010a) Sheep zoonoses: further information for readers. *Veterinary Times* 40, 31.

Harwood, D.G., McPherson, G.C. and Woodger, N.G.A. (2010b) Possible horse chestnut poisoning in a Cashmere goat. *Veterinary Record* 167, 461–462.

Hay, L. (1990) Prevention and treatment of urolithiasis in sheep. *In Practice* 12, 87–91.

Head, K. (1990) Tumours in sheep. *In Practice* 12, 68–80.

Hoinville, L.J., Tongue, S.C. and Wilesmith, J.W. (2010) Investigation of maternal transmission of scrapie in naturally-infected sheep flocks. *Preventive Veterinary Medicine* 93, 121–128.

Hubbs, J.C. (1947) Deadly nightshade poisoning. *Veterinary Medicine* 42, 428–429.

Hughes, L.E., Kershaw, G.F. and Shaw, I.G. (1959) "B" or border disease. An undescribed disease of sheep. *Veterinary Record* 71, 313.

Hughes, Ted (1984) *What is the Truth*. Faber and Faber, London and Boston.

Ingoldby, L. and Jackson, P. (2001). Induction of parturition in sheep. *In Practice* 23, 228–231.

Jackson, P. (1986) Skin diseases of goats. *In Practice* 8, 5–10.

Jeffery, M. (1993) Sarcocystosis of sheep. *In Practice* 15, 2–8.

Kawaji, S., Begg, D.J., Plain, K.M. and Whittington, R.J. (2011) Use of faecal quantitative PCR testing to detect Johne's disease in sheep. *Journal of Veterinary Microbiology* 148, 35–44.

Keen, J.E. and Elder, R.O. (2002) Isolation of Shigatoxigenic *Escherichia coli* O157 from hide surfaces and the oral cavity of finished beef feedlot cattle. *Journal of American Veterinary Medical Association* 220, 756–763.

Kerry, J.B. and Craig, G.R. (1979) Field studies in sheep with multicomponent clostridial vaccines. *Veterinary Record* 105, 551–554.

Koop, G., Rietman, J.F. and Pieterse, M.C. (2010) *Staphylococcus aureus* mastitis in Texel sheep associated with suckling twins. *Veterinary Record* 167, 868–869.

Lomax, S., Dickson, H., Sheil, M. and Windsor, P.A. (2010) Topical anaesthesia in lambs undergoing castration and tail docking. *Australian Veterinary Journal* 88, 67–72.

MacDougall, D.F. (1991) Diagnosis, monitoring and prognosis of renal disease. *In Practice* 13, 250–256.

Martínez-de la Puente, J., Moreno-Indias, I., Morales-Delanuez, A., Ruiz-Díaz, M.D., Hernández-Castellano, L.E., Castro, N. and Argüello, A. (2011) Effects of feeding management and time of day on the occurrence of self-suckling in dairy goats. *Veterinary Record* 168, 378.

Mitchell, E.S.E., Hunt, K.R., Wood, R. and McLean, B. (2010) Anthelmintic resistance on sheep farms in Wales. *Veterinary Record* 166, 651–652.

Michell, S., Mearns, R., Richards, I., Donnan, A.A. and Bartley, D.J. (2011) Benzimidazole resistance in *Nematodirus battus*. *Veterinary Record* 168, 623.

Mueller, K. (2009) Common surgical procedures in goats. *Goat Veterinary Society Journal* 26, 9–14.

Mutayoba, B.M., Meyer, H.H.D., Osaso, J. and Gombe, S. (1989) Trypanosome-induced increase in prostaglandin F2alpha and its relationship with corpus luteum function in the goat. *Theriogenology* 32, 545–555.
Nodelijk, G., van Roermund, H.J.W., van Keulen, L.J.M., Engel, B., Vellema, P. and Hagenaars, T.J. (2011) Assessment of a genetic breeding control strategy for scrapie. *Veterinary Research* 42, 5.
Ortin, A., Verde, M.T., Ramos, J.J., Fernandez, A., Loste, A., Ferrer, L.M., Lacasta, D. and Bueso, J.P. (2010) *Staphylococcus chromogenes* – induced folliculitis in goat kids. *Veterinary Record* 166, 273–274.
Payne, J. and Liversey, C. (2010) Lead poisoning in cattle and sheep. *In Practice* 32, 64–69.
Petridou, E.J., Gianniki, Z., Giadinis, N.D., Filioussis, G., Dovas, C.I. and Psychas, V. (2011) Outbreak of polyarthritis in lambs attributed to *Pasteurella multocida*. *Veterinary Record* 168, 50.
Philbey, A.W. and Morton, A.G. (2001) Paraquat poisoning in sheep from contaminated water. *Australian Veterinary Journal*, 79, 842–843.
Quintas, H., Reis, J., Pires, I. and Alegria, N. (2010) Tuberculosis in goats. *Veterinary Record* 166, 437–438.
Razavi, S.M. and Hassanvand, A. (2007) A survey on prevalence of different *Eimeria* spp. in goats in Shiraz suburbs. *Journal of the Faculty of Veterinary Medicine of the University of Tehran* 61, 373–376.
Richardson, C., Taylor, W.P., Terlecki, S. and Gibbs, E.P.J. (1985) Observations on transplacental infection with bluetongue virus in sheep. *American Journal of Veterinary Research* 46, 1912–1922.
Rifatbegovic, M., Maksimovic, Z. and Hulaj, B. (2011) *Mycoplasma ovipneumoniae* associated with severe respiratory disease in goats. *Veterinary Record* 168, 565.
Roberts, H., Carbon, M., Hartley, M. and Sabirovic, M. (2011) Assessing the risk of disease introduction in imports. *Veterinary Record* 168, 447–448.
Saegerman, C., Bolkaerts, B., Baricalla, C., Raes, M., Wiggers, L., de Leeuw, I., Vandenbussche, F., Zimmer, J.Y., Haubruge, E., Cassart, D., De Clercq, K. and Kirschvink, N. (2011) The impact of naturally-occurring, trans-placental bluetongue virus serotype-8 infection on reproductive performance in sheep. *Veterinary Journal* 167, 72–80.
Sargison, N. (1995) Differential diagnosis and treatment of sheep scab. *In Practice* 17, 3–9 and 467–469.
Sargison, N. (2001) Copper poisoning in sheep and cattle. *UKVet* 6, 54–58.
Sargison, N. and Edwards, G. (2009) Tick infestations in sheep in the UK. *In Practice* 31, 58–65.
Sargison, N.D. and Scott, P.R. (2011) Diagnosis and economic consequences of triclabendazole resistance in *Fasciola hepatica* in a sheep flock in south-east Scotland. *Veterinary Record* 168, 159.
Scott, P. (2000) Ultrasonography of the urinary tract in male sheep with urethral obstruction. *In Practice* 22, 329–334.
Scott, P.R. (2007) *Sheep Medicine*. Manson Publishing Ltd, London, pp. 256–260 and 315.
Scott, P. (2010) Intussusception in neonatal lambs. *UKVet* 15, 39–40.
Scott, P. (2011) Uterine torsion in the ewe. *UKVet* 16, 37–39.
Scott, W.A. (2010) Apparent low toxicity of yew in munjac deer and Soay sheep. *Veterinary Record* 166, 246.
Sharpe, A.E., Brady, C.P., Johnson, A., Byrne, W., Kenny, K. and Costello, E. (2010) Concurrent outbreak of tuberculosis and caseous lymphadenitis in a goat herd. *Veterinary Record* 166, 591–592.
Stevenson, M.J. (2010) Apparent low toxicity of yew in grazing animals. *Veterinary Record* 166, 307.
Stratton, M.R. (1919) Water hemlock poisoning. *Colorado Medicine* 16, 104–111.
Swarbrick, O. (2010) Apparent low toxicity of yew in grazing animals. *Veterinary Record* 166, 307.
Taylor, M. (2002) Parasites of goats: a guide to diagnosis and control. *In Practice* 24, 76–89.
Terlecki, S., Richardson, C., Done, J.T., Harkness, J.W., Sands, J.J., Shaw, I.G., Winkler, C.E., Duffell, S.J., Patterson, D.S. and Sweasey, D. (1980) Pathogenicity for the sheep foetus of Bovine Virus Diarrhoea-mucosal disease virus of bovine origin. *British Veterinary Journal* 136, 602–611.
Uzal, F.A., Paulson, D., Eigenheer, A.L. and Walker, R.L. (2007) *Malassezia slooffiae*-associated dermatitis in a goat. *Veterinary Dermatology* 18, 348–352.
Van der Burgt, G. (2010) *Mycobacterium bovis* causing clinical disease in adult sheep. *Veterinary Record* 166, 306.
Watson, P. (2004) Differential diagnosis of oral lesions and FMD in sheep. *In Practice* 26, 182–191.
Wessels, M.E., Payne, J., Willmington, J.A., Bell, S.J. and Davies, I.H. (2010) *Yersinia pseudotuberculosis* as a cause of ocular disease in goats. *Veterinary Record* 166, 699–670.
Wilsmore, A. (1989) Birth injury and perinatal loss in lambs. *In Practice* 11, 239–243.
Winter, A.C. (1995) Problems of extensive farming systems. *In Practice* 17, 217–220.
Winter, A. (2004) Lameness in sheep. 2. Treatment and control. *In Practice* 26, 130–139.
Woods, L.W., Puschner, B., Filigenzi, M.S., Woods, D.M. and George, L.W. (2011) Evaluation of the toxicity of *Adonis aestivalis* in sheep. *Veterinary Record* 168, 49.

Index

Note: page numbers in **bold** refer to figures and tables.